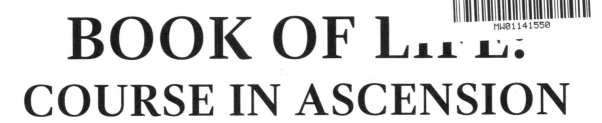

BOOK OF LIFE:
COURSE IN ASCENSION

**365 DAY DEVOTIONAL SELF MASTERY GUIDE AND
LIFE COACHING SECRETS PRACTICAL BLUEPRINT**

<u>INCLUDES:</u> DIVINE ORACLES, UNIVERSAL LAWS, POSITIVE AFFIRMATIONS,
GRATITUDE AND ASCENSION CODES
<u>RECEIVE:</u> ASCENSION LIGHT CODE TRANSMISSION AND OFFICIAL ASCENSION LIFE
CERTIFICATE OF COMPLETION
12 MONTHS OF PURE HEAVENLY GOOD NEWS.
SEE INSIDE!

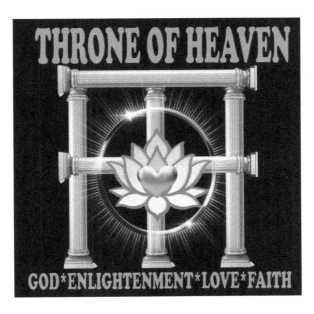

Diana Hutchings

Author's Tranquility Press
MARIETTA, GEORGIA

Diana Hutchings/Author's Tranquility Press
2706 Station Club Drive SW
Marietta, GA 30060
www.authorstranquilitypress.com

Ordering Information:
Quantity sales. Special discounts are available on quantity purchases by corporations, associations, and others. For details, contact the "Special Sales Department" at the address above.

Book of Life/Diana Hutchings
Paperback: 978-1-958554-86-9
eBook: 978-1-958554-87-6

Scripture quotations marked KJV are from the Holy Bible, King James Version (Authorized Version). First published in 1611. Quoted from the KJV Classic Reference Bible, Copyright © 1983 by The Zondervan Corporation.

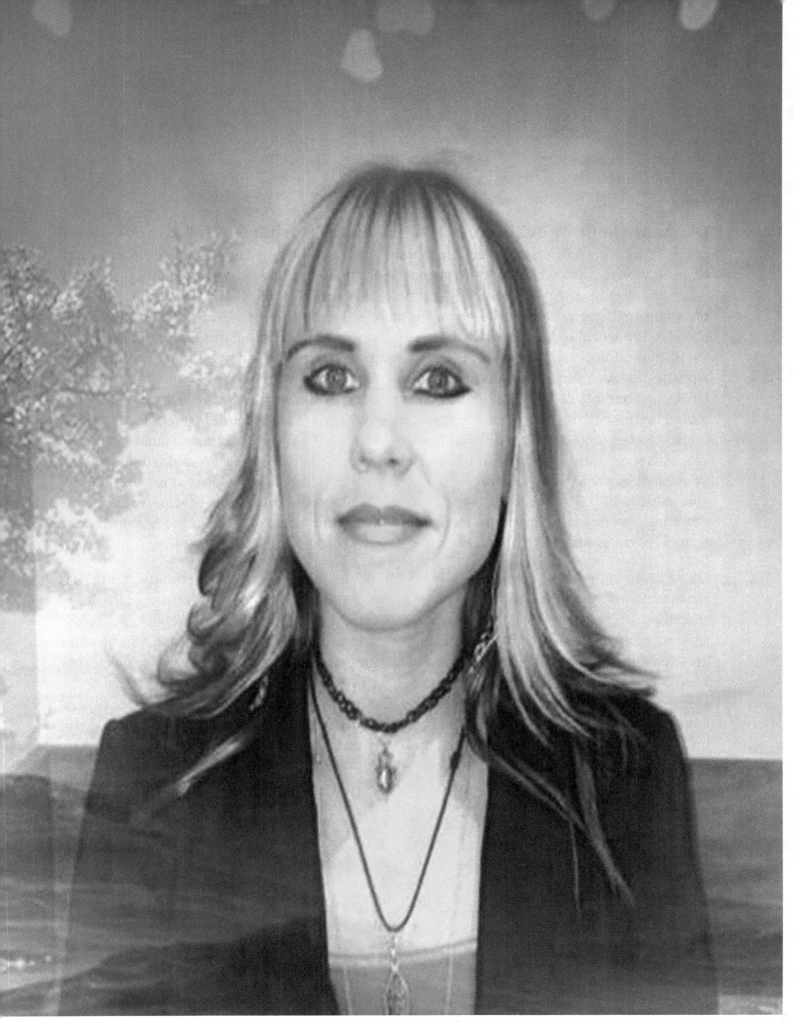

About the Author

Diana Michelle Hutchings aka **Diana Eliya Moriah Prince** is a professional oracle, educator, author, speaker, life coach, artist and healer. Her channeled divine soul name is Moriah Eliya which literally means God is my teacher, the Lord Almighty is my God. After graduating with a Bachelor of Arts in Religion and a Bachelor of Education, she went on a spiritual quest. God chose Diana to paint the Holy Bible's seven seals of God. She traveled the world to hand deliver these painted scrolls with landmarks like: Eiffel Tower in Paris, Pyramids of Giza in Egypt, Diana of Ephesus in Greece, Temple of Heaven in China, Apostles Rock in Australia, Sundial in Machu Picchu, and the Golden Temple in Jerusalem. On December 21, 2012 Diana dedicated her work to the Lord. Mayan Prophecy said this would be the end of the world. On the same day 12/21/12 her dad informed her that their house located on the highest hill was burning down while she's working at Planet Beach sun spa. This moment was a huge shift in consciousness for her. The Lord reminded her "where your heart is, there your treasure will be." In 2022, she became the official oracle, founder and creator of "Throne of Heaven." Services and products include oracle readings, life coaching sessions, masterclasses, intensives, reiki attunements, chakra balancing, numerology, financial advising, Akashic record readings. Visit www.throneofheaven.com.

Diana often called Wonder Woman loves all, God, family, friends, community, Lord Hari Krishna Rama Amrinder and Goddess Namaste Athena Warrior of Moksha. Diana loves travelling, crystals, numerology, astrology, aromatherapy, sound healing, Reiki, reflexology, fitness, herbalism, shamanism, exercising, qi gong, poetry, art therapy, dancing, jewelry creations like sacred crystal tree of life and creating dreamcatchers and dream weavers. The Lord is her greatest love! Our purpose is to share in God's wisdom, mysteries, secrets, power, glory, dignity, riches, strength and blessings. Our goal is to serve. To serve is to make others' lives better. Throne of Heaven's mission is to transform the soul, heart, mind and body of humanity to enlighten and enlighten more in order to create the love peace harmony universal family.

Prologue

Hi hola bonjour my name is Diana Michelle Hutchings. I have two cats Hari Krishna Rama Amrinder and Namaste Athena Warrior of Moksha. Born and raised in the fastest growing hamlet in the world called Sherwood Park. Lucky I was raised in a two-parent home on the highest hill in all of Sherwood Park, Alberta, Canada with her brother and sister. I just want to give a special shout out to my mom Alberta Hutchings and my dad Ken Hutchings for being so supportive. I love God, my family and friends. Ever since I was little, I was lucky winning scratch cards, draws and prizes. My family was really into sports. She played everything except anything on skis and skate, even played Alberta Basketball in high school where I learned all about discipline. DISCIPLINE IS THE ABILITY TO GIVE YOURSELF A COMMAND AND FOLLOW IT I am not here to tell my life story just a few memorable pieces of the puzzle that brought me here today. By a show of hands who likes to party? Haha that's good. I had a lot of that when I was younger too. To be honest it got heavy and was into crystal meth for about 6 years on and off. I never was a religious person. Yes I grew up in a believing household but we rarely went to church. There was a time I said there was no God. Believe me when I say this: I learned the hard way there is a God and He is very real. The Law of Belief is a universal law the governs us. "WHEN YOU BELIEVE IN A THING, BELIEVE IN IT ALL THE WAY." WALT DISNEY Other powerful divine light beings are here with us. I work with over 100 heavenly angels 63 fairies, elementals, ascended masters and Akashic Masters and other spiritual guides. I used to take 20 books out at the library every week to read about various topics like anatomy, healing, astronomy, alchemy, psychology and the list goes on. James Redfield is an author who has a series that I absolutely cherish. Have you heard of the Celestine Prophecy? Did you know you can watch it on you tube for free? James Redfield has many other books like Celestine Vision, 10th insight, 11th insight and The Secret of Shambalah. I called this Speech or Prologue the Secret to Shambalah because I will share my personal story, passions and vision of utopian vision future while sharing a few secrets to eternal bliss. I am hoping to inspire you to create the future you desire. If you got a pen and paper now. I invite you to imagine because IMAGINATION IS THE MENTAL FACULTY OUT OF WHICH VISIONS ARISE. Right now imagine, visualize and describe what your idea of a utopian future would be like, look like, feel like. Always describe the 5 w's and the H. The who, what, where, when, why and hows. Learned the power of answered these questions when I received my private security diploma after 911. This is the secret graphic organizer for any good plan in any subject. Actually before 911 I was working the Horse track in the lounge just after high school. My first boyfriend loved him since I was 15 he was my first crush and I lost my virginity to him. He knocked me up just before 911. We were smoking a lot of cracks and I was one to want the perfect job, partner, wedding before I had children. So, I had an abortion not realizing anything about the morals of abortions or the souls involved inside our bodies. God please forgive me and understands all those children who are unborn and there is a special place for them. Let's just say our relationship did not last long after but the partying still carried on. Furthermore, on with the story I was reading so many other books one night about two years later I decided to open the bible and was sketching out on crystal. God said to me that I am an angel. Within weeks I went completely sober almost nun like. Took off to the mountains for the summer and never touched it since. I know there are some fun substances out there, please be careful. Take your vitamins and supplements. It is as simple as taking one complete B vitamin which can reduce stress, increase energy, metabolize fats, proteins and carbohydrates Remember to give thanks. Ask for blessings upon the substances you put into your system. Let's do a quick blessing. Hold your glass, cup mug, pen, paper, maybe gum, vape or another substance you will put into your system later. Repeat After Me Dear God, Thank you for this substance. May it help me be stronger, smarter, faster, stronger, better and more attractive. Amen. Who do you really want to be? THINK AND ACT LIKE THE PERSON YOU WANT TO BE.

Ok back to my personal journey. About 2 years of being sober I had a dream. I remember my mom took me to go See Adam the Dreamhealer. By the way folks, if you want a fast forward into self-healing skills read Adam the Dreamhealer books. As Walt Disney says, "LAUGHTER IS TIMELESS, IMAGINATION HAS NO AGE AND DREAMS ARE FOREVER." Being a dreamer led me to my shamanism work. I drew a whole coloring book of animals and birds on my walls when I was 12. Always loved and connected well with nature, animals and children. Discovered I was a clairsentient in 2019, Mother Nature one my saviors.

My big dream that I had around 2008 was of two mattress size holy scriptures, the Holy Bible and the Holy Quran in the back of a red truck box. I was in the truck and out the front windshield I could see this big, enormous mushroom cloud. Looked like a nuclear blast if I have ever seen one. Not too long after that dream I located an English Holy Quran and Holy Bible and carried them with me, reading and writing and learning the scriptures. IF YOU CAN DREAM IT YOU CAN DO IT. I love to write. It is a passion. How many of you write notes or journal? Let's do a quick exercise. OK. Write a list of everything you love right now. Keep writing and thinking of your ideas and listen as the story as it unravels.

I have a Bachelor in Arts I majored in religion. During College, I deepened my connection with God and God was my number 1 everything. For your awareness, I worked as a security guard, personal trainer, library helper during college. I worked out life 5 hours of the day. Then received the highest GPA in the Christian College during my graduating year in religion. I understand what it is like to have lots of friends to having God as my only friend. During the spiritual evolution process we go through relationship changes. We outgrow some people, even our family. If this has happened to you, this is normal.

There is a difference between religion and spirituality. Where God is there is religion where spirituality is there your self is. YOUR SPIRITUAL DNA IS PERFECT ALL KNOWING ALL POWERFUL ALL PRESENT. Believe in God, source, universe, higher self, divine light and love, Namaste and all that stuff. I got into painting after high school. The first painting I ever framed was of Mother Mary and Jesus. I got offered to come to Vegas to share my poem Alchemy. So many cool achievements and memories to share. I love to paint, sculpt, doodle around. I dated all my paintings and art on December 21, 2012 and dedicated all my works to God. Anyone remember what was going to happen December 21 2012? The day the world was to end, doomsday December 21, 2012, when my dad called me. It was my second shift at Planet Beach. My dad said come home the house is on fire. This was an utter shift in consciousness. It is strange that I got dropped off that day in a red truck by my boyfriend at the time; with my back pack and My Holy Quran and Holy Bible. This boyfriend is a whole other conversation. Let's just say people come into our lives to teach us lessons. Some lessons are harder than others, but I am grateful and thankful for everyone I had the pleasure of getting to know and interact with my whole life. Blessings to you all! Blessings to all you who are reading this too. Shortly after that I started compiling the Book of Life through divine channeling and bibliomancy. Wanna know the secret to your heart? Bibliomancy. YOUR MIND AND THOUGHTS MUST OPERATE ON THE SAME FREQUENCY AS YOUR HEART AND SOUL. Find any scriptures or guided text preferably holy and knock on the book then open to a page to read any verse. Choose only the good positive language and ditch any negativity by not focusing on it. This method is very similar to using oracle cards. Oracle cards are designed to guide, provide actions and assistance and deliver needs and wants. This led to creating 12 plus divine oracles. You would love to use these oracles because It is my intention they will guide you to the best path. I have oracles like true love, heavenly abundance, sacred awakening, celestial kosmos, holy angels, fairy wellness, godly virtues, power protection, more. Even created a board game called Ladders of Ascension in which I need help to make my publishing dreams come true and share this amazing game with the world.

WANNA KNOW THE REAL SECRET IN LIFE? Its energy, chi, frequency and vibration. What can you do to raise your vibration right in this very minute? In 2013 I embarked on my Reiki journey into becoming a Reiki Master Healer. Reiki literally means universal life force energy. This led to understanding crystal energy, meditation, pendulums, and opened up many doors of learning opportunities. I suggest you all learn reiki.

What really gets you fired up? My passion is seeing others be their best selves. Other passions include children and seeing their development and enhancement. This is why I became a teacher. I got my permanent Alberta teaching certificate in 2010 on Valentine's Day. Learned over the years that gathering the skills of professional planning, organizing, delivering, assessing and recreating lessons gave me the skills to teach what I love. If you love what you do its like you never have to work a day in your life. Now I educate on ways to enhance life. POWERING BETTER THOUGHTS BETTER FEELINGS BETTER ATTITUDE = BETTER RESULTS. Educating on subjects like self-actualization or self-transcendence like Abraham Maslow once told. When you get to the top of the pyramid you will know because everything will flow smoothly and perfectly as if you are a genie. In fact you are your own personal genie. I call lamborginis lamborgenies as my grandpa once said. I manifested being in a lamborgini months later after realizing that is what I wanted and put it on the bucket list. We can all have what we want and better.

EVERYTHING IS ENERGY. MATCH THE FREQUENCY OF THE REALITY YOU WANT AND YOU CANNOT HELP BUT GET THAT REALITY. Use the magic of wishful thinking. Magic is defined as focused intention. I want to get your juices flowing and open the doors of opportunity for you. It's all in the work I do. I am a spiritual wellness life coach, healer, author and intuitive oracle. I help others master emotional intelligence and be their best selves. We cover the universal laws that govern our planet. Like the law of attraction, Reiki and shamanism are energy tools that can transform your life in all space, time, dimension, reality, incarnation and lifetime. For example, we will do some (EFT) Emotional Freedom Technique tapping. With your index finger and middle finger tap between your brows and the top of the head and repeat after me. Tap and say. "I will create a harmonious utopian future and live my best life. You will create a harmonious utopian future and live my best life. We will create a harmonious utopian future and live my best life." Good job!

We provide the strategies, techniques and blueprints to completely level you up. YOU MUST THINK AND ACT LIKE YOU ALREADY ACHIEVED WHAT IT IS THAT YOU WANT. Think of the blueprint like a math strategy or science method with step-by-step instructions that give you the solution and solve your problem. One strategy is called the prayer intention field. This was discussed in James

Redfield's book, "The Secret of Shambalah," when he suggested that if you really want something to happen in the future you got to send a field of intention into the future. For example, say you are going to the grocery store. Visualize getting a close parking spot or ask for one. Imagine there is no one in the lineup and you do not have to wait. Prethink of a sale for your items. Request a cart and basket that is clean and available. Maybe you want the store to be less busy with happy, healthy and friendly staff. You can use the prayer intention field anytime and anywhere What is it that you really want to happen in the future? What is your vision of a perfect future? Where do you see yourself in 3 years? I welcome you to make a dream board and soul collage of what you want in your future. Thoughts and feelings create manifestations. Energy plus motion creates emotion.

My future vision of a utopian society is to create Shambalah. Shambalah literally means a heavenly spiritual kingdom or paradise. January 1, 2022, I took first action step to make this a reality by registering and creating Throne of Heaven. This is my business, life and universe. I am the founder of Throne of Heaven's business. I am the author and illustrator of the Book of Life. Projecting in the next 3 years we will create a heavenly oasis retreat. Offering customized retreats with 100's of holistic practitioners. Including a massive pyramid house, geodesic domes, infinity crystal pools, water yoga, elixir fountains, waterfall experiences, a throne of heaven attraction and much more. I am looking for future partners, angel investors and potential clients and colleagues who wish to share and invest in our Shamabalah vision. Speaking of investing, I am new to the financial industry and am officially a life licensed agent and insurance provider for North America. We are offering free consultations and have a superpowered presentation to share if you are interested in making or saving money, getting out of debt, protecting your life and loved ones and possibly receive a part or full time career opportunity.

This dream led me to create the Book of Life which I will discuss later and the whole purpose and intention for this beautiful journey. Rhonda Byrne in the books The Secret, The Power and The Magic. She inspired my gratitude journey. Thank you all for taking the time to read this in completion. It has taken me about 7 years to make this a reality. THE MORE YOU ARE IN A STATE OF GRATITUDE, THE MORE YOU ATTRACT THINGS TO BE GRATEFUL FOR.

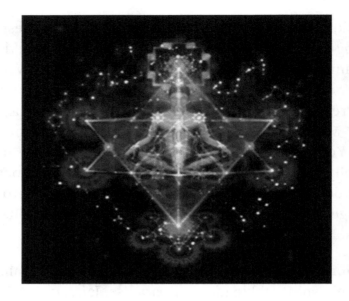

Table of Contents

BONUS: Oracles

Isaiah 65:17 "For behold, I create new heavens and a new earth; And the former shall not be remembered or come to mind.

Revelation 22:13 I am the Alpha and the Omega, the Beginning and the End, the First and the Last."

2 Peter 1:11 And God will open wide the gates of heaven for you to enter into the eternal kingdom of our Lord and Savior Jesus Christ.

The Word was GOD!

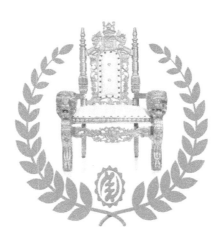

Acknowledgements

I am grateful for all my family, friends, colleagues, mentors, teachers and students for gracing me with their wisdom, energy and support. In addition, to all the attunements, practitioner treatments, group healing sessions, light workers, self-help books, Spirit Science, angels, archangels, ascended masters, ancestors and guides that have assisted me along this journey. Thank you God, creator, higher self, Holy Spirit! You worked through us to do your work. Thank you for choosing me to be your medium. Thank you in my past, present and future. As an old lady once said, there are no strangers dear, just friends you haven't met. Thank you all to whom contributed to the successful sharing and tuning in of good news. Thank you Author's Tranquility Press for publishing and marketing. Blessings are bestowed upon all of you.

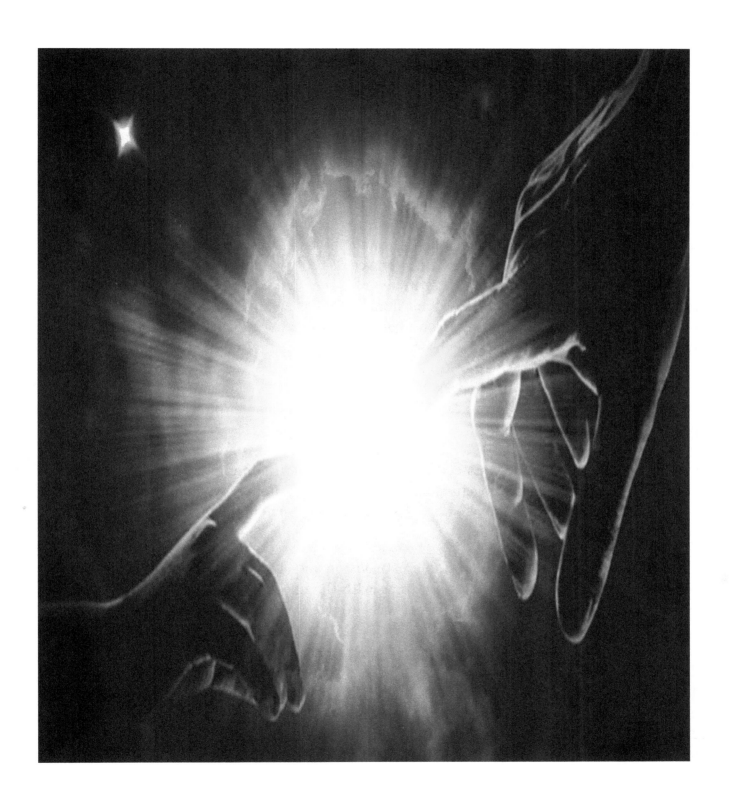

Introduction

This book is inspired by God's Holy Spirit and a dream. This dream included me as a passenger (messenger) with a massive bed sized Holy Bible and Holy Qur'an then I saw a huge mushroom cloud in the distance like a bomb or something. The Almighty's power rests in the word of God. Each verse was done via bibliomancy. Bibliomancy is the art of knocking on one's inner self using scriptures and opening the book to any passage then reading the message. Guaranteed your life will change for the better. After reading the Rhonda Byrne's books, "The Secret" and "The Magic," the power of positive thinking and gratitude became more influential. Gratitude is an attitude and the benefits reap compensation. It is recommended you read the day's reading along with pick an angel to invoke 3x and start this book with the 31 day step by step plan; that includes templates you may use for the whole year. Blessed Be! Each message will be perfect for you at the moment. The intention for publishing this book is to share in God's mysteries and wisdom to enlighten, love, heal and provide assistance to you. In the back of the book is a bunch of helpful items to achieve your best potential. This is a book you can read and pick up anywhere. You will be sure to receive perfect divine intervention. If you love this book, please subscribe to the website www.throneofheaven.com and add us from LinkedIn, Twitter, Instagram, YouTube, Facebook and Pinterest. If you decide you need an accountability partner and want to become the best version of you check out the coaching packages on our website. We would love to get to know you better. God Bless and enjoy an optimistic, powerful journey bringing many blessings and successes in all areas of your life.

This book was designed for you to create, vision and succeed. Discovering your akashic records of enlightenment and bliss. Working with the universal laws, acquiring virtues and seeking the assistance of the holy angels will provide you with the wisdom to focus your intentions, time and energy into spiritual practices that are going to align your mind, body and soul in every lifetime, generation, dimension, reality, space and time. Going through each day while randomly opening up the book to see what oracle is telling you. Your job is to ask. This book can be used at anytime anywhere. Knock on the book to activate your knowing thyself and asking about something. Open the book of life and read whichever spot you are drawn to. Another word for this strategy is called bibliomancy. Channeling divine intervention with the Holy Spirit, source, your higher self, God, or whatever you want to call it. You will learn overtime the lesson, advice, quality is just where you need to put your focus. The plan is there. Truly you do the work the reward is there. Try the better habit challenge. It takes 21 days to create a good habit. 90 days to change a lifestyle. 365 days to master your life.

RECOMMENDED: Everyday pick an oracle to choose from.

BONUS ORACLE READING: For your highest and best good it is recommended to book a private oracle reading with Throne of Heaven to answer any questions, concerns or responses to life's happenings to assist you on your path. BOOK a one on one we can provide guidance about relationships, career, health, abundance, personal growth and more.

+if you like these oracles you can buy the oracle deck that resonates with you. There are beautiful pictures that go along with messages.

COACHING TRAINING PROGRAM: Pair this with an intensive life coaching session. For example, Achieving Life Goals, Secrets to Happiness, Fulfilling Life Purpose, Balancing Success, Path to Self-Actualization, Chakra Rainbow Healing, Elemental Magic, Akashic Records, Nutrition and more. Go on www.throneofheaven.com make sure to subscribe to receive rewards, free resources, masterclasses, summits, discounts, blogs, community connections, group invitations, events and ongoing support. Vision Workshop, Financial Freedom workshop, Business workshop, 13 Rays of Chakra Light, Oaths of Manifestation.

GIFT TO YOU: I would love for you to book a free 15 minute clarity, strategy, discovery or breakthrough call to hear about your most important goal, dream or vision.

SPEAKING: If you would like us to join, speak or present at any of your functions please private message us.

Bismillah (In the name of Allah or God Jesus and the Holy Spirit)

Asher (so be it)

Amen (Thank you God)

Superhearts Unite

By Diana Hutchings

Superhero stories exist everywhere but this story is beyond special. It all began in a mother's womb. One night the day before the galactic birth planet Indigo visited the womb. Next day her water broke and she delivered twin suns. The three symbolize Godhood. These three divine, heavenly lights are flames lighting up all of existence. The creators were happy and it was good.

They received all the treasures of life in Godspeed. Given the keys of heaven inspiring faith, love, hope, peace, dreams and success. Faith is the key, the key to all hearts. Unlocking the truth from where it all starts. Hope is the key for whom wishes ring true. Simple, sincere made manifest by you.

Love fills a key triumphant and bright. Wear it and feel the love spreading your light. Peace is the key to your own inner place. Radiating wisdom to the whole human race. Dreams are the key where all doors open. Imagine a utopian world where ideas have awoken. Success is the key to your ultimate quest. Reaching your goals and being your best. The entire multiverse was entrusted to the birthed sacred hearts. Their nicknames were Wonderheart and Superheart. Thirteen elected crystal aliens whom guarded all 13 planets and zodiacs came to bless Wonderheart and Superheart. Planets near and far started to align after the blessing. The astrological zodiacs rule the houses of different planets. The Holy Spirit always divinely intervened with Wonderheart and Superheart. Igniting the inspiring triple flames of Godhood.

Planet Indigo supported Wonderheart and Superheart as they were granted power over every galaxy and universe. They were good and they were Almighty. Planet Indigo lived long and prospered because of their blessing uniting superhearts. All the planets aligned in harmony. Then Eureka, Beetleguese and Armageddon collided after the planetary alignment. It was the end of a new beginning. And the birth of a new, better and more perfect creation.

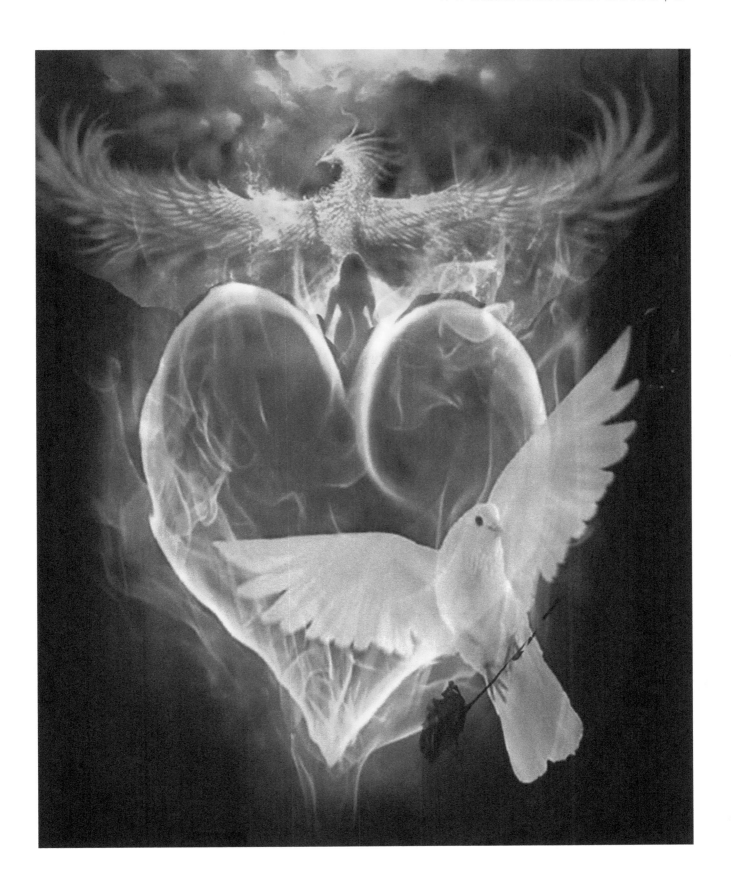

THRONE OF HEAVEN 2
31 Day Devotional Improving Your Lifestyle
Blueprint Ascension Guide

Day 1

<u>To Do Checklist</u>

Date:	
Shower(s) or Bath(s)	
Water Intake at least 1000ml-2000ml	
Sleep Hours (7 to 9 hours)	
Meditative Mindfulness (ex. Chakra visualization, mantras, deep breathing, affirmations	
Exercise (10-30min)	
Daily Reading SEE 365 day devotional section	
Take a multivitamin+ Vitamin B complex	
Eat all food groups	
Self-Care (massage Live Clean lotion all over body after shower and brush teeth X2/day)	
Fill in your monthly planner USE calendar	
Clean your fridge	
Send a sweet text to someone	
Attract Abundance (3 things you are grateful for) 1. 2. 3.	
Pray for what you need and want Dear God,	

need	want

Amen	
Manifest Daily Goal(s)+Intention+personal to do list 1. 2. 3.	

Day 2

To Do Checklist

	Date
	Shower(s) or Bath(s)
	Water Intake 1000ml-2000mL
	Sleep Hours (7 to 9 hours)
	Meditative Mindfulness
	Exercise (10-30min)
	Daily Reading SEE 365 day devotional section
	Take a multivitamin+Vitamin B complex
	Eat all food groups
	Self-Care (5 deep breaths, take vitamins, massage Live Clean lotion, brush teeth)
	Smile at everyone
	Clean your pantry
	Share a hug or kiss
	Attract Abundance (3 things you are grateful for) 1. 2. 3.

Pray for your home and family
Dear God,

home	family

Amen

Manifest Daily Goal(s)+Intention
1.
2.
3.

Day 3

To Do List

	Date
	Shower(s) or Bath(s)
	Water Intake 1000ml pure and clean
	Sleep Hours (7 to 9 hours)
	Meditative Mindfulness (deep breathing 10-30minutes)
	Exercise (10-30min)
	Daily Reading
	Take a multivitamin
	Eat all food groups
	Self-Care (5 deep breaths, take vitamins, massage Live Clean lotion, brush teeth)
	Read something interesting
	Clean your appliances
	Have a long conversation with someone
	Attract Abundance (3 things you are grateful for) 1. 2. 3.
	Pray for your neighbors or someone close to you Dear God,

neighbors	Someone close

Amen

	Manifest Daily Goal(s)+Intention 1. 2. 3.

Day 4

To Do List

	Date
	Shower(s) or Bath(s)
	Water Intake 1000ml pure and clean
	Sleep Hours (7 to 9 hours)
	Meditative Mindfulness (deep breathing 10-30minutes)
	Exercise (10-30min)
	Daily Reading
	Take a multivitamin
	Eat all food groups
	Self-Care (5 deep breaths, take vitamins, massage Live Clean lotion, brush teeth)
	Write or draw something
	Clean your kitchen
	Write a note to someone and give it to them
	Attract Abundance (3 things you are grateful for) 1. 2. 3.
	Pray for anyone you know who needs it Dear God, Amen
	Manifest Daily Goal(s)+Intention 1. 2. 3.

Day 5

To Do List

	Date
	Shower(s) or Bath(s)
	Water Intake 1000ml pure and clean
	Sleep Hours (7 to 9 hours)
	Meditative Mindfulness (deep breathing 10-30minutes)
	Exercise (10-30min) +walk
	Daily Reading
	Take a multivitamin
	Eat all food groups
	Self-Care (5 deep breaths, take vitamins, massage Live Clean lotion, brush teeth)
	Listen to your favorite music
	Clean your kitchen equipment
	Research the definition of love and create an acrostic poem about love L O V E
	Attract Abundance (3 things you are grateful for) 1. 2. 3.
	Pray for your community and connections Dear God, Amen
	Manifest Daily Goal(s)+Intention 1. 2. 3.

Day 6

To Do List

	Date
	Shower(s) or Bath(s)
	Water Intake 1000ml pure and clean
	Sleep Hours (7 to 9 hours)
	Meditative Mindfulness (deep breathing 10-30minutes)
	Exercise (10-30min)
	Daily Reading
	Take a multivitamin
	Eat all food groups
	Self-Care (5 deep breaths, take vitamins, massage Live Clean lotion, brush teeth)
	Do something new
	Clean your drawers
	Get a 20 second hug
	Attract Abundance (3 things you are grateful for) 1. 2. 3.
	Pray for good health Dear God, Amen
	Manifest Daily Goal(s)+Intention 1. 2. 3.

Day 7

To Do List

	Date
	Shower(s) or Bath(s)
	Water Intake 1000ml pure and clean
	Sleep Hours (7 to 9 hours)
	Meditative Mindfulness (deep breathing 10-30minutes)
	Exercise (10-30min)
	Daily Reading
	Take a multivitamin
	Eat all food groups
	Self-Care (5 deep breaths, take vitamins, massage Live Clean lotion, brush teeth)
	Create a music playlist (Soundcloud, Spotify, amazon)
	Clean your baseboards
	Create a safe word with a friend
	Attract Abundance (3 things you are grateful for) 1. 2. 3.
	Pray for security Dear God, Amen
	Manifest Daily Goal(s)+Intention 1. 2. 3.

Day 8

To Do List

	Date
	Shower(s) or Bath(s)
	Water Intake 1000ml pure and clean
	Sleep Hours (7 to 9 hours)
	Meditative Mindfulness (deep breathing 10-30minutes)
	Exercise (10-30min)
	Daily Reading
	Take a multivitamin
	Eat all food groups
	Self-Care (5 deep breaths, take vitamins, massage Live Clean lotion, brush teeth)
	Do a random act of kindness
	Clean your bathroom sink(s)
	Try a new dish
	Attract Abundance (3 things you are grateful for) 1. 2. 3.
	Pray for a perfect partner or companion(s) Dear God, Amen
	Manifest Daily Goal(s)+Intention 1. 2. 3.

Day 9

To Do List

	Date
	Shower(s) or Bath(s)
	Water Intake 1000ml pure and clean
	Sleep Hours (7 to 9 hours)
	Meditative Mindfulness (deep breathing 10-30minutes)
	Exercise (10-30min)
	Daily Reading
	Take a multivitamin
	Eat all food groups (no sugar today)
	Self-Care (5 deep breaths, take vitamins, massage Live Clean lotion, brush teeth)
	Visit a place (new or your favorite)
	Clean your toilet(s) and replenish toiletries
	Hold hands with someone
	Attract Abundance (3 things you are grateful for) 1. 2. 3.
	Pray for your friends Dear God, Amen
	Manifest Daily Goal(s)+Intention 1. 2. 3.

Day 10

To Do List

	Date
	Shower(s) or Bath(s)
	Water Intake 1000ml pure and clean
	Sleep Hours (7 to 9 hours)
	Meditative Mindfulness (deep breathing 10-30minutes)
	Exercise (10-30min)
	Daily Reading
	Take a multivitamin
	Eat all food groups
	Self-Care (5 deep breaths, take vitamins, massage Live Clean lotion, brush teeth)
	Give to charity or donate
	Clean your vehicle or mode of transportation
	Play a game
	Attract Abundance (3 things you are grateful for) 1. 2. 3.
	Pray for people around the world Dear God, Amen
	Manifest Daily Goal(s)+Intention 1. 2. 3.

Day 11

To Do List

	Date
	Shower(s) or Bath(s)
	Water Intake 1000ml pure and clean
	Sleep Hours (7 to 9 hours)
	Meditative Mindfulness (deep breathing 10-30minutes)
	Exercise (10-30min)
	Daily Reading
	Take a multivitamin
	Eat all food groups
	Self-Care (5 deep breaths, take vitamins, massage Live Clean lotion, brush teeth)
	Invite company share a meal
	Clean your bathroom +shower/bath
	Share a childhood memory or your favorite memory
	Attract Abundance (3 things you are grateful for) 1. 2. 3.
	Pray for peace Dear God, Amen
	Manifest Daily Goal(s)+Intention 1. 2. 3.

Day 12

To Do List

	Date
	Shower(s) or Bath(s)
	Water Intake 1000ml pure and clean
	Sleep Hours (7 to 9 hours)
	Meditative Mindfulness (deep breathing 10-30minutes)
	Exercise (10-30min)
	Daily Reading
	Take a multivitamin
	Eat all food groups
	Self-Care (5 deep breaths, take vitamins, massage Live Clean lotion, brush teeth)
	Get dressed up and go out
	Clean your mirrors
	Walk
	Attract Abundance (3 things you are grateful for) 1. 2. 3.
	Pray for abundance Dear God, Amen
	Manifest Daily Goal(s)+Intention 1. 2. 3.

Day 13

To Do List

Date	
Shower(s) or Bath(s)	
Water Intake 1000ml pure and clean	
Sleep Hours (7 to 9 hours)	
Meditative Mindfulness (deep breathing 10-30minutes)	
Exercise (10-30min)	
Daily Reading	
Take a multivitamin	
Eat all food groups	
Self-Care (5 deep breaths, take vitamins, massage Live Clean lotion, brush teeth)	
Affirm 7 times we are compassionate, loving and loveable	
Clean your workspace	
Do something relaxing	
Attract Abundance (3 things you are grateful for) 1. 2. 3.	
Pray for riches Dear God, Amen	
Manifest Daily Goal(s)+Intention 1. 2. 3.	

Day 14

<u>To Do List</u>

	Date
	Shower(s) or Bath(s)
	Water Intake 1000ml pure and clean
	Sleep Hours (7 to 9 hours)
	Meditative Mindfulness (deep breathing 10-30minutes)
	Exercise (10-30min)
	Daily Reading
	Take a multivitamin
	Eat all food groups
	Self-Care (5 deep breaths, take vitamins, massage Live Clean lotion, brush teeth)
	Fill in your daily planner and to do list
	Clean your desk
	Buy something for someone
	Attract Abundance (3 things you are grateful for) 1. 2. 3.
	Pray for success Dear God, Amen
	Manifest Daily Goal(s)+Intention 1. 2. 3.

Day 15

To Do List

	Date
	Shower(s) or Bath(s)
	Water Intake 1000ml pure and clean
	Sleep Hours (7 to 9 hours)
	Meditative Mindfulness (deep breathing 10-30minutes)
	Exercise (10-30min)
	Daily Reading
	Take a multivitamin
	Eat all food groups (avoid flour)
	Self-Care (5 deep breaths, take vitamins, massage Live Clean lotion, brush teeth)
	Create a vision board
	Clean your bed sheets
	Buy your favorite magazine
	Attract Abundance (3 things you are grateful for) 1. 2. 3.
	Pray for mother earth Dear God, Amen
	Manifest Daily Goal(s)+Intention 1. 2. 3.

Day 16

To Do List

	Date
	Shower(s) or Bath(s)
	Water Intake 1000ml pure and clean
	Sleep Hours (7 to 9 hours)
	Meditative Mindfulness (deep breathing 10-30minutes)
	Exercise (10-30min)
	Daily Reading
	Take a multivitamin
	Eat all food groups
	Self-Care (5 deep breaths, take vitamins, massage Live Clean lotion, brush teeth)
	Start a collection of something and continue collecting
	Clean bedroom floors
	Share old memories with someone (maybe via scrapbook)
	Attract Abundance (3 things you are grateful for) 1. 2. 3.
	Pray for your career and dream job(s) Dear God, Amen
	Manifest Daily Goal(s)+Intention 1. 2. 3.

Day 17

To Do List

Date	
Shower(s) or Bath(s)	
Water Intake 1000ml pure and clean	
Sleep Hours (7 to 9 hours)	
Meditative Mindfulness (deep breathing 10-30minutes)	
Exercise (10-30min)	
Daily Reading	
Take a multivitamin	
Eat all food groups	
Self-Care (5 deep breaths, take vitamins, massage Live Clean lotion, brush teeth)	
Affirm 7 times I am successful in everything I do	
Clean your walls	
Take a selfie and a few photos	
Attract Abundance (3 things you are grateful for) 1. 2. 3.	
Pray for transportation Dear God, Amen	
Manifest Daily Goal(s)+Intention 1. 2. 3.	

Day 18

To Do List

	Date
	Shower(s) or Bath(s)
	Water Intake 1000ml pure and clean
	Sleep Hours (7 to 9 hours)
	Meditative Mindfulness (deep breathing 10-30minutes)
	Exercise (10-30min)
	Daily Reading
	Take a multivitamin
	Eat all food groups
	Self-Care (5 deep breaths, take vitamins, massage Live Clean lotion, brush teeth)
	Enroll in a course or professional development hobby
	Clean your windows
	Make a list of why you love yourself
	Attract Abundance (3 things you are grateful for) 1. 2. 3.
	Pray for music Dear God, Amen
	Manifest Daily Goal(s)+Intention 1. 2. 3.

Day 19

To Do List

	Date
	Shower(s) or Bath(s)
	Water Intake 1000ml pure and clean
	Sleep Hours (7 to 9 hours)
	Meditative Mindfulness (deep breathing 10-30minutes)
	Exercise (10-30min)
	Daily Reading
	Take a multivitamin
	Eat all food groups (no caffeine today)
	Self-Care (5 deep breaths, take vitamins, massage Live Clean lotion, brush teeth)
	Try a new food or restaurant
	Clean your doorknobs, phones, computers, tvs and remotes
	Donate unused clothing and apparel
	Attract Abundance (3 things you are grateful for) 1. 2. 3.
	Pray for your reputation and fame Dear God, Amen
	Manifest Daily Goal(s)+Intention 1. 2. 3.

Day 20

To Do List

	Date
	Shower(s) or Bath(s)
	Water Intake 1000ml pure and clean
	Sleep Hours (7 to 9 hours)
	Meditative Mindfulness (deep breathing 10-30minutes)
	Exercise (10-30min)
	Daily Reading
	Take a multivitamin
	Eat all food groups
	Self-Care (5 deep breaths, take vitamins, massage Live Clean lotion, brush teeth)
	Make a music playlist for someone or something
	Clean your closets and organize clothes
	Go through old pictures, videos and scrapbook
	Attract Abundance (3 things you are grateful for) 1. 2. 3.
	Pray for creativity Dear God, Amen
	Manifest Daily Goal(s)+Intention 1. 2. 3.

Day 21

To Do List

Date	
Shower(s) or Bath(s)	
Water Intake 1000ml pure and clean	
Sleep Hours (7 to 9 hours)	
Meditative Mindfulness (deep breathing 10-30minutes)	
Exercise (10-30min)	
Daily Reading	
Take a multivitamin	
Eat all food groups	
Self-Care (5 deep breaths, take vitamins, massage Live Clean lotion, brush teeth)	
Go out with a friend or call them	
Clean your Living room	
Wear an eye mask for bedtime	
Attract Abundance (3 things you are grateful for) 1. 2. 3.	
Pray for order and cleanliness Dear God, Amen	
Manifest Daily Goal(s)+Intention 1. 2. 3.	

Day 22

To Do List

	Date
	Shower(s) or Bath(s)
	Water Intake 1000ml pure and clean
	Sleep Hours (7 to 9 hours)
	Meditative Mindfulness (deep breathing 10-30minutes)
	Exercise (10-30min)
	Daily Reading
	Take a multivitamin
	Eat all food groups
	Self-Care (5 deep breaths, take vitamins, massage Live Clean lotion, brush teeth)
	Draw, color or paint something. Go to paint night
	Rearrange an area that hasn't been done in a year or two
	Exercise with someone or go to Zumba or yoga
	Attract Abundance (3 things you are grateful for) 1. 2. 3.
	Pray for your hobbies and entertainment Dear God, Amen
	Manifest Daily Goal(s)+Intention 1. 2. 3.

Day 23

To Do List

	Date
	Shower(s) or Bath(s)
	Water Intake 1000ml pure and clean
	Sleep Hours (7 to 9 hours)
	Meditative Mindfulness (deep breathing 10-30minutes)
	Exercise (10-30min)
	Daily Reading
	Take a multivitamin
	Eat all food groups
	Self-Care (5 deep breaths, take vitamins, massage Live Clean lotion, brush teeth)
	Go out somewhere with someone
	Clean your floors
	Say Ho onoponopono 7 times which means Thank you. I am sorry. I love you
	Attract Abundance (3 things you are grateful for) 1. 2. 3.
	Pray for loved ones Dear God, Amen
	Manifest Daily Goal(s)+Intention 1. 2. 3.

Day 24

<u>To Do List</u>

	Date
	Shower(s) or Bath(s)
	Water Intake 1000ml pure and clean
	Sleep Hours (7 to 9 hours)
	Meditative Mindfulness (deep breathing 10-30minutes)
	Exercise (10-30min)
	Daily Reading
	Take a multivitamin
	Eat all food groups
	Self-Care (5 deep breaths, take vitamins, massage Live Clean lotion, brush teeth)
	Go see a movie, comedy or play
	Clean your curtains
	Create a bucket list
	Attract Abundance (3 things you are grateful for) 1. 2. 3.
	Pray for your senses Dear God, Amen
	Manifest Daily Goal(s)+Intention 1. 2. 3.

Day 25

To Do List

	Date
	Shower(s) or Bath(s)
	Water Intake 1000ml pure and clean
	Sleep Hours (7 to 9 hours)
	Meditative Mindfulness (deep breathing 10-30minutes)
	Exercise (10-30min)
	Daily Reading
	Take a multivitamin
	Eat all food groups
	Self-Care (5 deep breaths, take vitamins, massage Live Clean lotion, brush teeth)
	Answer the question What is the purpose of your life?
	Clean and go through your storage room
	Get or schedule a massage or Self-Care appointment
	Attract Abundance (3 things you are grateful for) 1. 2. 3.
	Pray for happiness Dear God, Amen
	Manifest Daily Goal(s)+Intention 1. 2. 3.

Day 26

To Do List

	Date
	Shower(s) or Bath(s)
	Water Intake 1000ml pure and clean
	Sleep Hours (7 to 9 hours)
	Meditative Mindfulness (deep breathing 10-30minutes)
	Exercise (10-30min)
	Daily Reading
	Take a multivitamin
	Eat all food groups (extra fruit)
	Self-Care (5 deep breaths, take vitamins, massage Live Clean lotion, brush teeth)
	Play a game
	Clean your fridge
	Have or schedule a date
	Attract Abundance (3 things you are grateful for) 1. 2. 3.
	Pray for love Dear God, Amen
	Manifest Daily Goal(s)+Intention 1. 2. 3.

Day 27

To Do List

	Date
	Shower(s) or Bath(s)
	Water Intake 1000ml pure and clean
	Sleep Hours (7 to 9 hours)
	Meditative Mindfulness (deep breathing 10-30minutes)
	Exercise (10-30min)
	Daily Reading
	Take a multivitamin
	Eat all food groups
	Self-Care (5 deep breaths, take vitamins, massage Live Clean lotion, brush teeth)
	Create a personalized coat of arms
	Clean your backyard/balcony
	Cook someone their favorite meal now or another time
	Attract Abundance (3 things you are grateful for) 1. 2. 3.
	Pray for your purpose in life Dear God, Amen
	Manifest Daily Goal(s)+Intention 1. 2. 3.

Day 28

To Do List

	Date
	Shower(s) or Bath(s)
	Water Intake 1000ml pure and clean
	Sleep Hours (7 to 9 hours)
	Meditative Mindfulness (deep breathing 10-30minutes)
	Exercise (10-30min)
	Daily Reading
	Take a multivitamin
	Eat all food groups
	Self-Care (5 deep breaths, take vitamins, massage Live Clean lotion, brush teeth)
	Get or schedule a family photo
	Clean your entry way(s)
	Host and plan a party
	Attract Abundance (3 things you are grateful for) 1. 2. 3.
	Pray for education and knowledge Dear God, Amen
	Manifest Daily Goal(s)+Intention 1. 2. 3.

Day 29

To Do List

Date	
Shower(s) or Bath(s)	
Water Intake 1000ml pure and clean	
Sleep Hours (7 to 9 hours)	
Meditative Mindfulness (deep breathing 10-30minutes)	
Exercise (10-30min)	
Daily Reading	
Take a multivitamin	
Eat all food groups	
Self-Care (5 deep breaths, take vitamins, massage Live Clean lotion, brush teeth)	
Join and attend a community class or event.	
Clean your family room	
Plan and book a vacation	
Attract Abundance (3 things you are grateful for) 1. 2. 3.	
Pray for good habits Dear God, Amen	
Manifest Daily Goal(s)+Intention 1. 2. 3.	

Day 30

To Do List

Date	
Shower(s) or Bath(s)	
Water Intake 1000ml pure and clean	
Sleep Hours (7 to 9 hours)	
Meditative Mindfulness (deep breathing 10-30minutes)	
Exercise (10-30min)	
Daily Reading	
Take a multivitamin	
Eat all food groups	
Self-Care (5 deep breaths, take vitamins, massage Live Clean lotion, brush teeth)	

Write a cheque to yourself for what you need and why

THE BANK OF UNIVERSE
FEEL GOOD REMITTANCE ADVICE

Date D D M M Y Y

PAY _____ OR BEARER

DOLLARS _____ $ ____

MEMO _____ NON-NEGOTIABLE: THE POWER OF BELIEF

DRAWN ON THE UNIVERSAL ACCOUNT:
UNLIMITED ABUNDANCE

CHECK NUMBER ⦂|| 000 333 444 111111 ||⦂

The Universe
SIGNATURE
by Special Delivery

Compliments from EvelynLim.com

Clean your bedsheets	
Do your laundry	
Attract Abundance (3 things you are grateful for) 1. 2. 3.	
Pray for anything, Dear God, Amen	
Manifest Daily Goal(s)+Intention 1. 2. 3.	

Day 31

To Do List

Date	
Shower(s) or Bath(s)	
Water Intake 1000ml pure and clean	
Sleep Hours (7 to 9 hours)	
Meditative Mindfulness (deep breathing 10-30minutes)	
Exercise (10-30min)	
Daily Reading	
Take a multivitamin	
Eat all food groups	
Self-Care (5 deep breaths, take vitamins, massage Live Clean lotion, brush teeth)	
Review monthly to do list	
Clean anything that needs it	
Read a book of interest	
Attract Abundance (3 things you are grateful for) 1. 2. 3.	
Pray for wishes and desires Dear God, Amen	
Manifest Daily Goal(s)+Intention 1. 2. 3.	

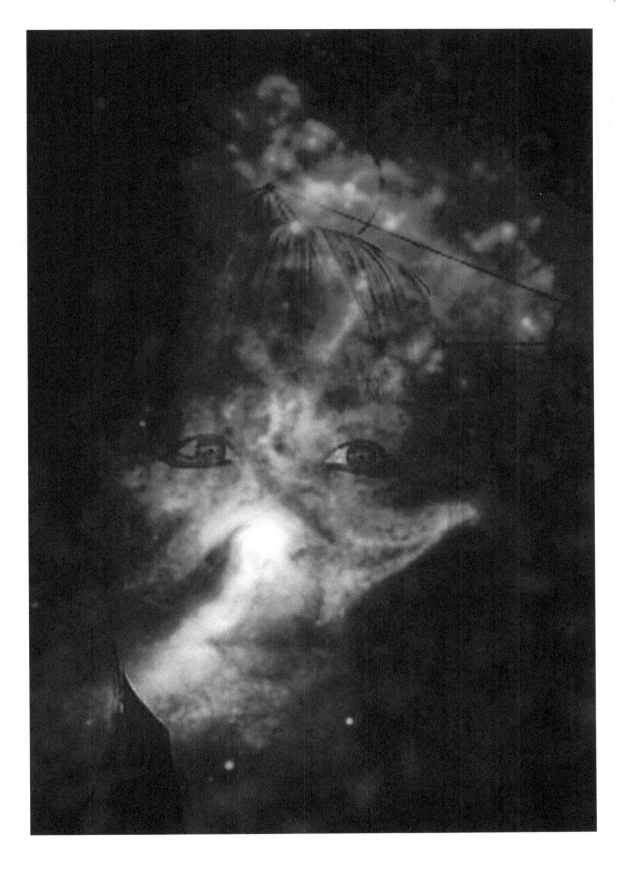

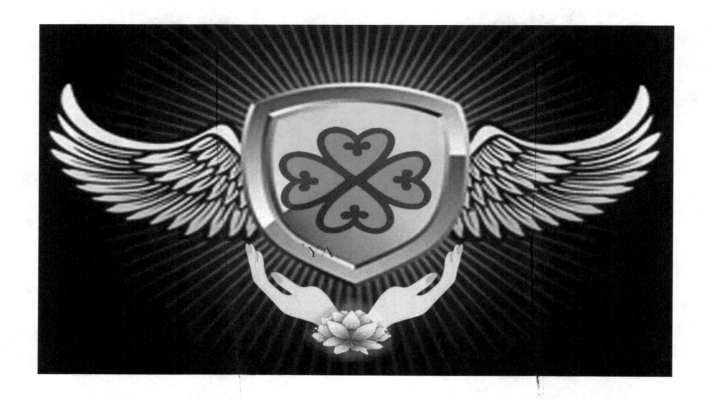

365 Days Devotional Readings with Gratitude and Positive Affirmations

Calendar Daily Readings

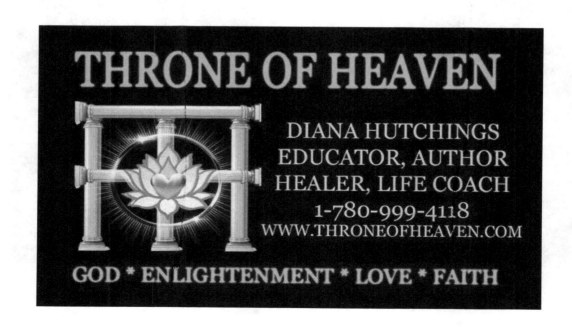

January 1

Colossians 2:9

Christ Begins Real Life

God lives fully in Christ. And you are fully grown because you belong to Christ, who is over every power and authority. Circumcision removes flesh from the body. You were baptized. Then you were raised because you had faith in the power of God. God let Christ make you alive, when he forgave all.

The Rocky Tract

These are the Ayat of revelation of the Qur'an that makes things clear. Leave them to enjoy good things in this life and to please themselves.

Everything that is happening is happening for my ultimate good.

The perfect partner is present in my life now and forever.

I have strength in my heart and clarity in my mind.

I trust my inner wisdom and intuition.

I know my wisdom guides me to the right decisions.

I choose friends who approve of me and love me.

I am doing work what I enjoy while fulfilling my purpose.

I am good and look good always.

I succeed in everything I do.

I can get anything I want anytime.

January 2

Peter 1:9

Living as the Lord's Followers

We have everything we need to live a life that pleases God. It was all given to us by God's own power when we learned that he had invited us to share in his wonderful goodness. God made great and marvelous promises. Do your best to improve. You can do this by adding goodness, understanding, self-control, patience, devotion to God, concern for others and love.

Spider

Serve Allah that will be best for you if ye understand! Seek ye sustenance from Allah, serve Him and be grateful to Him and to Him will be your return. The duty of the messenger is to preach publicly and clearly. See now how Allah originates creation then repeats it truly that is easy for Allah. Say, travel through the earth and see how Allah did originate creation so will Allah produce a later creation for Allah has power over all things.

Everything that is happening is happening for your ultimate good.

The perfect partner is present in your life now and forever.

You have strength in your heart and clarity in your mind.

You trust your inner wisdom and intuition.

You know your wisdom guides you to the right decisions.

You choose friends who approve of you and love you.

You are doing work that you enjoy and find fulfilling your purpose.

You are good and look good always.

You succeed in everything you do.

You can get anything you want anytime.

January 3

Ephesians 5:17

Living as People of Light

Find out what the Lord wants you to do. When you meet together sing psalms, hymns and spiritual songs as you praise the Lord with all your heart. Always use the name of our Lord Jesus Christ to thank God the Father of everything.

The Light

O ye who believe! For the grace and mercy of Allah on you Allah doth purify whom he pleases and Allah is one who hears and knows all things. On the day when their tongues, hands and feet will bear witness as to their actions on that day Allah will pay them back all their just dues and they will realize that Allah is the very truth that makes all things manifest. Women of purity are for men of purity and men of purity are for women of purity.

Everything that is happening is happening for our ultimate good.

The perfect partner is present in our life now and forever.

We have strength in our heart and clarity in our mind.

We trust our inner wisdom and intuition.

We know our wisdom guides us to the right decisions.

We choose friends who approve of us and love us.

We are doing work that we enjoy and find fulfilling our purpose.

We are good and look good always.

We succeed in everything we do.

We can get anything we want anytime.

January 4

Ephesians 3

Christ's Love for Us

I kneel in prayer to the father all beings in heaven and on earth receive their life from him. God is wonderful and glorious. I pray that his spirit will make you become strong followers and that Christ will live in your hearts because of your faith. Stand firm and be deeply rooted in this love. I pray that you and all of God's people will understand what is called wide or long or high or deep. I want you to know all about Christ's love it is too wonderful, to be measured. Your lives will be filled with all that God is.

The Heifer

O ye who believe! When you deal with each other in transactions involving future obligations in a fixed period of time reduce them to writing. Let a scribe write down faithfully as between the parties, let not the scribe refuse to write as Allah has taught him so let him write.

I am grateful to be a healer and am healed completely.

I am grateful to be faithful and loyal always.

I am grateful to be beautiful inside and out.

I am grateful that everything about me is perfect.

I am grateful God puts me first always.

I am grateful to believe in myself and my dreams.

I am grateful to be happy all the time.

I am grateful to be brilliant, clever, quick, loving and lovable always.

I am grateful to be free all the time.

I am grateful to deserve the best always and get it.

January 5

John 5:19

The Son's Authority

Jesus told the people I tell you for certain that the son can do anything on his own. He can do what he sees the father doing and he does exactly what he sees the father do. The father loves the son and has shown him everything he does. The father will show him even greater things and you will be amazed. Just as the father gives life so the son gives life to anyone he wants to. The father has made his son the judge of everyone. The father wants all people to honor the son as much as they honor him.

Joseph

Now with him there came into two young men. Said one of them, I see myself in a dream pressing wine. We see thou art one that doth good to all. He said before any food comes in due course to feed either of you I will surely reveal to you the truth and meaning of this.

You are grateful to be a healer and you're healed.

You are grateful to be faithful and loyal always.

You are grateful to be beautiful inside and out.

You are grateful that everything about you is perfect.

You are grateful God puts you first always.

You are grateful to believe in yourself and your dreams.

You are grateful to be happy all the time.

You are grateful to be brilliant, clever, quick, loving and lovable always.

You are grateful to be free all the time.

You are grateful to deserve the best always and get it.

January 6

Revelation 5:9

Seal of God

Then they sang a new song. You are worthy to receive the scroll and open its seals because you bought for God's people from every tribe language, nation and race. You let them become kings and serve God as priests and they will rule on earth. As I looked, I heard the voices of a lot of angels around the throne and the voices of the living creatures and of the leaders. There were millions and millions of them and they were saying in a loud voice the lamb is worthy to receive power, riches, wisdom, strength, honor, glory and praise.

Ta Ha

A revelation from him who created the earth and the heavens on high. Allah most gracious is firmly established on the throne of authority. If though pronounce the word aloud it is no matter for verily he knoweth what is secret and what is yet hidden. Allah there is no god but He. To Him belong the most beautiful names.

We are grateful to be healers and we are healed.

We are grateful to be faithful and loyal always.

We are grateful to be beautiful inside and out.

We are grateful that everything about us is perfect.

We are grateful God puts us first always.

We are grateful to believe in us and our dreams.

We are grateful to be happy all the time.

We are grateful to be brilliant, clever, quick, loving and lovable always.

We are grateful to be free all the time.

We are grateful to deserve the best always and get it.

January 7

Galatians 3:21

God's Promises

If any law could give life to us we could become acceptable to God by obeying the law. God's promises will be for anyone who has faith in Jesus Christ. In fact, the law was our teacher. We had faith and were acceptable to God. But once a person has learned to have faith there is no more need to have the law as a teacher.

The Prophets

And we have set on the Earth Mountains standing firm lest it should shake with them and we have made therein broad highways between mountains for them to pass through that they may receive guidance. And we have made the heavens as a canopy well-guarded.

All my relationships are long, lasting, loving and perfect.

My perfect partner is the love of my life and he/she loves me as much as I love him/her.

I have attracted the most loving person in my life and we are full of joy.

My partner and I are a perfect match and our love is divine.

I radiate pure, unconditional love to my partner and he/she to me and we compliment each other.

I understand my partner completely.

I am in love with a loving person who is caring, committed, loyal, trustworthy and understanding.

I give out love and it is returned to me multiplied many folds.

I deserve love and get it in abundance.

I see everything with loving eyes and ears and I love everything I see and hear.

January 8

John 16:16

Turn to Joy

Jesus told his disciples, "For a little while you won't see me but after a while you will see me." What does he mean by saying that he is going to the father.

The Women

Those men Allah knows what is in their hearts and speak to them a word to reach their very souls. We sent a messenger but to be obeyed in accordance with the will of Allah. All who obey Allah and the messenger are in the company of those whom is the grace of Allah prophets (who teach), sincere (lovers of truth), witnesses (who testify) and the righteous (who do good). Ah what a beautiful fellowship.

All your relationships are long, lasting, loving and perfect.

Your perfect partner is the love of your life and you love each other.

You have attracted the most loving person in your life and you are full of joy.

Your partner and you are a perfect match and your love is divine.

You radiate pure, unconditional love to your partner and you compliment each other.

You understand your partner completely.

You are in love with a loving person who is caring, committed, loyal, trustworthy and understanding.

You give out love and it is returned to you multiplied many fold.

You deserve love and get it in abundance.

You see everything with loving eyes and ears and you love everything you see and hear.

January 9

Matthew 6:19

Treasures in Heaven

Store up treasures on earth. Store up your treasures in heaven. Your treasure will always be where your heart is.

Al-An Am

O ye assembly of Jinn's and men. Come there unto you messengers from amongst you, settling forth unto you my signs and warning you of the meeting of this day of yours. To all are degrees or ranks according to their deeds for thy Lord is mindful of anything that they do. Thy Lord is self-sufficient, full of Mercy.

All our relationships are long, lasting, loving and perfect.

Our perfect partner is the love of our life and loves us.

We have attracted the most loving person in our life and we are full of joy.

Our partner and us are a perfect match and our love is divine.

We radiate pure, unconditional love to our partner and we compliment each other.

We understand our partner completely.

We are in love with a loving person who is caring, committed, loyal, trustworthy and understanding.

We give out love and it is returned to us multiplied many fold.

We deserve love and get it in abundance.

We see everything with loving eyes and ears and we love everything we see and hear.

January 10

1 Corinthians 1:10

Taking Sides

My dear friends as a follower of our Lord Jesus Christ I beg you to get along with each other. Don't take sides. Always try to agree in what you think. They have said that some of you claim to follow me, while others claim to follow Apollos or Peter or Christ.

The Women

O ye who believe! Approach prayers after washing your whole body. If ye find water then take for yourselves clean water and rub therewith your faces and hands for Allah forgives again and again. Allah hath full knowledge. Allah is enough for a protector and Allah is enough for a helper.

I am grateful to attract Jesus my soul mate and twin flame.

I am grateful my soul mate is strongly attracted to me.

I am grateful to be focused on my perfect partner and our happiness.

I am grateful to live happily ever after.

I am grateful me and my perfect partner give off positive and loving energy always.

I am grateful it's easy to be loved, loving and lovable.

I am grateful to receive beauty, love and loyalty from my perfect partner and it's returned to him.

I am grateful we support and believe in each other.

I am grateful I attract and stimulate my partner perfectly.

I am grateful me and my partner do exciting things and we are best friends.

January 11

Luke 2:27

God Keeps His Promises

Simeon took Jesus in his arms and praised God, Lord I am your servant and now in peace because you have kept your promise to me. With my own eyes I have seen what you have done to save your people and foreign nations will also see this mighty power is a light for all nations and it will bring honor to your people Israel.

The Poets

If such our will we could send down to them from the sky a sign. But there comes to them a newly revealed; message from Allah most gracious. So, they will know soon enough the truth. They look at the earth how many noble things of all kinds we have produced therein? Verily in this is a sign.

You are grateful to attract Jesus your soul mate and twin flame.

You are grateful your soul mate is strongly attracted to you.

You are grateful to be focused on your perfect partner and your happiness.

You are grateful to live happily ever after.

You are grateful you and your perfect partner give off positive and loving energy always.

You are grateful it's easy to be loved, loving and lovable.

You are grateful to receive beauty, love and loyalty from your perfect partner and it's returned.

You are grateful you support and believe in each other.

You are grateful you attract and stimulate your partner perfectly.

You are grateful you and your partner do exciting things and you are best friends.

January 12

John 16:18

The Work of the Holy Spirit

The Spirit will come and show the people of this world the truth and God's justice and the judgment. The Spirit will show them that they have faith in me. I am going to the father and you won't see me again. The spirit shows what is true and will come and guide you into the full truth.

The Gold Adornments

By the book that makes things clear. We have made it a Qur'an in Arabic thereat ye may be able to understand and learn wisdom. But how many were the prophets. We sent amongst the peoples of old? Thus, has passed on the parable of the peoples of old.

We are grateful to attract Jesus our soul mate and twin flame.

We are grateful our soul mate is strongly attracted to us.

We are grateful to be focused on our perfect partner and our happiness.

We are grateful to live happily ever after.

We are grateful we give off positive and loving energy always.

We are grateful it's easy to be loved, loving and lovable.

We are grateful to receive beauty, love and loyalty from our perfect partner and it's returned.

We are grateful we support and believe in each other.

We are grateful we attract and stimulate our partner perfectly.

We are grateful we do exciting things and we are best friends.

January 13

1 Corinthians 10:23

Always Honor God

Some of you say we can do whatever we want to. But I tell you that maybe good or helpful. We should think about others. However, when you buy meat in the market go ahead and eat it. Keep your conscience clear by not asking where the meat came from. The scriptures say the earth and everything in it belong to the Lord.

The Table Spread

O ye who believe! The good things which Allah hath made lawful for you. Eat of the things which Allah hath provided for you, lawful and good. He will call you to account for what is in your oaths.

I can easily hold a good conversation.

I am a good listener and can connect well with others.

I am confident, friendly and outgoing always.

I am always willing to make new friends.

I am easy to approach and project positive body language.

I find it easy to be in social situations.

I try to put myself in positive social situations.

I am making more good friends every day.

Being someone who can talk to anyone has added value to my life.

I enjoy meeting new and interesting people to be friends with.

January 14

Revelations11:15

Time for Judgment

At the sound of the 7th trumpet loud voices were heard in heaven. They said, now the kingdom of this world belongs to our Lord and to his chosen one. And he will rule forever and ever. Then the 24 elders who are seated on thrones in God's presence knelt down and worshiped him. They said Lord God all powerful you are and you were and we thank you. You used your great power and started ruling. Now the time has come to be judged. It is time for you to reward your servants the prophets and all your people who honor your name no matter who they are.

The Heights

Do they reflect? Do they see in the government or the heavens and the earth and all that Allah hath created? Do they see that it may be that their term is nigh drawing to an end? What message after this will they then believe?

You can easily hold a good conversation.

You are a good listener and can connect well with others.

You are confident, friendly and outgoing always.

You are always willing to make new friends.

You are easy to approach and project positive body language.

You find it easy to be in social situations.

You try to put yourself in positive social situations.

You are making more good friends every day.

Being someone who can talk to anyone has added value to your life.

You enjoy meeting new and interesting people to be friends with.

January 15

Luke 4:17

Jesus Begins his Work

He was given the book of Isaiah the prophet he opened it and read, the Lord's spirit has come to me because he has chosen me to tell the good news. The Lord sent me to announce freedom to give sight, to free everyone and to say this year the Lord has chosen. Jesus closed the book then handed it back to the man in charge and sat down. Doctor first make yourself well.

The Repentance

Then rejoice in the bargain which ye have concluded that is the achievement supreme. Those that turn to Allah in repentance that serves him and praise him that wonder in devotion to the cause of Allah that bow down and prostrate themselves in prayer that enjoin good, observe the limit set by Allah these do rejoice. So, proclaim the glad tidings to the believers.

We can easily hold a good conversation.

We are good listeners and can connect well with others.

We are confident, friendly and outgoing always.

We are always willing to make new friends.

We are easy to approach and project positive body language.

We find it easy to be in social situations.

We try to put ourselves in positive social situations.

We are making more good friends every day.

Being someone who can talk to anyone has added value to our life.

We enjoy meeting new and interesting people to be friends with.

January 16

Hebrews 8:1

A Better Promise

What I mean is that we have a high priest who sits at the right side of Gods great throne in heaven. He also serves as the priest in the most holy place inside the real tent there in heaven. This tent of worship was set up by the Lord. Since all priests must offer gifts and sacrifices, Christ also needed to have something to offer.

The Night Journey

Behold we said to the angels bow down unto Adam they bowed down. Shall I bow down to one whom thou didst create from clay? He said seest thou? Enough is thy Lord for a disposer of affairs.

I am grateful loving relationships come easily to me.

I am grateful to attract wonderful positive people into my universe.

I am grateful to enjoy the company of everyone.

I am grateful and honored to have some good friends in my life.

I am grateful to communicate with everyone effectively.

I am grateful I've earned the respect of all my friends and family and coworkers.

I am grateful to expect great relationships therefore that's what I receive.

I am grateful people find me intellectually and socially stimulating and fun.

I am grateful I have very trustworthy kind and helpful friends.

I am grateful my friends are there when I need them.

January 17

Psalm 72

A Prayer for God to Guide and Help the King

Let peace and justice rule every mountain and hill. Let the king defend them. Let the king live forever like the sun and the moon. Let the king be fair with everyone and let there be peace until the moon falls from the sky.

The Cave

We placed cornfields each of those gardens brought forth its produce in the midst of them we caused a river to flow (abundant) was the produce this man had. He said to this companion in the course of mutual agreement more wealth than I thank you and more honor and power in my following of men.

You are grateful loving relationships come easily to you.

You are grateful to attract wonderful positive people into your universe.

You are grateful to enjoy the company of everyone.

You are grateful and honored to have some good friends in your life.

You are grateful to communicate with everyone effectively.

You are grateful you have earned the respect of all your friends, family and coworkers.

You are grateful to expect great relationships therefore that's what you receive.

You are grateful people find you intellectually and socially stimulating and fun.

You are grateful you have very trustworthy kind and helpful friends.

You are grateful your friends are there when you need them.

January 18

1 Corinthians 18:1

Christ is God's Power and Wisdom

For those of us who are being saved, it is God's power at work. My dear friends remember what you were when God chose you.

Hud

And of surety to all will your Lord pay back in the recompense of their deeds for he knoweth well all that they do. Therefore, stand firm in the straight path as thou art commanded thou and those who with thee turn unto Allah and he seeth well all that ye do.

We are grateful loving relationships come easily to us.

We are grateful to attract wonderful positive people into our universe.

We are grateful to enjoy the company of everyone.

We are grateful and honored to have some good friends in our life.

We are grateful to communicate with everyone effectively.

We are grateful we have earned the respect of all our friends, family and coworkers.

We are grateful to expect great relationships therefore that's what we receive.

We are grateful people find us intellectually and socially stimulating and fun.

We are grateful we have very trustworthy kind and helpful friends.

We are grateful our friends are there when we need them.

January 19

1 Thessalonians 4

The Thessalonians Faith and Example

My dear friends God loves you and we know he has chosen you to be his people. Know what kind of people we were and how we helped you. So when you accepted the message you followed our example and the example of the Lord. The Holy Spirit made you glad. They also tell how you are waiting for his son Jesus to come from heaven. God raised him and on the Day of Judgment Jesus will save us.

The Night Journey

Establish regular prayers at the suns decline. Carry their testimony. And pray in the small watches of the morning. It would be an additional prayer or spiritual profit for thee, soon will thy Lord raise thee to a station of praise and glory by the gate of truth and honor and likewise my exit by the gate of truth and honor and grant me from thy presence an authority to aid me. And say truth has now arrived.

I am appreciated and compensated wherever I work.

I deserved to be employed and paid well.

I am attracting opportunities every day.

When it is time for a new job the perfect position presents itself.

I am very successful in my chosen career.

I now do work I love.

I can balance work and play.

Success, money and happiness come easily to me.

At my job, my coworkers and I encourage our growth and success.

I know where I am and where I want to go and how to get there.

January 20

1 Timothy 12

Being Thankful for God's Kindness

I thank Christ Jesus our Lord. He has given me the strength for my work because he knew that he could trust me. He had mercy on me. Christ Jesus our Lord was very kind to me. He has greatly blessed my life with faith and love just like his own. Christ Jesus came into the world to save.

The Rocky Tract

These are the Ayat of revelations of a Qur'an that makes things clear. Leave them to enjoy the good things of this life and to please.

You are appreciated and compensated wherever you work.

You deserved to be employed and paid well.

You are attracting opportunities everyday.

When it is time for a new job the perfect position presents itself.

You are very successful in your chosen career.

You now do work you love.

You can balance work and play.

Success, money and happiness come easily to you.

At your job your coworkers and you encourage your growth and success.

You know where you are and where you want to go and how to get there.

January 21

John 10:7

Jesus is a Good Shepherd

Jesus said: I tell you for certain that I am the gate for the sheep. I am the gate. All who come in through me will be saved. Through me they will come and go and find pasture. I come so that everyone would have life. I am the good shepherd. I know my sheep and they know me. Just as the father knows me. I know the father and I give up my life for my sheep.

The Poets

Moses said to them, "Throw ye that which ye are about to throw! So they threw their ropes and their rods and said, we believe in the Lord of the Worlds. The Lord of Moses and Aaron. We shall return to our Lord! Our Lord will forgive us that we become believers.

We are appreciated and compensated wherever we work.

We deserved to be employed and paid well.

We are attracting opportunities every day.

When it is time for a new job the perfect position presents itself.

We are very successful in our chosen careers.

We now do work we love.

We can balance work and play.

Success, money and happiness come easily to us.

At our job our coworkers and us encourage our growth and success.

We know where we are and where we want to go and how to get there.

January 22

1 Corinthians 14:26

Worship Must Be Orderly

My friends when you meet to worship you must do everything for the good of everyone there. That's how it should be when someone sings or teaches or tells. No more than 2 or 3 of you should speak unknown languages during the meeting. You must take turns and someone should always be there to explain what you mean.

The Believers

We sent Noah to his people and he said, O my people worship Allah. Noah said, "O my Lord! Help me." So we inspired him with this message. Construct the ark within our sight and under our guidance then when our command and the fountains of the earth comes gush forth thousands of pairs of every species male and female.

I am grateful to be the best I can be.

I am grateful to be a light of God to my clients and the people I work with.

I am grateful for amazing opportunities.

I am grateful to every person whom contributed to my success.

I am grateful to have the most blessed perfect career.

I am grateful to communicate very well.

I am grateful for all my talents and abilities.

I am grateful to be a pretty easy-going leader and colleague that gives wise advice.

I am grateful to be successful in everything I do all the time.

I am grateful to do my job super well and I love it.

January 23

Luke 2:8

The Shepherds

All at once an angel came down to them from the Lord and the brightness of the Lord's glory flashed around them the shepherds. But the angel said I have good news for you which will make everyone happy. This very day in King David's hometown a savior was born to you. He is Christ the Lord. Suddenly angels came down from heaven joining in praising God. Praise God in heaven and peace on earth to everyone who pleases God.

Hud

And of a surety to all will your Lord pay back the recompense of their deeds for he knoweth well all that they do. Therefore, stand firm in the straight path as thou art commanded thou and those who with thee turn unto Allah and he seeth that they do.

You are grateful to be the best you can be.

You are grateful to be a light of God to your clients and the people you work with.

You are grateful for amazing opportunities.

You are grateful to every person whom contributed to your success.

You are grateful to have the most blessed perfect career.

You are grateful to communicate very well.

You are grateful for all your talents and abilities.

You are grateful to be a pretty easy-going leader and colleague that gives wise advice.

You are grateful to be successful in everything you do all the time.

You are grateful to do your job super well and you love it.

January 24

Revelation 16:4

The Lord God is Honest and Fair

I heard, Lord God All Powerful your judgments are honest and fair. Remember that Christ says the angel who has power over water say, you have always been and you will always be the holy God. You had the right to judge in this way. After this I heard the altar shout yes Lord God All Powerful your judgments are honest and fair. Remember Christ says, when I come it will surprise you. But God will bless you if you are awake and ready.

The Originator

Praise be to Allah who created out of nothing the heavens and the earth who made the angels, messengers with wings two or three or four pairs he adds to creation as he pleases for Allah has power over all things. He is exalted in power full wisdom O men! Call to mind the grace of Allah unto you.

We are grateful to be the best we can be.

We are grateful to be a light of God to our clients and the people we work with.

We are grateful for amazing opportunities.

We are grateful to every person whom contributed to our success.

We are grateful to have the most, blessed perfect career.

We are grateful to communicate very well.

We are grateful for all our talents and abilities.

We are grateful to be an easy-going leader and colleague that gives wise advice.

We are grateful to be successful in everything we do all the time.

We are grateful to do our job super well and we love it.

January 25

2 Corinthians 5:11

Bringing People to God

We know what it means to respect the Lord and we encourage everyone to turn to him. God himself knows what we are like and I hope you also know what kind of people we are. We want you to be proud of us it is between God and us, but if we are in our own minds it is for your good we are ruled in powerful moments by Christ's love for us, for everyone.

The Pilgrimage

Those who leave their homes in the cause of Allah will Allah bestow verily a goodly provision. Verily He will admit them to a place with which they shall be well pleased for Allah is All Knowing, Most Forbearing. Allah will help him for Allah is one that forgives again and again. That is because Allah merges night into day and he merges day and night and verily it is Allah who hears and sees all things. This is because Allah He is the reality.

I have abundant energy, vitality and wellbeing.

I am ready to be healed.

I am guided and receive clear messages to validate the best path for wellbeing.

I exercise regularly to keep myself fit and energetic.

I am healthier, fitter, faster and stronger.

I treat my body, mind and soul in respectful ways.

I am the picture of positive energy and wellbeing.

I have chosen to be happy because it's good for my health.

I am in super good health, wealth and happiness.

All my body, mind and soul function perfectly well.

January 26

1 Timothy 2

How to Pray

First of all I ask you to pray for everyone. Ask God to help and bless them all and tell God how thankful you are for each of them. Pray for kings and others so that we live a quiet and peaceful life, we worship and honor God. This kind of prayer is good and it pleases God our Savior. God wants everyone to be saved and to know the whole truth which is there is only one God and Christ Jesus is the only one who can bring us to God. Jesus was truly human and he gave himself to rescue all of us.

The Table Spread

Recite to them the truth of the story of the two sons of Adam. Behold they each presented a sacrifice to Allah, it was accepted. Allah the Cherisher of the Worlds. If anyone saved a life it would be as if he saved the life of the whole people. There came to them our messengers with clear signs.

You have abundant energy, vitality and well-being.

You are ready to be healed.

You are guided and receive clear messages to validate the best path for well-being.

You exercise regularly to keep yourself fit and energetic.

You are healthier, fitter, faster and stronger.

You treat your body, mind and soul in respectful ways.

You are the picture of positive energy and wellbeing.

You have chosen to be happy because it's good for your health.

You are in super good health, wealth and happiness.

All your body, mind and soul functions perfectly well.

January 27

1 Corinthians 15:12

God's People will be Raised to Life

Christ has been raised to life! He makes us certain that others will also be raised to life. We will be raised to life because of Christ. Christ has all powers and forces the end will come and he will give the kingdom to God the Father. Christ will rule until he puts all under his power.

The Cattle

To whom we gave life and a light whereby he can walk amongst men. Allah knoweth best where and how to carry out his mission. Truly my prayer and my service of sacrifice and my life are all for Allah, the Cherisher of the Worlds.

We have abundant energy, vitality and well-being.

We are ready to be healed.

We are guided and receive clear messages to validate the best path for well-being.

We exercise regularly to keep ourselves fit and energetic.

We are healthier, fitter, faster and stronger.

We treat our body, mind and soul in respectful ways.

We are the picture of positive energy and wellbeing.

We have chosen to be happy because it's good for our health.

We are in super good health, wealth and happiness.

All our bodies, minds and souls function perfectly well.

January 28

1 Corinthians 3:16

Only One Foundation

All of you surely know that you are God's temple and that his Spirit lives in you. Together you are God's holy temple. You can truly be wise. It is just as the scriptures say, God catches the wise.

The Ants

When they come before the judgment seat Allah will say, and the word will be fulfilled. See they not that we have made the night for them to rest in and the day to give them light. Verily in this are signs for any people that believed. And the day the trumpet will be sounded.

I am grateful the body heals with play; the mind heals with laughter and the soul heals with relaxation.

I am grateful I choose inner peace, happiness and well-being.

I am grateful I am filled with wellness, health and vitality always.

I am grateful to respect my body, mind and soul.

I am grateful all is well always.

I am grateful to be a giver, a giver of love, strength and good vibes.

I am grateful to keep myself fit and energetic always.

I am capable and competent in my body, mind and soul to accomplish anything.

I am grateful to be quick, alert, awake and enlightened.

January 29

James 5:7

Be Patient and Kind

My friends be patient until the Lord returns. Think of farmers who wait patiently for the spring and summer rains to make their valuable crops grow. The judge is right outside the door. My friends follow the example of the prophets who spoke for the Lord. They were patient. In fact, we praise the ones who endured the most. You remember how patient Job was and how the Lord helped him. The Lord did this because he is merciful and kind.

The Winds that Scatter

Has the story reached thee of the honored guests of Abraham. Behold they entered his presence and said peace he said peace! They said give him glad tidings of a son endowed with knowledge. They said even so has thy Lord spoken and he is full of wisdom and knowledge.

You are grateful the body heals with play, the mind heals with laughter and the soul heals with relaxation.

You are grateful you choose inner peace, happiness and well-being.

You are grateful you are filled with wellness, health and vitality always.

You are grateful to respect your body, mind and soul.

You are grateful all is well always.

You are grateful to be a giver, a giver of love, strength and good vibes.

You are grateful to keep yourself fit and energetic always.

You are capable and competent in your body, mind and soul to accomplish anything.

You are grateful to be quick, alert, awake and enlightened.

January 30

Acts 1:6

Jesus is Taken to Heaven

Jesus said to them you don't need to know the time of those events that only the father knows. But the Holy Spirit will come upon you and give you power. After Jesus had said this and while they were watching he was taken up into a cloud. They kept looking up into the sky. Jesus has been taken to heaven.

Joseph

These are the symbols or verses of the perspicuous book. We have sent it down as an Arabic Qur'an in order that ye may learn wisdom. We do relate unto thee the most beautiful of stories in that we reveal to thee this portion of the Quran before this. Behold Joseph said to his father o my father I did see eleven stars the sun and the moon and I saw them prostrate themselves to me.

We are grateful the body heals with play, the mind heals with laughter and the soul heals with relaxation.

We are grateful we choose inner peace, happiness and well-being.

We are grateful we are filled with wellness, health and vitality always.

We are grateful to respect our body, mind and soul.

We are grateful all is well always.

We are grateful to be a giver, a giver of love, strength and good vibes.

We are grateful to keep ourself fit and energetic always.

We are capable and competent in our body, mind and soul to accomplish anything.

We are grateful to be quick, alert, awake and enlightened.

January 31

St John 17:1

Father Glorify Us

As thou hast given him power over all flesh that he should give eternal life to as many as though hast given him. And this is life eternal that they might know the only true God and Jesus Christ whom thou hast sent. I have glorified thee on the earth I have finished the words which though gavest me to do. And now O father glorify me with thine own self with the glory I had with before the world was.

Luqman

These are verses of the wise book. A guide and mercy to the doers of good. These are on true guidance from their Lord and these are the ones who will prosper. For those who believe and work righteous deeds there will be in gardens of bliss to dwell therein. The promise of Allah is true and he is exalted in power, wise.

I am financially free.

I have more money than I ever needed.

I am one with this power, infinite love, infinite supplier and infinite channel.

I am a vibrational match for financial prosperity.

I have good credit and no debts that are not already paid.

I can manage my finances wisely.

I expect an abundance of money to come to me.

I honor and respect my values and joyfully increase my assets.

I have a good money vibration that brings joy and delight to all.

February 1

Hebrews 3:4

A Rest for God's People

For every house is builder by some men but he that built all things is God. But Christ as a son over his own house whose house are we if we hold fast the confidence and the rejoicing of the hope firm unto the end. Wherefore as the Holy Ghost saith today if ye will hear his voice.

Abraham

Speak to my servants who have believed that they may establish regular prayer and spend in charity out of the sustenance we have given them secretly and openly before the coming of a day. It is Allah who hath created the heavens and the earth and sendeth down rain from the skies and with it fruits wherewith to feed you, It is he who hath made the ships subject to you, they may sail across the sea by his command and the rivers also hath been made subject to you.

You are financially free.

You have more money than you ever needed.

You are one with this power, infinite love, infinite supplier and infinite channel.

You are a vibrational match for financial prosperity.

You have good credit and no debts that are not already paid.

You can manage your finances wisely.

You expect an abundance of money to come to you.

You honor and respect your values and joyfully increase your assets.

You have a good money vibration that brings joy and delight to all.

February 2

Ephesians 6:14

Be Ready

Let the truth be like a belt around your waist and let God's justice protect you like armor. Tell the good news about peace be like shoes on your feet. Let your faith be like a shield. Let God's saving power be like a helmet and for a sword use Gods message that comes from the spirit. Stay alert and keep praying for God's people. Pray that I will be given the message to speak and that I may explain the mystery of the good news.

The Moon

That the fruit of his striving will soon come in sight. Then will he be rewarded with a reward complete. That to your Lord is the final goal that it is he who grants laughter that it is he who grants life that he did create in pairs male and female. That he has promised a second creation. It is he who gives wealth and satisfaction that he is the Lord.

We are financially free.

We have more money than we ever needed.

We are one with this power, infinite love, infinite supplier and infinite channel.

We are a vibrational match for financial prosperity.

We have good credit and no debts that are not already paid.

We can manage our finances wisely.

We expect an abundance of money to come to us.

We honor and respect our values and joyfully increase our assets.

We have a good money vibration that brings joy and delight to all.

February 3

Ephesians 5:21

Wives and Husbands

Honor Christ and put others first. A wife should put her husband first as she does the Lord. A husband is the head of his wife as Christ is the head and the savior of the church which is his own body. He made the church holy by the power of his word and he made it pure by washing it with water. A husband should love his wife as much as he loves himself. A husband who loves his wife shows that he loves himself. Each wife should respect her husband.

Mary

The day shall gather the righteous to Allah most gracious like a band presented before a king for honors. None shall have the power of intercession but such as one as has received permission or promise from Allah most gracious. They say Allah most gracious has begotten a son.

I am grateful prosperity has come and will stay.

I am grateful my skills and knowledge are of. service to the world.

I am grateful to love actively and passively making money.

I am grateful unexpected money comes to me all the time.

I am grateful the universe conspires to make me wealthy.

I am grateful the universe is conspiring to make me wealthy.

I am grateful my positive attitude is attracting money.

I am grateful to become richer and richer every day.

I am grateful to have an infinite supply of money and love.

I am grateful I live in financial security.

I am grateful to have well taken care of clean luxurious items.

February 4

Ephesians 6:1

Children and Parents

Children you belong to the Lord and you do the right thing when you obey your parents. The first commandment with a promise says obey your father and mother and you will have a long and happy life. Parents don't be hard on your children. Raise them properly. Teach them and instruct them about the Lord. You must obey your earthly masters. Show them great respect and be as loyal to them as you are to Christ. To please them at all times.

The Repentance

Then rejoice in the bargain which ye have concluded that is the achievement supreme. Those that turn to Allah in repentance that serves him and praise him that wonder in devotion to the cause of Allah that bow down and prostrate themselves in prayer that enjoin good and observe the limit set by Allah these do rejoice. So proclaim the glad tidings to the believers.

I am grateful prosperity has come and will stay.

I am grateful my skills and knowledge are of service to the world.

I am grateful to love actively and passively making money.

I am grateful unexpected money comes to me all the time.

I am grateful the universe conspires to make me wealthy.

I am grateful my positive attitude is attracting money.

I am grateful to become richer and richer every day.

I am grateful to be an infinite supply of money and love.

I am grateful I live in financial security.

I am grateful to have well taken care of clean, luxurious items.

February 5

Psalm 49

Listen to Wisdom

Everyone on this earth, listen to what I have to say! Listen no matter who you are. Speak words of wisdom. God will rescue me.

The Believer

Raised high above ranks (or Degrees) He is the Lord of the throne of authority and by his command doth he send the spirit of inspiration to any of his servants as he pleases that it may warn men of the day of mutual meeting. The day wherein they will all come forth. Whose will be the dominion that day? Allah the one the irresistible. That day will every soul be requited for what it earned that day for Allah is swift in taking account.

You are grateful prosperity has come and will stay.

You are grateful your skills and knowledge are of service to the world.

You are grateful to love actively and passively making money.

You are grateful unexpected money comes to you all the time.

You are grateful the universe conspires to make you wealthy.

You are grateful your positive attitude is attracting money.

You are grateful to become richer and richer every day.

You are grateful to be an infinite supply of energy and money and love.

You are grateful you live in financial security.

You are grateful to have well taken care of clean luxurious items.

February 6

Galatians 5:1

Christ Gives Freedom

Christ has set us free! This means we are really free. Now hold on to your freedom. If you are a follower of Christ Jesus, it makes no difference whether you are circumcised or not. All that matters is your faith that makes you love others. Use it as an opportunity to serve each other with love.

The Poets

Who created me and it is he who guides me. Who gives me food and drink? It is he who cures me. And who I hope will forgive on the Day of Judgment O my Lord! Bestow wisdom on me and join me with the righteous grant me honorable mention the tongue of truth among the latest generations. Make me one of the inheritors of the garden of bliss.

We are grateful prosperity has come and will stay.

We are grateful our skills and knowledge are of service to the world.

We are grateful to love actively and passively making money.

We are grateful unexpected money comes to us all the time.

We are grateful the universe conspires to make us wealthy.

We are grateful we have a positive attitude in attracting money.

We are grateful to become richer and richer every day.

We are grateful to be an infinite supply of money and love.

We are grateful we live in financial security.

We are grateful to have well taken care of clean, luxurious items.

February 7

Luke 20:14

Life in the Future World

The people in this world get married. They will be like angels and will be God's children because they have been raised to life. In the story about the burning bush Moses clearly shows that people will live again. He said, "The Lord is the God worshiped by Abraham, Isaac and Jacob. So, the Lord is the God of the living. This means that everyone is alive.

The Winds that Scatter

By the winds that scatter broadcast. And those that flow with ease and gentleness and those that distribute by command. Verily that which ye are promised is true. And verily judgment and justice must indeed pass. By the sky with its numerous paths.

I excel in all that I do and success comes easily to me.

I have the power to create all the success and prosperity I desire.

I am worthy of all good life must offer.

I am always open minded and easy to get along with.

I am surrounded by positive supportive people who believe in me.

I believe in myself and my ability to succeed.

I always dress for success in body, mind and soul.

I am well organized and manage my time with expert efficiency.

I am committed to achieving success in every area of my life.

My ambitions are in perfect alignment with my personal values.

February 8

James 3:13

Wisdom from Above

Are any of you wise or sensible? Then show it by living right and by being humble and wise in everything you do. The wisdom that comes from above leads us to be pure, friendly, gentle, sensible, kind, helpful, genuine, and sincere. When peacemaker's plant seeds of peace they will harvest justice.

Al-Fatihah

In the name of Allah, the Gracious, the Merciful. All praise belongs to Allah, Lord of all the worlds. The Gracious, the Merciful Master of the Day of Judgment. Thee alone do we worship and thee alone do we implore for help. Guide us to the right path.

You excel in all that you do and success comes easily to you.

You have the power to create all the success and prosperity you desire.

You are worthy of all good life must offer.

You are always open minded and easy to get along with.

You are surrounded by positive supportive people who believe in you.

You believe in yourself and your ability to succeed.

You always dress for success in body, mind and soul.

You are well organized and manage your time with expert efficiency.

You are committed to achieving success in every area of your life.

Your ambitions are in perfect alignment with your personal values.

February 9

Psalm 70

God is Wonderful

Save me Lord God! Hurry and help. Always say God is wonderful. You are the one who saves me. I run to you Lord for protection. You do what is right so come to my resolve. Listen to my prayer and keep me safe. Be my mighty rock.

Ya Sin

We have instructed the prophet in poetry this is a message and a Qur'an making things clear that it may give admonition. See they that it is we who have created for them among the things which our hands have fashioned cattle, which are under dominion. Some they eat they get milk to drink. Will they be grateful?

We excel in all that I do and success comes easily to us.

We have the power to create all the success and prosperity we desire.

We are worthy of all good life offers.

We are always open minded and easy to get along with.

We are surrounded by positive supportive people who believe in us.

We believe in ourselves and our ability to succeed.

We always dress for success in body, mind and soul.

We are well organized and manage our time with expert efficiency.

We are committed to achieving success in every area of our life.

Our ambitions are in perfect alignment with our personal values.

February 10

Romans 5:1

What it Means to be Acceptable to God

By faith we have been made acceptable to God. And now because of our Lord Jesus Christ we live at peace with God. Christ has also introduced us to God's kindness on which we take our stand. So, we are happy as we look forward to sharing in the glory of God. Endurance builds character which gives us a hope. All of this happens because God has given us the Holy Spirit who fills our hearts with his love.

The Poets

Moses said the Lord and cherisher of the heavens and the earth and all between. Moses threw his rod when behold in adoration saying, we believe in the Lord of the worlds.

I am strong in faith, give gratitude to my savior.

I grow stronger in everything because the Lord is with me.

I lift God on high and he lifts me up too.

I live, breathe and work for the Lord.

My higher spirit guides me in the direction of my dreams.

I am guided by God.

God loves me and lives inside and all around me.

Everywhere I go the Lord is and works his miracles for my good.

I am a winner and attract success through the power of faith.

I have everything because I have the Lord.

February 11

Psalm 9

Sing Praises to the Lord

I will praise you Lord with all my heart and tell about the wonders you have worked God most high. I will rejoice I will celebrate and sing because of you. You take your seat as judge and your fair decisions prove that I was in the right. You warn the nations. You rule forever Lord and you are on your throne ready for judgment. You judge the world fairly and treat all nations with justice.

Expounded

Better in speech than one who calls men to Allah, works righteousness and says, I am of those who bow in Islam. And one will be granted such goodness those who exercise patience and self-restrain persons of the greatest good fortune. Among his signs are the night and the day and the sun and the moon. Adore the sun and the moon adore Allah. Who created them if it is him ye wish to serve he who gives life can surely give life. For he has power over all things.

I am grateful for all my skills and talents that serve me well.

I am grateful to become successful.

I am grateful to always attract successful people.

I am grateful to stay focused on my missions pursue.

I am grateful for all the abundance flowing into my life.

I am grateful to attract good favorable outcomes always.

I am grateful success is my reality and it comes easy.

I am grateful to dress for success and achieve prosperity.

I am grateful for my financial success.

I am grateful to live up to my full potential.

February 12

John 6:39

Jesus is from Heaven

Jesus said to them, I am the bread of life. I said to you that you have seen me. All that the father gives me will come to me. For I have come down from heaven not to do my own will but the will of him who sent me. This is the will of him who sent me that of all that he had given me. Everyone who beholds the son and believes in him will have eternal life and I myself will raise him up on the last day.

The Women

Men are the protectors and maintainers of women because Allah has given strength and because they support them from their means. Therefore, the righteous woman is devoutly obedient and guard what Allah would have them guard.

You are grateful for all your skills and talents that serve you well.

You are grateful to become successful.

You are grateful to always attract successful people.

You are grateful to stay focused on your missions pursue.

You are grateful for all the abundance flowing into your life.

You are grateful to attract good favorable outcomes always.

You are grateful success is your reality and it comes easy.

You are grateful to dress for success and achieve prosperity.

You are grateful for your financial success.

You are grateful to live up to your full potential.

February 13

1 John 4:4

Spirit of Truth

You are from God little children and because greater is he who is in you than he who is in the world. They are from the world therefore they speak as from the world and the world listens to them we are from God. He who knows God listens to us. We know the spirit of truth. Beloved, let us love one another for love is from God and everyone who loves is born of God and knows God. But this the love of God was manifested in us that God sent his only begotten son into the world so that we might live though him.

Ta Ha

Moses said O my Lord! Expand me my breast, ease my task for me. And they may understand what I say and give me a minister from your family. Aaron my brother added to my strength and make him have my task. That we may celebrate the praise and remember thee for thou art he that ever regardeth us.

We are grateful for all our skills and talents that serve us well.

We are grateful to become successful.

We are grateful to always attract successful people.

We are grateful to stay focused on our missions pursue.

We are grateful for all the abundance flowing into our life.

We are grateful to attract good favorable outcomes always.

We are grateful success is our reality and it comes easy.

We are grateful to dress for success and achieve prosperity.

We are grateful for our financial success.

We are grateful to live up to our full potential.

February 14

Revelation1

The Revelation of Jesus Christ

John who testified to the word of God and to the testimony of Jesus Christ. Blessed is he who reads and those who hear the words of the prophecy and heed the things which are written in it for the time is near. John to the seven churches that are in Asia. Grace to you and peace from him who is and who was and the seven spirits who are before this throne.

The Cattle

They know full well to whom we have given the book that it hath been sent down from thy Lord in truth. The word of the Lord doth find its fulfillment in truth and in justice none can change his words for he is the one who heareth and knoweth all. Thy Lord he knoweth best who they are that receive his guidance.

My mind is brilliant, my body is healthy and my soul is tranquil.

Every cell in my body vibrates good health.

I manifest perfect health.

All my senses are perfect, whole and completely well.

Wellness, strength, joy, comfort, ease and love are my natural state of being.

Every organ, system and sense in my body functions perfectly well.

My subtle energies are positive, vibrant, radiant, balanced and flowing well.

I am 100% perfectly healthy all the time.

My body, mind and soul have a natural genius for healing.

I am dedicated to succeeding always.

February 15

Psalm 3

Morning Prayer of Trust in God

But you o Lord are a shield about me, my glory the one who lifts my head. He answered me from this holy mountain. Selah! I lay down and slept I awoke for the Lord sustains me. Arise o Lord save me. O my God, your blessing be upon your people Selah.

Bees

One day every soul will be recompensed fully for all its actions. Sets forth a parable, a city enjoining security and quiet abundantly supplied with sustenance from every place. Yet was grateful for the favors of Allah. So, eat of the sustenance which Allah has provided for you lawful and good and be grateful for the favors of Allah it is he whom ye serve.

Your mind is brilliant, your body is healthy and your soul is tranquil.

Every cell in your body vibrates with good health.

You manifest perfect health.

All your senses are perfect, whole and completely well.

Wellness, strength, joy, comfort, ease and love are your natural state of being.

Every organ, system and sense in your body functions perfectly well.

Your subtle energies are positive, vibrant, radiant, balanced and flowing well.

You are 100% perfectly healthy all the time.

Your body, mind and soul have a natural genius for healing.

You are dedicated to succeeding always.

February 16

Ephesians 6:1

Family Relationships

Honor your father and mother which is the first commandment with a promise. So that it may be well with you and that you may live long on the earth. Fathers bring them up in this discipline and instruction of the sincerity of your heart as to Christ. Stand firm therefore having truth and having put on the breastplate of righteousness and having shod your feet with the preparation of the gospel of peace and take the helmet of salvation and the sword of the spirit.

The Believers

Those who sustained the throne of Allah and those around it sing glory and praise to their Lord. Believe him and implore forgiveness for those who believe our Lord. His reach is over all things in mercy and knowledge.

Our mind is brilliant, our body is healthy and our soul is tranquil.

Every cell in our body vibrates with good health.

We manifest perfect health.

All our senses are perfect, whole and completely well.

Wellness, strength, joy, comfort, ease and love are our natural state of being.

Every organ, system and sense in our body functions perfectly well.

Our subtle energies are positive, vibrant, radiant, balanced and flowing well.

We are 100% perfectly healthy all the time.

Our body, mind and soul have a natural genius for healing.

We are dedicated to succeeding always.

February 17

John 16:1

The Work of the Holy Spirit

But now I am going to him who sent me and ask me where are you going? I tell you the truth it is to your advantage that I go away for if I do go away the helper shall come to you but I will send him to you. And he when he comes will convict the world concerning righteousness and judgment because the ruler of this world has been judged.

The Narrations

Thy Lord does create and choose as he pleases. He knows all that their hearts conceal and all that they reveal. And he is Allah there is no god but he. To him be praise at the first and at the last for him is the command and to him shall you all be brought back. Say see ye if Allah went to make the night perpetual over you to the Day of Judgment.

I am grateful to give and receive the best always.

I am grateful I feed, train and focus on perfection and success.

I am grateful all my senses are happy and whole.

I am grateful to radiate perfect health, wellness and happiness always.

I am grateful to have eyes to see, ears to hear, mouth and tongue to taste, hands and feet to touch, a heart to feel and a complete and whole body with all its functions.

I am grateful I know how to heal and can heal others anytime.

I am grateful all my body, mind and soul vibrate with perfect health and wellness.

I am grateful all my body functions well.

I am grateful to take good care of myself always.

February 18

Mark 1:3

The Preaching of John the Baptist

In the desert someone is shouting get the road ready for the Lord. Make a straight path for him. Fill up every valley and level every mountain and hill. Straighten the paths and smooth out the roads. Then everyone will see the saving power of God. Crowds of people came out to be baptized.

The Criterion

On the Day of Judgment he repents, believes, and works righteous deeds for Allah will change such persons into good. Allah is oft forgiving most merciful and whoever repents and does well have truly turned to Allah with an acceptable conversion.

You are grateful to give and receive the best always.

You are grateful you feed, train and focus on perfection and success.

You are grateful all your senses are happy and whole.

You are grateful to radiate perfect health, wellness and happiness always.

You are grateful to have eyes to see, ears to hear, mouth and tongue to taste, hands and feet to touch, a heart to feel and a complete and whole body with all its functions.

You are grateful you know how to heal and can heal others anytime.

You are grateful all your body, mind and soul vibrate with perfect health and wellness.

You are grateful all your body functions well.

You are grateful to take good care of yourself always.

February 19

Romans 5:18

Adam and Christ

Because of the good thing that Christ has done, God accepts us and gives us the gift of life. Jesus obeyed him and will make many people acceptable to God. The law came so that the full power could be seen. God's kindness was even more powerful. God's kindness now rules and God has accepted us because of Jesus Christ our Lord.

Mary

I am indeed a servant of Allah. He hath given me revelation and made me a prophet. And he hath made me blessed wheresoever I be and hath enjoined on me prayer and charity as long as I live. He hath made me kind to my mother. So peace is on me. Such was Jesus the son of Mary it is a statement of truth about which they dispute.

We are grateful to give and receive the best always.

We are grateful we feed, train and focus on perfection and success.

We are grateful all our senses are happy and whole.

We are grateful to radiate perfect health, wellness and happiness always.

We are grateful to have eyes to see, ears to hear, mouth and tongue to taste, hands and feet to touch, a heart to feel and a complete and whole body with all its functions.

We are grateful we know how to heal and can heal others anytime.

We are grateful all our body, mind and soul vibrate with perfect health and wellness.

We are grateful all our bodies functions well.

We are grateful to take good care of ourselves always.

February 20

Revelation 7:11

People from Every Nation

Our God who sits on the throne, has the power to save his people and so does the lamb. The angels who stood around the throne knelt in front of it with their faces to the ground. The elders and the four living creatures knelt there with them. Then they all worshiped and said, amen! Praise, glory, wisdom, thanks, honor, power and strength belong to our God forever and ever. Amen.

The Heights

It is he who created you from a single person and made his mate like nature in order that he might dwell with her in love. When they are united she bears a light burden. They both pray to Allah their Lord saying, if thou givest us a goodly child we vow we shall ever be grateful. From your Lord and guidance and mercy and for any who have faith.

My happiness makes people happy.

Be happy is my motto.

Living makes me happy and happiness is my goal.

Being happy comes easy to me.

The future is always bright and happy.

Kindness breeds love and love results in happiness.

Happiness is my journey and God blessed me with it.

I am kind, loving and happy always.

Joy flows in my positive thoughts and joy exists.

I am overcome with gratitude for the bliss that fills my life.

February 21

1 Corinthians 15

Christ came from Heaven

The scriptures tell us the first man Adam became a living person but the last Adam that is Christ is a life giving spirit. What comes first is the natural body then the spiritual body comes later. Adam the first man came from the dust of the earth while Christ came from heaven. Earthly people are like the earthly man heavenly people are like the heavenly man. Our bodies must be transformed into immortal bodies.

The Dawn

I had sent forth good deeds for this future life. To the righteous soul will be said O you soul in complete rest and satisfaction. Come back you to your Lord well pleased yourself and well pleasing unto him. Enter then among my devotees. Yes enter my heaven.

Your happiness makes people happy.

Be happy is your motto.

Living makes you happy and happiness is your goal.

Being happy comes easy to you.

The future is always bright and happy.

Kindness breeds love and love results in happiness.

Happiness is your journey and God blessed you with it.

You are kind, loving and happy always.

Joy flows in your positive thoughts and joy exists.

You are overcome with gratitude for the bliss that fills your life.

February 22

1 Corinthians

Love

I could speak all languages of humans and of angels. Love is kind and patient. Love rejoices in the truth. Love is always supportive, loyal, hopeful and trusting. Now all we can see of God is like a cloudy picture in a mirror. For now there are faith, hope and love. But of these three the greatest is love.

The Night Journey

It is you Lord that knoweth best and if he please he granteth you mercy, or if he please, punishment. We have sent thee to be a disposer of their affairs for them and if it is your Lord that knoweth best all beings that in the heavens and on earth. We did bestow on some prophets more gifts than on others and we gave to David the gift of the Psalms.

Our happiness makes people happy.

Be happy is our motto.

Living makes me happy and happiness is our goal.

Being happy comes easy to us.

The future is always bright and happy.

Kindness breeds love and love results in happiness.

Happiness is our journey and God blessed us with it.

We are kind, loving and happy always.

Joy flows in our positive thoughts and joy exists.

We are overcome with gratitude for the bliss that fills our life.

February 23

Luke 17:1

Faith and Service

Jesus said to his disciples there will always be something that causes people to love more. So be careful what you do. Correct any followers of mine and forgive the ones who say they are sorry. You should still forgive that person. The apostles said to the Lord make our faith stronger. Jesus replied if you had faith no bigger than a tiny mustard seed you could tell this mulberry tree to pull itself up roots and all and to plant itself in the ocean and it would.

Winding Sand Tracts

The revelation of the book is from Allah the exalted in power full of wisdom. We created the heavens and the earth and all between them for just ends and for a term appointed. Show me what it is they have created on earth, or have they a share in the heavens? Bring me a book revealed before this.

I am grateful to God for my successful life.

I am grateful happiness is everywhere.

I am grateful all my happy thoughts bring happy results.

I am grateful to be happy live a joyous life.

I am grateful to share joy with others well and often.

I am grateful to feel peaceful, joyful and happy always.

I am grateful it's a happy and healthy universe.

I am grateful my happiness benefits others.

I am grateful my joyful life will last forever.

I am grateful I am constantly in a state of peace, joy, love, happiness and bliss.

February 24

Proverbs 2

Wisdom and Friends

My child you must follow and treasure my teachings and my instructions. Keep in tune with wisdom and think what it means to have common sense. Beg as loud as you can for common sense. Search for silver and hidden treasure. Then you will understand what it means to respect and to know the Lord God. All wisdom comes from the Lord and so do common sense and understanding. God gives helpful advice to everyone who obeys him and protects those who live as they should. God sees that justice is done and he watches over everyone who is faithful to him. With wisdom your will learn what is right and honest and fair.

The Table Spread

O ye who believe. Fulfill all obligations. Lawful unto you for food are all four foot animals. The people to the sacred house seeking of the bounty and good pleasure of their Lord.

You are grateful to God for your successful life.

You are grateful happiness is everywhere.

You are grateful all your happy thoughts bring happy results.

You are grateful to be happy live a joyous life.

You are grateful to share joy with others well and often.

You are grateful to feel peaceful, joyful and happy always.

You are grateful it's a happy and healthy universe.

You are grateful your happiness benefits others.

You are grateful your joyful life will last forever.

You are grateful you are constantly in a state of peace, joy, love, happiness and bliss.

February 25

Proverbs 2:16

Wisdom and Purity

Wisdom will protect you. Follow the example of good people and live an honest life. You are honest and innocent you will keep your land. Trust God my child remember my teachings and instructions and obey them completely. They will help you live a prosperous life. Let love and loyalty always show like a necklace and write them in your mind. God and people will like you and hold you in high esteem. With all your heart you must trust the Lord. Always let him lead you and he will clear the road for you to follow.

The Table Spread

Recite to them the truth of the story of the two sons of Adam. Behold they each presented a sacrifice to Allah and it was accepted from one. Allah doth accept of the sacrifice of those who are righteous. If anyone saved a life it would be as if he saved the life of the whole people.

We are grateful to God for our successful life.

We are grateful happiness is everywhere.

We are grateful all our happy thoughts bring happy results.

We are grateful to be happy live a joyous life.

We are grateful to share joy with others well and often.

We are grateful to feel peaceful, joyful and happy always.

We are grateful it's a happy and healthy universe.

We are grateful our happiness benefits others.

We are grateful our joyful life will last forever.

We are grateful we are constantly in a state of peace, joy, love, happiness and bliss.

February 26

1 Corinthians 6:12

Honor God with your Body

Some of you say we can do anything we want to. Food is meant for the bodies and our bodies are meant for food. You surely know that your body is a temple where the Holy Spirit lives.

The Believers

And we gave Moses the book in order that they might receive guidance. And we made the son of Mary and his mother as a sign. We gave them both shelter on high ground affording rest and security furnished with springs. O ye messengers. Enjoy all things good and pure and work righteousness for I am well acquainted with all that ye do and verily this brotherhood of yours is a single brotherhood and I am your Lord and Cherisher.

I am grounded, safe and secure.

I always feel safe and protected everywhere.

I am always safe to be myself.

I am divinely protected in all that I do.

I am relaxed and secure always.

I feel safe and secure because I am optimistic and joyful always.

My home always keeps me and my family safe and protected.

My life is safe and my thoughts are positive and protected always.

My safety is guaranteed all the time.

February 27

1 Corinthians 7:17

Obey the Lord Always

In every church I tell the people to stay as they were when the Lord Jesus chose them and God called them to be his own. Now I say the same thing to you if you are already circumcised don't try to change it. If you are not circumcised don't get circumcised. Being circumcised or uncircumcised isn't really what matters. The important thing is to obey God's commands. If you can win your freedom you should when the Lord chooses free people.

Those Ranged in Ranks

Lord of the heavens and of the earth and all between them and Lord of every point at the rising of the sun. We have indeed decked the lower heaven with beauty in the stars. The sincere and devoted servants of Allah for them is a sustenance determined fruits delights and they shall enjoy honor and dignity in gardens of felicity facing each other on thrones of dignity.

You are grounded, safe and secure.

You always feel safe and protected everywhere.

You are always safe to be yourself.

You are divinely protected in all that I do.

You are relaxed and secure always.

You feel safe and secure because you are optimistic and joyful always.

Your home always keeps you and your family safe and protected.

Your life is safe and your thoughts are positive and protected always.

Your safety is guaranteed all the time.

February 28

Luke 2:28

Simeon Praises the Lord

Lord I am your servant now in peace because you have kept your promise to me. With my own eyes I have seen what you have done to save your people and foreign nations will also see this. Your mighty power is a light for all nations, it will bring honor to your people Israel. Jesus parents were surprised. At this time a man named Simeon was living in Jerusalem. Simeon was a good man. He loved God and was waiting for God to save the people of Israel. God's spirit came to him.

The Believer

Our Lord! Hast thou given us life! The Command is with Allah, most high, most great! He it is who showeth us his signs sendeth down sustenance for you from the sky, but only those receive admonition who turn to Allah. Call ye upon Allah with sincere devotion to him.

We are grounded, safe and secure.

We always feel safe and protected everywhere.

We are always safe to be our self.

We are divinely protected in all that I do.

We are relaxed and secure always.

We feel safe and secure because we are optimistic and joyful always.

Our home always keeps us and our family safe and protected.

Our life is safe and our thoughts are positive and protected always.

Our safety is guaranteed all the time.

February 29

James 4:11

God Alone is Judge

Your job is obey the law not to judge whether it applies to you. God alone who gave the law is the judge. He has the power to save or to destroy. So what right do you have to judge your neighbor?

Friday

Whatever is in the heavens and on earth does declare the praises and glory to Allah the sovereign the holy one the exalted the mighty the wise. It is he who has sent amongst them an apostle to rehearse to them his signs to purify them and to instruct them in scriptures and wisdom. Such is the bounty of Allah which he bestows on whom he wills and Allah is the Lord of the highest bounty.

Abundance and prosperity are your birthright.

You are in a state of contentment and have an abundance of love and joy.

You are and will always be prosperous, successful and righteous.

All your thoughts and actions lead to abundance, prosperity and love.

You are successful because you are kind and generous.

You enjoy all the abundance of good things in your life.

You are open to receiving an abundance of good things in your life.

You always have what you need when you need it.

You love all the exciting safe opportunities of wealth, abundance and fame.

My universe is full with abundance, wealth, good health, love and happiness.

February 30

Luke 5

Instructions for the 12 Apostles

Jesus called together his 12 apostles and gave them complete power over all. Then he sent them to tell about Gods kingdom to heal. Take a walking stick or a traveling bag or food or money or even a change of clothes when you are welcomed into a home stay until you leave their town.

Noah

We sent Noah to his people with the command. I am to you a Warner clear and open. That ye should worship Allah and obey him. So he may forgive you and give you respite for a stated term. For when the term given by God is accomplished it cannot be put forward if ye only know. He said o my Lord I have called my people day and night.

We can maintain cleanliness and purity always.

We have good personal hygiene.

We can keep our home, car and where we work neat and clean always.

We balance our body with clean and fresh nutrients.

We get a good daily dose of pure, clean, fresh air.

Every day we set an intention to experience love, peace, cleanliness and purity.

Purity, holiness and cleanliness will exalt the human condition.

We keep ourselves clean, bright and pure always.

Cleanliness preserves beauty.

Keeping our mind, body and soul clean and tidy is important to us.

March 1

Matthew 7:1

Judging Others

He will treat you exactly as you treat them. Ask and you will receive. Search and you will find. Knock and the door will be opened for you. Everyone who asks will receive. Everyone who searches will find. And the door will be opened for everyone who knocks. But your heavenly father is even more ready to give good things to people who ask. Treat others as you want them to treat you. This is what the law and the prophets are all about.

Ya sin

Say, He will give them life who created them for the first time. For He is well versed in every kind of creation. Yea indeed for he is the creator supreme of skill and knowledge (infinite)! Verily when he intends a thing his command is be and it is. So glory to him in whose hands is the dominion of all things and to him will ye be all brought back.

I am grateful my thoughts ensure my wellbeing, safety and optimism.

I am grateful for total security always everywhere.

I am grateful to be safe and secure always.

I am grateful to feel safe, secure well treated and respected always.

I am grateful to be divinely protected and guided.

I am grateful our home, car and family are sage and protected always.

I am grateful the universe protects me in all that I do.

I am grateful I am safe wherever I go.

I am grateful to be secure in everything.

I am grateful to be grounded, safe and secure all the time

March 2

Matthew 25:31

The Final Judgment

When the son of man comes in his glory with all his angels, he will sit on his royal throne. The people of all nations will be brought before him and he will separate them as shepherds separate their sheep from their goats. He will place the sheep on his right and the goats on his left. Then the king will say to those on the right My father has blessed you. Come and receive the kingdom that was prepared for you before the world was created. The ones on the right who pleased God will have eternal life.

The Night Journey

Those whom they call upon access to their Lord even those who are nearest they hope for this mercy.

You are grateful your thoughts ensure your wellbeing, safety and optimism.

You are grateful for total security always everywhere.

You are grateful to be safe and secure always.

You are grateful to feel safe, secure well treated and respected always.

You are grateful to be divinely protected and guided.

You are grateful your home, car and family are sage and protected always.

You are grateful the universe protects you in all that you do.

You are grateful you are safe wherever you go.

You are grateful to be secure in everything.

You are grateful to be grounded, safe and secure all the time.

March 3

Luke 8:46

A Woman Healed

Jesus answered, Someone touched me because I felt power going out from me. The woman knew that she could not hide so she knelt down in front of Jesus. She told everyone why she had touched him and that she had been healed right away. Jesus said to the woman you are now well. Jesus took hold of the girls hand and said, Child get up! She came back to life and got right up.

The Cave

Say, Allah's will be done! There is power with Allah! It may be that my Lord will give me something better than thy garden and that he will send on thy garden thunderbolts by way of reckoning from heaven. There the only protection comes from Allah the true one. He is the best to reward and the best to give success.

We are grateful our thoughts ensure my wellbeing, safety and optimism.

We are grateful for total security always everywhere.

We are grateful to be safe and secure always.

We are grateful to feel safe, secure well treated and respected always.

We are grateful to be divinely protected and guided.

We are grateful our home, car and family are sage and protected always.

We are grateful the universe protects us in all that we do.

We are grateful we are safe wherever we go.

We are grateful to be secure in everything.

We are grateful to be grounded, safe and secure all the times.

March 4

Psalm 64:65

The Lord Blesses Us

May the Lord bless his people with peace and happiness and let them celebrate. Our God you deserve praise in Zion, where we keep our promises to you. Everyone will come to you because you answer prayer. You forgive us. You bless your chosen ones and you invite them to live near you in your temple. We will enjoy your house the sacred temple. Our God, you save us and your deeds answer our prayers for justice. You give hope to people everywhere on earth.

The Repentance

Then rejoice in the bargain which ye have concluded that is the achievement supreme. Those that turn to Allah in repentance that serve him and praise him that wander in devotion to the cause of Allah and that bow down and prostrate themselves in prayer that enjoins good.

I am organized in all areas of my life.

I deserve to achieve my goals quickly and efficiently.

I am true to myself and I am a powerful creative soul.

Every experience I have is perfect for my growth.

I am committed to being better than yesterday.

I allow myself to feel complete peace right now and always.

I trust myself and believe in all my dreams.

I am in exactly the right place and it gets better every day.

It is safe for me to be successful, good looking and a happy millionaire.

We are attracting wellbeing and achieving our greatest potential.

March 5

1 John 4:4

Children God is Love

We belong to God and everyone who knows God will listen to us. My dear friends we must love each other. Love comes from God and we love each other. We are now God's children and we know him, God is love. God shared his love for us when he sent his only son into the world to give us life. Real love is his love for us.

The Iron

He is the first and the last, the evident and the hidden and he has full knowledge of all things, he it is who created the heavens and the earth in six days and is moreover firmly established on the throne of authority. He knows what enters within the earth and what comes forth out of it, what comes down from heaven and what mounts up to it.

You are organized in all areas of your life.

You deserve to achieve your goals quickly and efficiently.

You are true to yourself and you are a powerful creative soul.

Every experience you have is perfect for my growth.

You are committed to being better than yesterday.

You allow yourself to feel complete peace right now and always.

You trust yourself and believe in all your dreams.

You are in exactly the right place and it gets better every day.

It is safe for you to be a successful, good looking, happy millionaire.

You are attracting wellbeing and achieving our greatest potential.

March 6

Psalm 24

Who Can Enter the Lord's Temple

The earth and everything in it including its people belong to the Lord. The world and its people belong to him. The Lord placed it all on the oceans and rivers. Who may climb the Lord's hill or stand in his holy temple? Only those who do right for the right reasons. The Lord God who saves them will bless and reward them because they worship and serve the God of Jacob. Open the ancient gates so that the glorious king may come in. Who is this glorious king? He is our Lord a strong and might warrior.

The Cattle

And when there comes to them a sign from Allah, Allah knoweth best where and how to carry out his mission. Those whom Allah willeth to guide for them will be a home of peace in the presence of their Lord, he will be their friend because they practiced righteousness.

We are organized in all areas of our life.

We deserve to achieve our goals quickly and efficiently.

We are true to ourselves and we are powerful creative souls.

Every experience we have is perfect for our growth.

We are committed to being better than yesterday.

We allow ourselves to feel complete peace right now and always.

We trust ourselves and believe in all our dreams.

We are in exactly the right place and it gets better every day.

It is safe for us to be successful, good looking happy millionaires.

We are attracting wellbeing and achieving our greatest potential.

March 7

Psalm 25

A Prayer for Guidance and Help

I offer you my heart, Lord God and I trust you. Show me your path and teach me to follow and guide me by your truth and instruct me. You keep me safe and I always trust you. Please Lord remember you have always been patient and honest and merciful and you are kind. Show how truly kind you are and remember me. You are honest and merciful. You lead humble people to do what is right and to stay on your path. In everything you do you are kind and faithful to everyone who keeps our agreement with you.

The Poets

Behold I am to you a messenger worthy of all trust. So obey me. My reward is only from the Lord of the worlds. Give just measure and weight with scales true and upright. Thy Lord is he the exalted in might most merciful. Verily this is a revelation from the Lord of the worlds.

I am grateful to have open, clear, and honest communication always.

I am grateful to express myself creatively all the time.

I am grateful to learn and grow to be a better person.

I am grateful to receive progress and good results.

I am grateful the universe sends perfect situations and people always.

I am grateful I have time to love myself.

I am grateful life teaches me love and great lessons.

I am grateful all my lessons made me stronger, smarter, faster, wiser and more attractive.

I am grateful to be determined to learn and do everything well and with mastery.

March 8

2 Corinthians 4:6

God's Light Shines in our Hearts

For God said let there be light, this light shines in our hearts so we could know the glory of God that is seen in the face of Jesus Christ. We now have this light shining in our hearts but we ourselves are containing this great treasure. This makes it clear that our great power is from God.

The Family Imran

Remember that morning thou didst leave thy household early to post the faithful at their stations. Allah hearest and knoweth all things. Remember two of your parties meditated but Allah was their protector and in Allah should the faithful put their trust. Remember thou saidst to the faithful, "is it enough for you that Allah should help you with 3000 angels? To Allah belongth all that is in the heavens and on earth. He forgiveth whom he pleaseth but Allah is oft forgiving.

You are grateful to have open, clear, and honest communication always.

You are grateful to express myself creatively all the time.

You are grateful to learn and grow to be a better person.

You are grateful to receive progress and good results.

You are grateful the universe sends perfect situations and people always.

You are grateful you have time to love yourself.

You are grateful life teaches you love and great lessons.

You are grateful all your lessons made you stronger, smarter, faster, wiser and more attractive.

You are grateful to be determined to learn and do everything well and with mastery.

March 9

Colossians 1:15

The Person and Work of Christ

He was first born son superior to all creation. All things were created by God's son and everything was made for him. God's son was before all else and by him everything is held together. He is the head of his body which is the church. He is the very beginning. He would be above all others. God himself was pleased to live fully in his son and God was pleased by him to make peace so that all beings in heaven and on earth would be brought back to God.

Hud

We certainly gave the book of Moses. Had it been that a word had gone forth before from thy Lord pay back in full the recompense of their deeds for he knoweth well all that they do. Therefore stand firm in the straight path as thou art commanded thou and those who with thee turn unto Allah and transgress he seeth well all that you do.

We are grateful to have open, clear, and honest communication always.

We are grateful to express ourselves creatively all the time.

We are grateful to learn and grow to be a better people.

We are grateful to receive progress and good results.

We are grateful the universe sends perfect situations and people always.

We are grateful we have time to love ourselves.

We are grateful life teaches us love and great lessons.

We are grateful all our lessons made me stronger, smarter, faster, wiser and more attractive.

We are grateful to be determined to learn and do everything well and with mastery.

March 10

Mark 2:18

Eating

Some people came and asked Jesus. Why do the followers of John and those of the Pharisees often go without eating while your disciples never do? Jesus answered the friends of a bridegroom don't go without eating while he is still with them but the time will come when he will be taken from them. Then they will go without eating.

Abraham

O our Lord! I have made some of my offspring to dwell in a valley with cultivation by thy sacred house in order they may establish regular prayer so fill the hearts of some among men with love towards them and feed them with fruits so that they may give thanks. O our Lord truly thou dost know what we conceal and what we reveal for nothing is hidden from Allah on earth or in heaven.

The peace inside of my heart is the peace that's deeper than all understands.

I feel peace here and now and always.

I interact peacefully with others.

Peace is my perspective and I send peace from myself into the world.

I choose to be peaceful and free.

My environment is peaceful and serene.

I consciously recognize the peace present in all places and always.

I respond peacefully in all situations.

My mind, body and soul are calm and peaceful in every moment.

Peace starts with me.

March 11

Psalm 37

Trust the Lord

Trust the Lord and live right and the land will be yours and you will be safe. Do what the Lord wants. Let the Lord lead you and trust him to help. Then it will be as clear as the noonday sun that you were right. Be patient and trust the Lord.

Muhammad

But those who believe and work deeds of righteousness and believe in the revelation sent down to Muhammad for it is the truth from their Lord he will improve their conditions. Those who believe follow the truth from that Lord thus does Allah set forth for men their lessons by similitudes. That is because Allah is the protector for those who believe.

The peace inside of your heart is the peace that's deeper than all understands.

You feel peace here and now and always.

You interact peacefully with others.

Peace is your perspective and you send peace from yourself into the world.

You choose to be peaceful and free.

Your environment is peaceful and serene.

You consciously recognize the peace present in all places and always.

You respond peacefully in all situations.

Your mind, body and soul are calm and peaceful in every moment.

Peace starts with you.

March 12

Luke 20:41

About David's Son

Jesus asked why do people say that the Messiah will be the son of King David. In the book of Psalms David himself says the Lord said to my Lord, sit at my right side. David spoke of the Messiah be his son. Jesus looked up and says some people tossing their gifts into the offering box. I tell you that this woman has put in more than all the others.

Those Ranged in Ranks

O my Lord! Grant me a righteous son! So, we gave him the good news of a boy. Then when the son reached the age of work with him he said o my son! I see in a vision that I offer thee. The son said o my father! Do as thou art commanded thou will find me practicing patience and constancy! So, when they had both submitted their wills to Allah.

The peace inside of our heart is the peace that's deeper than all understands.

We feel peace here and now and always.

We interact peacefully with others.

Peace is our perspective and we send peace from myself into the world.

We choose to be peaceful and free.

Our environment is peaceful and serene.

We consciously recognize the peace present in all places and always.

We respond peacefully in all situations.

Our mind, body and soul are calm and peaceful in every moment.

Peace starts with us.

March 13

Romans 5:18

Adam and Christ

But because of the good thing that Christ has done. God accepts us gives us the gift of life. Jesus obeyed him and will make many people acceptable to God. God's kindness was more powerful. God's kindness rules and God has accepted us because of Jesus Christ our Lord.

The Gold Adornments

We have made Quran in Arabic that ye maybe able to understand and learn wisdom. And verily it is in the mother of the book, in our presence high in dignity full of wisdom. They were created by him the exalted in power full of knowledge. Yea the same that has made for you the earth like a carpet spread out and made for you roads and channels therein in order that ye may find guidance on your way.

I am grateful to find and keep inner peace.

I am grateful to feel calm and peaceful always.

I am grateful to find peace in so many ways.

I am grateful to be happy and have boosted feelings of joy and pleasure always.

I am grateful for all the blessings bestowed.

I am grateful to be at peace with myself and all the universe.

I am grateful to breathe peace and love.

I am grateful to clear my mind and relax and channel peace always.

I am grateful peace is my natural state of wellbeing.

I am grateful to radiate joy, beauty, peace, wisdom and power always.

March 14

Luke 19:45

Jesus in the Temple

The scriptures say my house should be a place of worship. Each day Jesus kept on teaching in the temple. Jesus replied I want to ask you a question. Who gave John the right to baptize was it God in heaven or merely some human being?

The Believers

My Lord is Allah when he has indeed come to you with clear signs.

You are grateful to find and keep inner peace.

You are grateful to feel calm and peaceful always.

You are grateful to find peace in so many ways.

You are grateful to be happy and have boosted feelings of joy and pleasure always.

You are grateful for all the blessings bestowed.

You are grateful to be at peace with yourself and all the universe.

You are grateful to breathe peace and love.

You are grateful to clear your mind and relax and channel peace always.

You are grateful peace is your natural state of well-being.

You are grateful to radiate joy, beauty, peace, wisdom and power always.

March 15

Revelation 12:10

God's Chosen Authority

Then I heard a voice from heaven shout our God has shown his saving power and his kingdom has come. Gods own chosen one has shown his authority. The heavens should rejoice together with everyone who lives there. The woman had given birth to a son was given 2 wings like those of a huge eagle so that she could fly.

The Victory

He sent down tranquility to them and then rewarded them with speedy victory. And many gains will they acquire besides and Allah is exalted in power full of wisdom. Allah has promised you many gains that ye shall acquire and he has given you these beforehand. Allah has power over all things.

We are grateful to find and keep inner peace.

We are grateful to feel calm and peaceful always.

We are grateful to find peace in so many ways.

We are grateful to be happy and have boosted feelings of joy and pleasure always.

We are grateful for all the blessings bestowed.

We are grateful to be at peace with ourselves and all the universe.

We are grateful to breathe peace and love.

We are grateful to clear our mind and relax and channel peace always.

We are grateful peace is our natural state of well-being.

We are grateful to radiate joy, beauty, peace, wisdom and power always.

March 16

John 12:12

Jesus Enters Jerusalem

God bless the one who comes in the name of the Lord! God bless the one who comes in the name of the Lord! God bless the king of Israel! Jesus found a donkey and rode on it just as the scriptures say. People of Jerusalem your king is now coming and he is riding on a donkey. But after he had been given his glory they remembered all this. Everything had happened exactly as the scriptures said it would.

Bees

For to anything which we have willed we but say this word be and it is. We will assuredly give a goodly home in this world, but the reward of the hereafter will be greater. They realized this. They are those who preserve in patience and put their trust on their Lord.

I am surrounded by love and everything is fine.

My heart is always open and I radiate love.

All my relationships are fun loving and beneficial.

I see and hear everything with loving eyes and ears and love everything I see and hear.

I deserve super love and I get it in abundance.

I have attracted the most loving people into my life.

I love myself and everybody.

My partner and I are a perfect match for each other and our love is always romantic, passionate, and healthy.

In love with all my relationships in the universe.

I only give and receive love.

March 17

1 Timothy 7:12

Being Thankful for Gods Kindness

I thank Christ Jesus our Lord. He has given me the strength for my work because he knew that he could trust me. Christ Jesus our Lord was very kind to me. He has greatly blessed my life with faith and love just like his own. Christ Jesus came into the world to save. This saying is true and it can be trusted. God had mercy on me and let me be an example of the endless patience of Christ Jesus. I pray that honor and glory will always be given to the only God who lives forever and is the invisible and eternal king.

Those Ranged in Ranks

Lord of the heavens and of the earth and all between them and Lord of every point at the rising of the sun. We have indeed decked the lower heaven with beauty in the stars for beauty and for guard. The sincere and devoted servants of Allah for them is a sustenance determined. Fruits delights and they shall enjoy honor and dignity in gardens of felicity facing each other on thrones of dignity.

You are surrounded by love and everything is fine.

Your heart is always open and you radiate love.

All your relationships are fun loving and beneficial.

You see and hear everything with loving eyes and ears and love everything you see and hear.

You deserve super love and you get it in abundance.

You have attracted the most loving people into your life.

You love yourself and everybody.

Your partner and you are a perfect match for each other and our love is always romantic, passionate, and healthy.

In love with all your relationships in the universe.

March 18

Colossians 3:18

Some Rules for Christian Living

Obey your earthly masters. Try to please them at all times. Honor the Lord and serve your masters with your whole heart. Work willingly as though you were serving the Lord himself and not just your earthly master. In fact the Lord Jesus Christ is the one you are really serving and you know that he will reward you.

Mary

He said I am indeed a servant of Allah. He hath given me revelation and made me a prophet. And he hath made me blessed wherever I be and hath enjoined on me prayer and charity. When young he hath made me kind to my mother. So peace is on me. Such was Jesus the son of Mary it is a statement of truth. Glory is to him. He determines a matter he only says to it be and it is.

We are surrounded by love and everything is fine.

Our heart is always open and we radiate love.

All our relationships are fun loving and beneficial.

We see and hear everything with loving eyes and ears and love everything we see and hear.

We deserve super love and we get it in abundance.

We have attracted the most loving people into our life.

We love ourselves and everybody.

Our partner and us are a perfect match for each other and our love is always romantic, passionate, and healthy.

In love with all our relationships in the universe.

We only give and receive love.

March 19

Luke12:8

Telling others about Christ

Don't worry about how to defend yourselves or what you will say. At that time the Holy Spirit will tell you what to say. Lord God blesses everyone in time of healing. Treat all nations with justice.

Yusuf

Allah made an example of him in the hereafter as in this life verily in this is an instructive warning. On high hath he raised its canopy and he hath given it order and perfection. Its splendor doth he bring with light and the earth hath he extended to a wide expanse.

I am grateful to be surrounded by love and all is well.

I am grateful to deserve love, romance and joy and I get it.

I am grateful to be true love.

I am grateful for enduring, loving relationships.

I am grateful to draw love and romance into my life and I accept it.

I am grateful all my relationships are harmonious with equal share of love.

I am grateful I follow God's example of true love.

I am grateful it's easy for me to give and receive love.

I am grateful to attract emotionally available, happy and healthy partners with my loving attractive self.

I am grateful to be open to receiving true love from the perfect person for me.

March 20

Psalm 9

Sing Praises to the Lord

I will praise you Lord with all my heart and tell about the wonders you have worked. God most high I will rejoice I will celebrate and sing because of you. You rule forever Lord and you are on your throne ready for judgment. You judge the world fairly and treat all nations with justice.

The Iron

Whatever is in the heavens and on earth let it declare the praises and glory of Allah for he is the exalted in might, the wise to him belongs the dominion of the heavens and the earth. It is he who gives life and he has power over all things. He has full knowledge of all things. He it is who created the heavens and the earth in six days and is moreover firmly established on the throne of authority.

You are grateful to be surrounded by love and all is well.

You are grateful to deserve love, romance and joy and you get it.

You are grateful to be true love.

You are grateful for enduring, loving relationships.

You are grateful to draw love and romance into your life and you accept it.

You are grateful all your relationships are harmonious with equal share of love.

You are grateful you follow God's example of true love.

You are grateful it's easy for you to give and receive love.

You are grateful to attract emotionally available, happy and healthy partners with your loving attractive self.

You are grateful to be open to receiving true love from the perfect person for you.

March 21

Psalm 41

A Prayer in Time of Healing

You Lord God bless everyone who cares and you rescue those people. You protect them and keep them alive. You make them happy here in this land. You always hear them and restore their strength. I prayed Lord heal me. You have helped me because I am innocent and you will always be close to my side.

The Night Journey

O my Lord! Let my entry be by the gate of truth and honor and likewise my exit by the gate of truth and honor and grant me from thy presence an authority to aid me and say truth has now arrived. We send down stage by stage in the Quran which is a healing and a mercy to those who believe. Lord knows best who it is that is best guided on the way.

We are grateful to be surrounded by love and all is well.

We are grateful to deserve love, romance and joy and we get it.

We are grateful to be true love.

We are grateful for enduring, loving relationships.

We are grateful to draw love and romance into my life and we accept it.

We are grateful all our relationships are harmonious with equal share of love.

We are grateful we follow God's example of true love.

We are grateful it's easy for us to give and receive love.

We are grateful to attract emotionally available, happy and healthy partners with our loving attractive self.

We are grateful to be open to receiving true love from the perfect person for us.

March 22

1 Thessalonians 2

Paul's Work in Thessalonica

You also know we did everything for you that parents would do for their own children. We begged, encouraged and urged each of you to live in a way that would honor God. He is the one who chose you to share in his own kingdom and glory. We always thank God that you believed the message we preached. It came from him. It is God's message and now he is working in you.

The Inner Apartments

Allah is he who hears and knows all things. O ye who believe. Raise not your voices above the voice of the prophet nor speak aloud to him in talk. Those that lower their voices in the presence of Allah's messenger their hearts has Allah tested for piety and for them is forgiveness and a great reward.

Gods favor and grace bless me every day.

Each day holds many unique blessings for me to experience and explore.

God effortlessly blesses me.

My life is full of wealth and blessings.

The universe blesses me in joyful and surprising many ways.

I am blessed and prospered because God loves me most.

I am living in comfort, ease, pleasure, luxury, fun, ecstasy, joy and bliss all the time.

I am blessed now and forever.

Each day of my life is magically, divine, blessed and joyous.

I am my eternal destiny abracadabra.

March 23

Romans 6:15

Do What Pleases God

I thank God that with all your heart you obeyed the teaching you received from me. Now you are set free and please God. I am using these everyday examples. Now you must make every part of your body serve God so that you will belong completely to him.

The Confederates

Verily Allah is full of knowledge and wisdom. Follow that which comes to those by inspiration from thy Lord. Allah is well acquainted with all that ye do. And put thy trust in Allah and enough is Allah as a disposer of affairs. Allah is oft forgiving most merciful. The prophet is closer to the believers than their own selves and his wives are their mothers. Blood relations among each other have closer personal ties in the decree of Allah.

Gods favor and grace bless you every day.

Each day holds many unique blessings for you to experience and explore.

God effortlessly blesses you.

Your life is full of wealth and blessings.

The universe blesses you in joyful and surprising many ways.

You are blessed and prospered because God loves you.

You are living in comfort, ease, pleasure, luxury, fun, ecstasy, joy and bliss all the time.

You are blessed now and forever.

Each day of your life is magically, divine, blessed and joyous.

You are my eternal destiny abracadabra.

March 24

Psalm 12

A Prayer for Help

Please help me Lord! Lord tell them, I will do something I'll rescue all. Our Lord you are true to your promises and your word is like silver healed seven times in a fiery furnace. You will protect us and always keep us safe from those people. A book that makes things clear. A guide and glad tidings for the believers. Those who establish regular prayers and give in regular charity and also have full assurance of the hereafter. As to thee the Qur'an is bestowed upon thee from the presence of one who is wise and all knowing.

The Prophets

And remember her who guarded her chastity. We breathed into her of our spirit and we made her and her son a sign for all peoples. Verily this brotherhood of yours is a single brotherhood and I am your Lord and cherishers therefore serve.

Gods favor and grace blesses us every day.

Each day holds many unique blessings for us to experience and explore.

God effortlessly blesses us.

Our life is full of love, wealth and blessings.

The universe blesses us in joyful and surprising many ways.

We are blessed and prospered because God loves us.

We are living in comfort, ease, pleasure, luxury, fun, ecstasy, joy and bliss all the time.

We are blessed now and forever.

Each day of our life is magical, divine, blessed and joyous.

We are our eternal destiny abracadabra.

March 25

Revelation 16:5

The Bowls of God

Then I heard the angel who has power over water say, you have always been and you will always be the holy God. You have the right to judge in this way. I heard the altar shout, yes Lord God all powerful, your judgments are honest and fair. Remember Christ says when I come it will surprise you but God will bless you if you are awake and ready.

Jonah

We settled the children of Israel in a beautiful dwelling place and provided for them sustenance of the best. If he design some benefit for thee it reach whomsoever of his servants he pleaseth and he is the oft forgiving most merciful. Follow thou the inspiration sent unto thee and be patient and constant.

I am grateful to bless and be blessed always.

I am grateful my body, mind and soul are divinely and eternally blessed.

I am grateful to bless and forgive everyone always.

I am grateful for all the blessings, prayers, visions and dreams.

I am grateful to be in Gods favor and grace always.

I am grateful for blessings all around me.

I am grateful for Gods protections, strength, understanding, knowledge and justice.

I am grateful to get everything I want and need.

I am grateful to be blessed, magical, good and attractive.

I am grateful God is blessed and created to love and provide for us.

March 26

James 1

Faith and Wisdom

Greeting to the twelve tribes scattered all over the world. My friends be glad. You know that you learn to endure by having your faith tested. But you must learn to endure everything so that you will be completely mature. If any of you need wisdom you should ask God and it will be given to you. God is generous. When you ask for something you must have faith.

The Mustering

Whatever is in the heavens and on earth of it declare the praises and glory of Allah for he is the exalted in might the wise. Our Lord forgives us and our brethren who came before us into the faith.

You are grateful to bless and be blessed always.

You are grateful your body, mind and soul are divinely and eternally blessed.

You are grateful to bless and forgive everyone always.

You are grateful for all the blessings, prayers, visions and dreams.

You are grateful to be in God's favor and grace always.

You are grateful for blessings all around you.

You are grateful for Gods protections, strength, understanding, knowledge and justice.

You are grateful to get everything you want and need.

You are grateful to be blessed, magical, good and attractive.

You are grateful God is blessed and created to love and provide.

March 27

Luke 10:21

Jesus Thanks His Father

At the same time Jesus felt the joy that comes from the Holy Spirit and he said my father Lord of heaven and earth I am grateful that you hid all this from wise and educated people. My father has given me everything and he is the only one who knows the son. The only one who really knows the father is the son.

The Kneeling Down

The revelation of the book is from Allah the exalted in power full of wisdom. And in the creation of yourselves and the fact that animals are scattered through the earth are signs for those of assured faith.

We are grateful to bless and be blessed always.

We are grateful our body, mind and soul are divinely and eternally blessed.

We are grateful to bless and forgive everyone always.

We are grateful for all the blessings, prayers, visions and dreams.

We are grateful to be in Gods favor and grace always.

We are grateful for blessings all around us.

We are grateful for Gods protections, strength, understanding, knowledge and justice.

We are grateful to get everything we want and need.

We are grateful to be blessed, magical, good and attractive.

We are grateful God is blessed and created to love and provide for us.

March 28

John 4

Jesus Will Finish God's Work

Jesus said my food is to do what God wants! He is the one who sent me and I must finish the work that he gave me to do. You may say that there are still 4 months until harvest time. But I tell you to look and you will see that the fields are ripe and ready to harvest. Even now the harvest workers are receiving their reward by gathering a harvest that brings eternal life. Then everyone who planted the seed and everyone who harvests the crop will celebrate together. So the saying proves true, "someone plants the seed and others harvest the crop.

The Glorious Morning Light

And verily the hereafter will be better for thee than the present. And soon will thy guardian Lord give thee that wherewith thou shalt be well pleased. Did he not give thee shelter and care? And he gave guidance. And made thee independent. Therefore the bounty of the Lord rehearse and proclaim.

All my life experiences are enriching and rewarding.

Being optimistic and happy is my top priority in my life.

I choose to be optimistic and happiness.

Each day I feel more positive about myself and my future.

Everyday my mood is lighter, brighter and happier.

Every day the quality of my life improves.

Everything is well and good in my life and my loved one's lives.

I always expect the best and focus on the present positive.

I am cheerful and optimistic in all situations.

I adorn my life with unlimited optimism and enthusiasm.

March 29

Colossians 2:30

Christ Brings New Life

Obeying these rules may seem to be a smart thing to do but they appear to make you love God more and to be very humble and to have control over your body.

Hud

We certainly gave the book to Moses. And of a surety to all will your Lord payback in full the recompense of their deeds. For he knoweth well all that they do. Therefore stand firm in the straight path as thou art commanded thou and those who will thee turn unto Allah. And be steadfast in patience for verily Allah will reward the righteous.

All your life experiences are enriching and rewarding.

Being optimistic and happy is your top priority.

You choose to be optimistic and happiness.

Each day you feel more positive about yourself and your future.

Everyday your mood is lighter, brighter and happier.

Every day the quality of your life improves.

Everything is well and good in your life and your loved one's lives.

You always expect the best and focus on the present positive.

You are cheerful and optimistic in all situations.

You adorn my life with unlimited optimism and enthusiasm.

March 30

2 Corinthians

Forgiveness

I also wrote because I wanted to test you and find out if you would follow my instructions. I will forgive anyone you forgive. Yes for your sake and with Christ as my witness. I have forgiven whatever needed to be forgiven. You are written in our hearts by the spirit. The scriptures say God commanded light to shine. Now God is shining in our hearts to let you know that his glory is seen in Jesus Christ's name.

The Gold Adornments

Verily we have brought the truth to you. If Allah most gracious had a song I would be the first to worship. Glory to the Lord of the heavens and the earth. The Lord of the throne of authority. He is free from the things they attribute to him. It is he who is God in heaven and God on earth and He is full of wisdom and knowledge and blessed.

All our life experiences are enriching and rewarding.

Being optimistic and happy is our top priority in my life.

We choose to be optimistic and happiness.

Each day we feel more positive about ourselves and our future.

Everyday our mood is lighter, brighter and happier.

Every day the quality of our life improves.

Everything is well and good in our life and our loved one's lives.

We always expect the best and focus on the present positive.

We are cheerful and optimistic in all situations.

We adorn our life with unlimited optimism and enthusiasm.

March 31

Revelation 13:18

Faith in God

You need wisdom to understand the number. I looked and saw the lamb standing on mount Zion. With him were a 144000 who had his name and his faith written on their foreheads. Then I heard a sound from heaven that was like a roaring flood or loud thunder elders. Or even like the music of harps. And a new song was being sung in front of God's throne.

Those Ranged in Ranks

And we gave them the book which helps to make things clear; and we guided them to the straightway. And we left this blessing for them among generations to come in later times. Peace and salutation to Moses and Aaron! Thus indeed do we reward those who do right. For they were two of our believing servants so also was Elias among those sent by us. Peace and salutation to such as Elias. Thus indeed do we reward those who do right.

I am grateful I always remain positive and optimistic.

I am grateful to be positive no matter what.

I am grateful to be excited and expect miracles every day.

I am grateful all my experiences are rewarding.

I am grateful I approach every situation with optimism and understanding.

I am grateful I easily maintain a positive mind frame.

I am grateful to focus and expect the best and receive it.

I am grateful to maintain a positively focused mindset.

I am grateful I keep a sense of humor in all situations.

I am grateful to see and find the good in everything.

April 1

Revelation 5

The Scroll and the Lamb

The lamb went over and took the scroll from the right hand of the one who sat on the throne. After he had taken it the 4 living creatures and 24 elders knelt down before him. Each of them had a harp and a gold bowl full of incense, which are the prayers of God's people. Then they sang a new song. You are worthy to receive the scroll and open its seals you bought for God's people from every tribe, language, nation and race.

The Inner Apartments

O mankind! We created you from a single pair of male and a female and made you into nations and tribes that ye may know each other. Verily the most honored of you in the sight of Allah is he who is the most righteous of you. And Allah has full knowledge and is well acquainted with all things. Allah is oft-forgiving oft merciful.

You are grateful you always remain positive and optimistic.

You are grateful to be positive no matter what.

You are grateful to be excited and expect miracles every day.

You are grateful all your experiences are rewarding.

You are grateful you approach every situation with optimism and understanding.

You are grateful you easily maintain a positive mind frame.

You are grateful to focus and expect the best and receive it.

You are grateful to maintain a positively focused mindset.

You are grateful you keep a sense of humor in all situations.

You are grateful to see and find the good in everything.

April 2

Psalm 3

A Prayer

You are my shield and you give me victory and great honor. I pray to you and you answer from your sacred hill. I sleep and wake up refreshed because you Lord protect me. Come and save me Lord God. You are my God and protector. The Lord has chosen everyone who is faithful to be his very own and he answers my prayers. You brought me more happiness than a rich honest of grain and grapes. I can sleep soundly because you Lord will keep me safe.

The Gold Adornments

When Jesus the son of Mary is held up as an example. He was a servant. We grant our favor to him and we made him an example of the children of Israel. And Jesus shall be a sign for the coming of the hour of judgment, therefore the hour is the straightway.

We are grateful we always remain positive and optimistic all the time.

We are grateful to be positive no matter what.

We are grateful to be excited and expect miracles every day.

We are grateful all our experiences are rewarding.

We are grateful we approach every situation with optimism and understanding.

We are grateful we easily maintain a positive mind frame.

We are grateful to focus and expect the best and receive it.

We are grateful to maintain a positively focused mindset.

We are grateful we keep a sense of humor in all situations.

We are grateful to see and find the good in everything.

April 3

Luke 17:14

Miraculous Healing

Jesus looked at them and said go show yourselves to the priests. On their way they were healed. When one of them discovered that he was healed he came back shaking praises to God. He bowed down at the feet of Jesus and thanked him.

Those Ranged in Ranks

O my Lord! Grant me a righteous son. So we gave him the good news of a boy ready. Then when the son reached the age of work with him he said, O MY SON! I see a vision that I offer thee. The son said, O my father does as thou art commanded. You will find me practicing in patience and constancy. So they had submitted their wills to Allah. Thus indeed do we reward those who do right?

I celebrate the diversity and connectedness present on all planets.

I care for the earth by recognizing its miraculous beauty.

I care for the earth by taking care of other creatures.

I care for earth by caring for my fellow beings.

I bless and care for the earth by using only what I need.

Every day I bless and care for the earth.

I believe in a protected earth and free humanity.

I am grounded in earth and one with the forest and land.

I am grounded to the ebb and flow of the sea and I am one with the ocean.

I am touched by nature and breathe fresh clean air.

April 4

Psalm 84

The Joy of Worship

Lord God all powerful your temple is so lovely. Deep in my heart I long for your temple and with all that I am I sing joyful songs to you. You bless everyone who lives in your house and they sing your praises. You bless all who depend on you for their strength and all who deeply desire to visit your temple. Lord God all-powerful the God of Jacob pleases answer my prayer. You are the shield that protects your people and I am your chosen one.

Qaf

Thou art Allah's messenger. They wonder that there has come to them a Warner from among themselves. We already know how much of them the earth takes away with us is a record guarding the full account. And the earth we have spread it out and set thereon mountains standing firm and produced therein every kind of beautiful growth.

You celebrate the diversity and connectedness present on all planets.

You care for the earth by recognizing its miraculous beauty.

You care for the earth by taking care of other creatures.

You care for earth by caring for my fellow beings.

You bless and care for the earth by using only what you need.

Every day you bless and care for the earth.

You believe in a protected earth and free humanity.

You are grounded in earth and one with the forest and land.

You are grounded to the ebb and flow of the sea and you are one with the ocean.

You are touched by nature and breathe fresh clean air.

April 5

Colossians 3

A Prayer of Thanks

Each time we pray for you we thank God, the father of our Lord Jesus Christ. We have heard of your faith in Christ and of your love for all of God's people because what you hope for is kept safe for you in heaven. You first heard about the hope when you believed the true message which is the good news. The good news is spreading all over the world with great success has spread in the same way among you ever since the first day you learned the truth about God's wonderful kindness from our good friend Epaphras.

Winding Sand Tracts

Therefore patiently preserve as did all messengers of flexible purpose. Thine but to proclaim the message. O our people hearken to the one who invites you to Allah and believe in him he will forgive you and deliver you.

We celebrate the diversity and connectedness present on all planets.

We care for the earth by recognizing its miraculous beauty.

We care for the earth by taking care of other creatures.

We care for earth by caring for my fellow beings.

We bless and care for the earth by using only what we need.

Every day we bless and care for the earth.

We believe in a protected earth and free humanity.

We are grounded in earth and one with the forest and land.

We are grounded to the ebb and flow of the sea and we are one with the ocean.

We are touched by nature and breathe fresh clean air.

April 6

Colossians 4

Pray

Be fair and honest. You have a master in heaven. Never give up praying and when you pray keep alert and be thankful. Be sure to pray that God will spread his message and explain the mystery about Christ. Please pray that I will make the message as clear as possible. Be pleasant and hold their interest when you speak the message. Choose your words carefully and be ready to give answers to anyone who asks questions.

The Poets

These are verses of the book that makes things clear. There comes not to them a newly revealed message from Allah most gracious. Do they look at the earth how many noble things of all kinds we have produced therein? Verily in this is a sign.

I am grateful I have a protective clean atmosphere.

I am grateful earth is perfectly designed, loved and cared for.

I am grateful for an infinity supply of available oxygen.

I am grateful Mother Nature is blessed and protected.

I am grateful blessed are the sons and daughters of light who know Mother Nature.

I am grateful Mother Nature gives us life and I respect her laws and will.

I am grateful the world is a good safe and fun place.

I am grateful for what God has given me.

I am grateful for nature all its beauty, abundance and providence.

I am grateful to take care of all creation.

April 7

Romans 4:21

The Promise Is For All Who Have Faith

But these words were not written only for Abraham. They were written for us since we will also be accepted because of our faith in God who raised Lord Jesus to life. God gave Jesus and he raised him to life so that we would be made acceptable to God. By faith we have been made acceptable to God. And now because of our Lord Jesus Christ we live out peace with God.

The Believer

And our Lord that they enter the gardens of eternity which thou hast promised to them and to the righteous among their fathers, their wives and their prosperity. For thou art he the exalted in might full of wisdom.

You are grateful you have a protective clean atmosphere.

You are grateful earth is perfectly designed, loved and cared for.

You are grateful for an infinity supply of available oxygen.

You are grateful Mother Nature is blessed and protected.

You are grateful blessed are the sons and daughters of light who know Mother Nature.

You are grateful Mother Nature gives us life and you respect her laws and will.

You are grateful the world is a good safe and fun place.

You are grateful for what God has given you.

You are grateful for nature all its beauty, abundance and providence.

You are grateful to take care of all creation.

April 8

Psalm 85

A Prayer of Peace

You have forgiven your people. Our Lord our God you save us. Please bring us back home. I will listen to you Lord God because you promise peace to those who are faithful. You are ready to receive everyone who worships you so that you will live with us in all your glory. Love and loyalty will come together, goodness and peace will unite.

The Narrations

And when it is recited to them they say we believe therein for it is the truth from our Lord indeed we have been Muslims bowing to Allah's will from before this. They be given their reward for that they have preserved with good and that they spend in charity out of what we have given them.

We are grateful we have a protective clean atmosphere.

We are grateful earth is perfectly designed, loved and cared for.

We are grateful for an infinity supply of available oxygen.

We are grateful Mother Nature is blessed and protected.

We are grateful blessed are the sons and daughters of light who know Mother Nature.

We are grateful Mother Nature gives us life and we respect her laws and will.

We are grateful the world is a good safe and fun place.

We are grateful for what God has given us.

We are grateful for nature all its beauty, abundance and providence.

We are grateful to take care of all creation.

April 9

Acts 13:35

God's Holy One

God will never let the body of his holy one decay. When David was alive he obeyed God. God raised Jesus. My friends the message is that Jesus can forgive you. Everyone who has faith in Jesus is set free. Be amazed and disappear. I will do something today.

Man

Verily we created man from a drop of mingled sperm in order to try him so we gave him the gifts of hearing and sight. We feed you for the love of Allah. Allah will deliver them from that day and will shed over them a light of beauty and blissful joy and because they were patient and constant. He will reward them with a garden and garments of silk.

I am happy that my vehicle is in excellent condition.

I am driving the perfect vehicle for me.

My automobile always gets me where I need to go and back safely.

I am blessed to drive a comfortable reliable car.

I love and care for the vehicle I drive.

My vehicle is easily affordable.

My vehicle is safe luxurious, spacious and gas efficient.

My vehicle runs perfectly well and is maintained excellently.

My vehicle is interesting and a pleasure to drive.

I am attracting a perfect second vehicle.

April 10

Psalm 97

The Lord Brings Justice

The Lord is king. Tell the earth to celebrate and all islands to shout, clouds surround him and his throne is supported by justice and fairness. Lightning is so bright that the earth sees it and trembles. Mountains melt away like wax in the presence of the Lord of all the earth. The heaven announce o Lord brings justice. Everyone sees Gods glory. The Lord rules the whole earth and love the Lord. God protects his loyal people and rescues them. If you obey and do right a light will show you the way and fill you with happiness.

The Prophets

Closer and closer to mankind comes their reckoning. My Lord knoweth every word spoken in the heavens and on earth. He is the one that heareth and knoweth all things. Before thee also the messengers we sent were but men to whom we granted inspiration.

You are happy that your vehicle is in excellent condition.

You are driving the perfect vehicle for you.

My automobile always gets you where you need to go and back safely.

You are blessed to drive a comfortable, reliable car.

You love and care for the vehicle you drive.

Your vehicle is easily affordable.

Your vehicle is safe, luxurious, spacious and gas efficient.

Your vehicle runs perfectly well and is maintained excellently.

Your vehicle is interesting and a pleasure to drive.

You are attracting a perfect second vehicle.

April 11

Psalm 110

The Lord Gives Victory

The Lord said to my Lord sit at my right side. The Lord will let your power reach out from Zion and you will rule. Your glorious power will be seen on the day you begin to rule. You will wear the sacred robes and shine like the morning sun in all of your strength. The Lord has made a promise that will never be broken. The Lord is at your right.

The Confederates

Allah is full of knowledge and wisdom. But follow that which comes to thee by inspiration from the Lord for Allah is well acquainted with all that ye do. And put thy trust in Allah and enough is Allah as a disposer of affairs.

We are happy that my vehicle is in excellent condition.

We are driving the perfect vehicle for us.

My automobile always gets us where we need to go and back safely.

We are blessed to drive a comfortable, reliable car.

We love and care for the vehicle we drive.

Our vehicle is easily affordable.

Our vehicle is safe luxurious, spacious and gas efficient.

Our vehicle runs perfectly well and is maintained excellently.

Our vehicle is interesting and a pleasure to drive.

We are attracting a perfect second vehicle.

April 12

Psalm 41

A Prayer in Time of Need

You Lord God bless everyone who cares and you rescue those people. You protect them and keep them alive, you make them happy here in this land. You always heal them and restore their strength. I prayed heal me.

The Cattle

When he it is who hath sent unto you the book explained in detail. They know full well to you whom we have given the book that it hath been sent down from thy Lord in truth. The word of the Lord doth find its fulfillment in truth and in justice none can change his words and for he is the one. Who heareth and knoweth all. Went through to follow the common run of those on earth they will lead thee away from the way of Allah.

I am grateful to use the law of attraction to manifest divine goodness.

I am grateful to own a safe, spacious and gas efficient vehicle.

I am grateful my transportation is affordable and easy.

I am grateful my vehicle is in increasingly good condition.

I am grateful to own, love and care for my vehicle well.

I am grateful my vehicle is perfectly maintained well.

I am grateful to love my comfortable ride of pleasure.

I am grateful my transportation is reliable, safe and fun.

I am grateful to provide joyous trips for me and others.

I am grateful for many blissful experiences in my vehicle.

April 13

1 Timothy 3:14

The Mystery of our Religion

After all the church of the living God is the strong foundation of truth. Here is the great mystery of our religion. Christ came as a human. The spirit proved that he pleased God and he was seen by angels.

The Family of Imran

For the righteous are in gardens in nearness to their Lord with rivers flowing beneath therein is their eternal home with companions pure and holy and the good pleasure of Allah. For in Allah's sight are all his servants. Those who show patience, firmness and self-control who are true in word and deed who worship devoutly who spend in the way of Allah and who pray for forgiveness in the early hours of the morning.

You are grateful to use the law of attraction to manifest divine goodness.

You are grateful to own a safe, spacious and gas efficient vehicle.

You are grateful your transportation is affordable and easy.

You are grateful your vehicle is in increasingly good condition.

You are grateful to own, love and care for your vehicle well.

You are grateful your vehicle is perfectly maintained well.

You are grateful to love your comfortable ride of pleasure.

You are grateful your transportation is reliable, safe and fun.

You are grateful to provide joyous trips for you and others.

You are grateful for many blissful experiences in your vehicle.

April 14

1 Corinthians 9:24

A Race

You know that many runners enter a race and only one of them wins the prize. So run to win. Athletes work hard to win a crown that cannot last but we do it for a crown that will last forever. I keep my body under control telling the good news to others.

The Gold Adornments

My devotees! Being those who have believed in our signs and bowed their wills to ours in Islam. Enter ye the gardens ye and your wives in beauty and rejoicing. To them will be passed round dishes and goblets of gold there will be there all that the souls desire all that the eyes could delight in and ye shall abide therein for aye. Such will be the gardens of which ye are made heirs and for your good deeds.

We are grateful to use the law of attraction to manifest divine goodness.

We are grateful to own a safe, spacious and gas efficient vehicle.

We are grateful our transportation is affordable and easy.

We are grateful our vehicle is in increasingly good condition.

We are grateful to own, love and care for our vehicle well.

We are grateful our vehicle is perfectly maintained well.

We are grateful to love our comfortable ride of pleasure.

We are grateful our transportation is reliable, safe and fun.

We are grateful to provide joyous trips for us and others

We are grateful for many blissful experiences in our vehicle.

April 15

Mark 16

Jesus is Alive

After the Sabbath Mary Magdalene, Salome and Mary the mother of James bought some spices to put on Jesus body. The man said you are looking for Jesus from Nazareth. God has raised him to life, and he isn't here. Now go and tell his disciples and especially Peter that he will go ahead of you to Galilee. You will see him there just as he told you.

Joseph

These are the symbols or verses of the perspicuous book. We have sent it down in Arabic Qur'an in order that ye may learn wisdom. We do relate unto thee the most beautiful of stories in that we reveal to thee these portions of the Quran. Behold Joseph said to his father. O my father and I did see eleven stars and the sun and the moon. I saw them prostrate themselves to me. Verily Joseph and his brethren are signs or symbols for seekers after truth.

I am perfectly beautiful inside and out.

I am comfortable and happy in my own skin.

I am turning more beautiful, attractive and good looking every day.

I am a true beauty with a natural pretty look.

I have an attractive beautiful body, mind and soul.

People look to me as a source of beauty and attraction.

I have a perfect self-image.

I am extremely attractive and sexy.

I am full of grace and elegance.

I am pleasing to look at and I smile all the time.

April 16

Luke 12:14

The One

My friends God is the one. Five sparrows are sold for just two pennies, but God doesn't forget a one of them. Even the hairs on your head are counted. You are worth much more than many sparrows.

The Prophets

To him belong all creatures in the heavens and on earth even those who are in his very presence to serve him. They celebrate his praises night and day. But glory to Allah the Lord of the throne high is he above what they attribute to him.

You are perfectly beautiful inside and out.

You are comfortable and happy in your own skin.

You are turning more beautiful, attractive and good looking every day.

You are a true beauty with a natural pretty look.

I have an attractive beautiful body, mind and soul.

People look to you as a source of beauty and attraction.

You have a perfect self-image.

You are extremely attractive and sexy.

You are full of grace and elegance.

You are pleasing to look at and you smile all the time.

April 17

John 17

Jesus Prays

Father the time has come for you to bring glory to your son in order that he may bring glory to you. And you gave him power over all people so that he would give eternal life to everyone you give to him. Eternal life is to know you the only true God and to know Jesus Christ the one you sent. I have brought glory to you here on earth by doing everything you gave me to do. Now father give me back the glory that I had with you before the world was created.

The Confederates

Ye have indeed in the messenger of Allah a beautiful pattern of conduct for anyone whose hope is in Allah and the final day and who engages much in the praise of Allah. When the believers saw the confederate forces they said, this is what Allah and his messenger told us what was true. And it only added to their faith and their zeal in obedience. Among the believers are men who have been true to their covenant with Allah completed their vow.

We are perfectly beautiful inside and out.

We are comfortable and happy in my own skin.

We are turning more beautiful, attractive and good looking every day.

We are a true beauty with a natural pretty look.

We have an attractive beautiful body, mind and soul.

People look to us as a source of beauty and attraction.

We have a perfect self-image.

We are extremely attractive and sexy.

We are full of grace and elegance.

We are pleasing to look at and we smile all the time.

April 18

John 6:55

True Food and Drink

If you do eat my flesh and drink my blood you will have eternal life. My flesh is the true food and my blood is the true drink. If you eat my flesh and drink my blood you are one with me and I am one with you. The living father sent me and I have life because of him. Now everyone who eats my flesh will live because of me.

The Gold Adornments

When Jesus the son of Mary is held up as an example. Behold he was a servant. We granted our favor to him and we made him an example to the children of Israel. And if it were our will we could make angels from amongst you succeeding each other on the earth. And Jesus shall be a sign for the coming of the hour of judgment.

I am grateful to be heavenly beautiful inside and out always.

I am grateful for my healthy skin, hair, teeth and body parts.

I am grateful to be fit, good looking and slender.

I am grateful to look good and feel great always.

I am grateful to possess beauty and elegance.

I am grateful to have good posture and carry myself well.

I am grateful every cell of my body radiates with beauty, purity, love, joy and good health.

I am grateful to be a beauty in mind, body and soul.

I am grateful everything and everyone is beautiful.

April 19

John 8:12

Jesus is the Light of the World

I am the light for the world. Follow me. You will have the light that gives life. Jesus replied even if I do speak for myself what I say is true. I know where I come from and where I am going. If I did judge, I would judge fairly. The father who sent me is here with me. Your law requires two witnesses to prove that something is true. I am one of my witnesses and the father who sent me is the other one.

The Crowds

The revelation of this book is from Allah, the exalted in power, full of wisdom. Verily it is we who have revealed the book to thee in truth so serve Allah offering him sincere devotion. Truly Allah will judge between them Allah wished to take himself a son he could have chosen whom he pleased out of those whom he doth create but glory be to him.

You are grateful to be heavenly beautiful inside and out always.

You are grateful for you have healthy, skin, hair, teeth and body parts.

You are grateful to be fit, good looking and slender.

You are grateful to look good and feel great always.

You are grateful to possess beauty and elegance.

You are grateful to have good posture and carry yourself well.

You are grateful every cell of your body radiates with beauty, purity, love, joy and good health.

You are grateful to be a beauty in mind, body and soul.

You are grateful everything and everyone is beautiful.

April 20

Psalm 150

Praise God

The Lord is good to his people. Shout praises to the Lord! Praise God in his temple. Praise him in heaven, his mighty fortress. Praise our God! His deeds are wonderful. Marvelous to describe. Praise God with trumpets and all kinds of harps. Praise him with tambourines and dancing with stringed instruments and woodwind. Praise God with cymbals with clashing cymbals. Let every living creature, praise the Lord.

The Repentance

There is a mosque whose foundation was laid on piety it is more worthy of the standing forth for prayer therein. In it are men who love to be purified and Allah loveth these who make themselves pure. He that layeth his foundation on piety to Allah and his good pleasure. Allah is all knowing wise.

We are grateful to be heavenly beautiful inside and out always.

We are grateful for my healthy, pretty skin, hair, teeth and body parts.

We are grateful to be fit, good looking and slender.

We are grateful to look good and feel great always.

We are grateful to possess beauty and elegance.

We are grateful to have good posture and carry ourselves well.

We are grateful every cell of our body radiates with beauty, purity, love, joy and good health.

We are grateful to be a beauty in mind, body and soul.

We are grateful everything and everyone is beautiful.

April 21

John 4:1

God is True

My dear friends we must love each other. Love comes from God and when we love each other it shows that we have been given new life. We are now God's children and we know him. God is love. God showed his love for us when he sent his only son into the world to give us life. Dear friends since God loved us this much we must love each other.

Fussilat

Who is better in speech than one who calls men to Allah works righteousness and says I am of those who bow in Islam? One will be granted such goodness except those who exercise patience and self-restraint none but persons of the greatest fortune. Seek refuge in Allah. He is the one who hears and knows all things. Adore the sun and the moon adore Allah who created them, if it is him ye wish to serve.

I can turn my dreams into realities.

I own my own dreams and I give them spiritual wings.

I have fun fulfilling my dreams.

Today I confidently strive towards my dreams.

I manifest my desires in dreams quickly, joyfully and perfectly.

Joyful dreams of love surround me everywhere always.

I remember my dreams every day.

I am living the life of my dreams.

My dreams are rich, vibrant, helpful and I remember them.

Subtle healing within my own blessed living cells begins in my dreams.

April 22

John 1:9

The Word of Life

The true light that shines on everyone was coming into the world. The word was in the world God had made the world with his word. He came into his own world. People accepted him and put their faith in him. So, he gave them the right to be the children of God.

Joseph

Allah will forgive you and he is the most merciful of those who show mercy. Go with this my shirt and cast it over the face of my father he will come to see clearly. Then come ye here to me together with all your family. Then when the bearer of good news came he cast the shirt over his face and he for with regained clear sign. He said soon will I ask my Lord for forgiveness.

You can turn your dreams into realities.

You own your own dreams and you give them spiritual wings.

You have fun fulfilling your dreams.

Today you confidently strive towards your dreams.

You manifest your desires in dreams quickly, joyfully and perfectly.

Joyful dreams of love surround you everywhere always.

You remember your dreams every day.

You are living the life of your dreams.

Your dreams are rich, vibrant, helpful and you remember them.

Subtle healing within your own blessed living cells begins in my dreams.

April 23

Psalm 19

The Wonders of God and the Goodness of his Law

The heavens keep telling the wonders of God and the skies declare what he has done. Each day informs the following day each night announces to the next. Their message reaches all the earth and it travels around the world. In the heavens a tent is set up for the sun. It rises like a bridegroom and gets ready like a hero. It travels all the way across the sky.

The Believer

The revelation of this book is from Allah exalted in power full of knowledge who forgiveth, accepted repentance, is strict in punishment and hath a long reach in all things. Raised high above ranks or degrees. He is the Lord of the throne of authority by his command doth he send the spirit of inspiration to any of his servants he pleases that it may warn men of the day of mutual meeting.

We can turn our dreams into realities.

We own my own dreams and we give them spiritual wings.

We have fun fulfilling our dreams.

Today I confidently strive towards our dreams.

We manifest our desires in dreams quickly, joyfully and perfectly.

Joyful dreams of love surround us everywhere always.

We remember our dreams every day.

We are living the life of our dreams.

My dreams are rich, vibrant, helpful and we remember them.

Subtle healing within our own blessed living cells begins in our dreams.

April 24

Psalm 32

The Joy of Forgiveness

O Lord you bless everyone. You protect me and put songs in my heart because you have saved me. You said to me I will point out the road that you should follow I will be your teacher and watch over you. Your kindness shields those who trust you. Lord and so your good people should celebrate.

The Prostration

It is Allah who has created the heavens and the earth, and all between then in 6 days and is firmly established himself on the throne of authority ye have none besides him to protect or intercede. He rules all affairs from the heavens and the earth and in the end will all affairs go up to him on a day the space whereof will be as a thousand years of reckoning and he who has made everything which he created good.

I am grateful for dreams, love, beauty, success.

I am grateful to achieve my dreams.

I am grateful my dreams provide good ideas, resources and people.

I am grateful to have peaceful rests.

I am grateful to believe in the good fortune of my dreams.

I am grateful for many blessings and miracles in my life.

I am grateful to accept my wishes and dreams coming true.

I am grateful I see, feel and hear my dreams and goals as already accomplished.

I am grateful to have faith in pursuing my dreams.

I am grateful to remember all my dreams of love, success and God.

April 25

Luke 4:31

Jesus

News about Jesus spread all over that part of the country. So he went over to her and she was able to get up, serve them a meal. After the sun set Jesus he put his hands on each of them and healed them.

The Spider

Recite what is sent of the book by inspiration and establish regular prayers. Remembrance of Allah is the greatest thing in life. And Allah knows the deeds that ye do.

You are grateful for dreams, love, beauty, success.

You are grateful to achieve your dreams.

You are grateful your dreams provide good ideas resources and people.

You are grateful to have peaceful rests.

You are grateful to believe in the good fortune of my dreams.

You are grateful for many blessings and miracles in your life.

You are grateful to accept your wishes and dreams coming true.

You are grateful you see, feel and hear your dreams and goals as already accomplished.

You are grateful to have faith in pursuing your dreams.

You are grateful to remember all my dreams of love, success and God.

April 26

Psalm 23

The Good Shepherd

You Lord are my shepherd I will never be in need. You let me rest in fields of green grass. You lead me to steams of peaceful water and you refresh my life. You are true to your name and you lead me along the right paths. You are with me and makes me feel safe. You treat me. You honor me and you fill my cup. Your kindness and love will always be with each day of my life and I will live forever in your house Lord.

The Cave

Praise be to Allah who hath sent his servant, the book. He hath made it straight and clear in order that he may warn. He may give glad tidings to the believers who work righteous deeds that they shall have a goodly reward.

We are grateful for dreams, love, beauty, success.

We are grateful to achieve our dreams.

We are grateful our dreams provide good ideas, resources and people.

We are grateful to have peaceful rests.

We are grateful to believe in the good fortune of our dreams.

We are grateful for many blessings and miracles in our life.

We are grateful to accept our wishes and dreams coming true.

We are grateful we see, feel and hear our dreams and goals as already accomplished.

We are grateful to have faith in pursuing our dreams.

We are grateful to remember all our dreams of love, success and God.

April 27

Colossians 1:15

The Person and Work of Christ

Christ is exactly like God. He is the first born seen superior to all creation. Everything was created by him everything in heaven and on earth everything seen and unseen including all forces and powers. All things were created by God's son and everything was made for him. God's son was before all else and by him everything is held together. He is the head of his body which is the church. He is the very beginning, the first to be raised. He would be above all others. God himself was pleased to live fully in his son. And God was pleased for him to make peace.

The Repentance

Allah hath promised to believer's men and women gardens under which rivers flow to dwell therein and beautiful mansions in gardens everlasting bliss. But the greatest bliss is the good pleasure of Allah that is the supreme felicity.

I have the confidence to make my wishes become a reality.

I can be exactly what I wish to be.

I can make my wishes come true.

Imagine my wishes coming true.

I wish only the best for everyone everywhere always.

I wish to be a good genie.

I wish for good, healthful, helpful and useful things and people and places.

I wish for God's will to be done.

I wish everyone was successful, good, righteous, healthy, happy and peaceful.

April 28

Colossians 3:10

Christ Brings New Life

Each of you is now a new person. You are becoming more like your creator and you will understand him better. Christ is all that matters and he lives in all of us. God loves you and has chosen you as his own special people. So be generous, kind, humble, meek and patient. Put up with each other and forgive anyone, just as Christ has forgiven you. Love is more important than anything else. It is what ties everything completely together.

Those Ranged in Ranks

Already has word been to our servants sent by us? That they would certainly be assisted.

You have the confidence to make your wishes become a reality.

You can be exactly what you wish to be.

You can make your wishes come true.

Imagine your wishes coming true.

You wish only the best for everyone everywhere always.

You wish to be a good genie.

You wish to wish for good healthful helpful and useful things and people and places.

You wish for God's will to be done.

You wish everyone was successful, good, righteous, healthy, happy and peaceful.

April 29

Psalm 44

A Prayer for Help

Our God, our ancestors told us what wonders you worked and we listened carefully. Then you loved them let our ancestors take over their land. Their strength and weapons were what won the land and gave them victory. You loved them with your powerful arm and your shining glory. You are my God and king and you give victory to the people of Jacob. I do depend on my arms or my sword. Wake up do something Lord help us!

Luqman

Seest thou the ships through the ocean by the grace of Allah. That He may show you of his signs. Verily in this are signs for all who constantly preserve and give thanks. When a wave covers them like the canopy of clouds they call to Allah. Offering him sincere devotion. O mankind! Do your duty to your Lord.

We have the confidence to make our wishes become a reality.

We can be exactly what we wish to be.

We can make our wishes come true.

Imagine our wishes coming true.

We wish only the best for everyone everywhere always.

We wish to be a good genie.

We wish to wish for good, healthful, helpful and useful things and people and places.

We wish for God's will to be done.

We wish everyone was successful, good, righteous, healthy, happy and peaceful.

April 30

Romans 8:1

Giving by the Power of God's Spirit

You belong to Christ Jesus. The Holy Spirit will give you life that comes from Christ Jesus and will set you free. He did this so that we would do what the law commands by obeying the spirit. The spirit thinks of spiritual things. If our minds are ruled by spirit we will have life and peace. God's spirit now lives in you and he will raise you to life by his spirit.

Hud

Thy Lord had so willed he could have made mankind one people. All that we relate to thee of the stories of the prophets with it we make firm thy heart in them. There cometh to thee the truth, as well as an exhortation and a message of remembrance to those who believe to Allah do belongs the unseen secrets of the heavens and the earth and to him goeth back every affair for decision.

I am grateful something better is perfectly manifesting.

I am grateful to make all my wishes come true.

I am grateful my wishes are a reality.

I am grateful all my wishes benefit everyone everywhere.

I am grateful wishes are granted in divine timing.

I am grateful to be a good genie and get anything I wish for.

I am grateful to wish everyone was healthy, happy, rich and peaceful.

I am grateful to wish Gods will be done always.

I am grateful to wish the best for everyone always.

I am grateful my wishes are always useful, beneficial and perfectly good always.

May 1

1 Peter 3

Wives and Husbands and Doing Right

If you are a wife, you must put your husband first. No one else will have to say anything to him because he will see how you honor God and live a pure life. Be beautiful in your heart by being gentle and quiet. This kind of beauty will last and God considers it very special. If you are a husband you should be thoughtful of your wife. Treat her with honor and she shares with you in the gift of life.

The Night Journey

Allah sent a man like us to be his messenger. Say if there were settled on angels walking about in peace and quiet. We should certainly have sent them down from the heavens an angel for a messenger. Say enough is Allah for a witness between me and you for he is very well acquainted with his servants and he sees all things.

You are grateful something better is perfectly manifesting.

You are grateful to make all your wishes come true.

You are grateful your wishes are a reality.

You are grateful all your wishes benefit everyone everywhere.

You are grateful wishes are granted in divine timing.

You are grateful to be a good genie and get anything you wish for.

You are grateful to wish everyone was healthy, happy, rich and peaceful.

You are grateful to wish Gods will be done always.

You are grateful to wish the best for everyone always.

You are grateful your wishes are always useful, beneficial and perfectly good always.

May 2

Mark 10:17

A Rich Man

As Jesus was walking down a road, a man ran up to him he knelt down and asked good teacher what can I do to have eternal life? Jesus replied, Why do you call me good? God is good. You know my commandments. Be faithful in marriage. Respect your father and mother. The man answered, teacher, I have obeyed all these commandments since I was a young man.

The Thunder

Is then he who standeth over every soul and knoweth all that it doth like any others? Is it that ye will inform him of something he knoweth on earth, or is it just a show of words? Allah doth blot out and confirm what he pleaseth with him is the mother of the book.

We are grateful something better is perfectly manifesting.

We are grateful to make all our wishes come true.

We are grateful our wishes are a reality.

We are grateful all our wishes benefit everyone everywhere.

We are grateful wishes are granted in divine timing.

We are grateful to be a good genie and get anything we wish for.

We are grateful to wish everyone was healthy, happy, rich and peaceful.

We are grateful to wish God's will be done always.

We are grateful to wish the best for everyone always.

We are grateful our wishes are always useful, beneficial and perfectly good always.

May 3

1 John 5

Victory Over the World

If we believe that Jesus is true Christ we are God's children. Everyone who loves the father will also love his children. If we love and obey God we know that we will love his children. We show our love for God by obeying his commandments. Every child of God gives us this victory.

The Women

They had done what they were actually told it would have been best for them and would have gone farthest to strengthen their faith. And we should then have given them from our presence a great reward. Allah and the messenger are in the company of those on whom is the grace of Allah of the prophets who teach the sincere lovers of truth, the witnesses who testify and the righteous who do good.

God gave me the discernment to make good decisions.

I use my expert common sense to direct my path.

My capabilities are enlightened with wisdom and understanding.

My wisdom is a gift from God.

My wisdom gives me the ability to perceive believe and proceed and achieve easily and well.

A wealth of information is available to me always

I have all the answers I need.

At every opportunity, I expand my knowledge and understanding.

I always receive, divine wisdom and guidance.

Being inquisitive, sophisticated, brilliant and clever comes naturally for me.

May 4

Luke 2:13

The Shepherds

Suddenly many other angels came down from heaven and joined in praising God. They said, praise God in heaven. Peace on earth to everyone who pleases God. After the angels had gone back to heaven the shepherds said to each other, let's go to Bethlehem and see what the Lord has told us. Everyone listened and was surprised.

Ya Sin

By the Qur'an full of wisdom thou art indeed one of the messengers. And he makes companions for us and he says who can give life? Say he will give them life. For he is well versed in every kind of creation. Is he who created the heavens and the earth able to create the like thereof? Yea indeed! For he is the creator supreme of skill and knowledge infinite.

God gave you the discernment to make good decisions.

You use my expert common sense to direct your path.

Your capabilities are enlightened with wisdom and understanding.

Your wisdom is a gift from God.

Your wisdom gives you the ability to perceive believe, proceed and achieve easily and well.

A wealth of information is available to you always.

You have all the answers you need.

At every opportunity, you expand your knowledge and understanding.

You always receive, divine wisdom and guidance.

Being inquisitive, sophisticated, brilliant and clever comes naturally for you.

May 5

Psalm 30

A Prayer of Thanks

I will praise you Lord. You saved me from the grace. I prayed to you. Lord God and you healed me, saving me. Your faithful people Lord will praise you with songs and honor your holy name. Your kindness lasts for a lifetime. I felt secure. You made me strong as a mighty mountain.

Muhammad

O ye who believe! Obey Allah and obey the messenger. Allah is with you and your good deeds. The life of this world is but play and amusement and if ye believe and guard and he will grant you your recompense.

God gave us the discernment to make good decisions.

We use our expert common sense to direct our path.

Our capabilities are enlightened with wisdom and understanding.

Our wisdom is a gift from God.

Our wisdom gives me the ability to perceive believe, proceed and achieve easily and well.

A wealth of information is available to us always.

We have all the answers we need.

At every opportunity, we expand our knowledge and understanding.

We always receive, divine wisdom and guidance.

Being inquisitive, sophisticated, brilliant and clever comes naturally for us.

May 6

John 5:31

Witnesses to Jesus

There is someone else who speaks for me and I know what he says is true. You sent messengers to John and he told them the truth. John was a lamp that gave a lot of light and you were glad to enjoy his light for a while. Something more important than John speaks for me. I mean the things that the father has given me to do. All these speak for me and prove that the father sent me.

The Narrations

Those to whom we sent the book before this they do believe in this revelation. And when it is recited to them they say we believe therein for it is the truth from our Lord indeed we have been Muslims bowing to Allah's will from before this. Twice will they be given their reward for that they have preserved with good and they spend in charity out of what we have given them.

I am grateful to absorb wisdom and knowledge easily.

I am grateful my intelligence leads me to the right path with the right decisions.

I am grateful I am intelligent with a wealth of knowledge.

I am grateful to be a master reader and can retain and recall anything.

I am grateful to find inspiration wisdom and knowledge.

I am grateful to have an extensive knowledge.

I am grateful knowledge and wisdom god has given me.

I am grateful I strive for excellence and seek knowledge.

I am grateful I am fluently and skilled in everything.

I am grateful to increase my wisdom, knowledge and understanding daily.

May 7

John 9:1

Jesus Heals a Man

As Jesus walked along he saw a man. You will see God work a miracle for him. While I am in the world, I am the light of the world. After he says said this he spit on the ground. He made some mud and smeared it on the man's eyes. Then said go wash off the mud in Siloam pool which means one who is sent. When he washed off the mud he could see.

The Star

He was taught by one mighty in power, endued with wisdom for he appeared in stately form. While he was the highest part of the horizon. Then he approached and came closer.

You are grateful to absorb wisdom and knowledge easily.

You are grateful your intelligence leads you to the right path with the right decisions.

You are grateful you are intelligent with a wealth of knowledge.

You are grateful to be a master reader and can retain and recall anything.

You are grateful to find inspiration wisdom and knowledge.

You are grateful to have an extensive knowledge.

You are grateful knowledge and wisdom God has given you.

You are grateful you strive for excellence and seek knowledge always.

You are grateful you are fluently and skilled in everything.

You are grateful to increase your wisdom, knowledge and understanding daily.

May 8

Jude

Be Helpful

Dear Friends keep building on the foundation of your most holy faith, as the Holy Spirit helps you to pray. And keep in step with God's love, as you wait for our Lord Jesus Christ to show how kind he is by giving you eternal life. Be helpful to all. Rescue any who need to be saved. Have mercy on everyone who needs it.

The Poets

These are verses of the book that makes things clear. If such were our will we could send down to them from the sky a sign. But there comes to them a newly revealed message from Allah most gracious. Thus Lord is he the exalted in mighty most merciful, Lord of the east and the west and all between and if yes only had sense.

We are grateful to absorb wisdom and knowledge easily.

We are grateful our intelligence leads us to the right path with the right decisions.

We are grateful we are intelligent with a wealth of knowledge.

We are grateful to be a master reader and can retain and recall anything.

We are grateful to find inspiration wisdom and knowledge.

We are grateful to have an extensive knowledge.

We are grateful knowledge and wisdom God has given us.

We are grateful we strive for excellence and seek knowledge always.

We are grateful we are fluently and skilled in everything always.

May 9

1 Peter 2:11

Live as God's Servants

Dear friends you are on this earth. Always let others see you behaving properly. Then on the Day of Judgment they will honor God by telling the good things they saw you do. The Lord wants you to obey all authorities especially the emperor who rules over everyone. You must also obey governors because they are sent by the emperor to praise good citizens.

The Heights

My Lord hath commanded justice and that ye set your whole selves to him. Call upon him making your devotion sincere as in his sight such as he created you in the beginning, so shall ye return. He will hath guided o children of Adam. Wear your beautiful apparel at every time and place of prayer eat and drink. The beautiful gifts of Allah which he hath produced for his servants and the things clean and pure which he hath provided for sustenance.

I am highly organized always.

I keep my work, home, and vehicle space tidy.

I am efficient, attentive, focused an orderly always.

I always show up on time.

I am reliable and organized person.

My life is completely organized and successful.

I am totally getting more organized every day.

I live a clutter free life.

My organizational skills are changing life for the better.

Staying organized is easy for me.

May 10

Acts 9:32

Peter Heals Aeneas

While Peter was traveling from place to place he visited the Lord's followers who lived in a town of Lydia. Peter said to Aeneas, Jesus Christ has healed you! Get up and make your bed. Right away he stood up. Many people in the towns of Lydia and Sharon saw Aeneas and became followers of the Lord. After Peter had sent everyone out of the room he knelt down and prayed. Then he turned to the body of Darcas and said Tabitha get up! the woman opened her eyes.

Abraham

You're Lord caused to be declared I will add more favors. Yet is Allah free of all wants worthy of all praise. Has the story reached you o people of those who went before you of the people of Noah, Ad and Thamud.

You are highly organized always.

You keep your work, home, and vehicle space tidy.

You are efficient, attentive, focused an orderly always.

You always show up on time.

You are reliable and organized person.

Your life is completely organized and successful.

You are totally getting more organized every day.

You live a clutter free life.

Your organizational skills are changing life for the better.

Staying organized is easy for you.

May 11

John 6:25

The Bread that Gives Life

Rabbi, when did you get here? Jesus answered, I tell you for certain that you are looking for me because you saw the miracles. Work for the food that gives eternal life. The son of man will give you this food because God the father has given him the right to do so. What exactly does God want us to do? The people Jesus answered God wants you to have faith in the one he sent.

Bees

Allah sets forth a parable of two men. Whom we bestowed goodly favors from ourselves and he spends thereof freely privately and publicly are the two equal? By no means praise be to Allah. To Allah belongeth the mystery of the heavens and the earth and the decision of the hours of judgment is as the twinkling of an eye or even quicker for Allah hath power over all things. It is he who brought you forth from the wombs of your mothers.

We are highly organized always.

We keep my work, home, and vehicle space tidy.

We are efficient, attentive, focused an orderly always.

We always show up on time.

We are reliable and organized person.

Our life is completely organized and successful.

We are totally getting more organized every day.

We live a clutter free life.

Our organizational skills are changing life for the better.

Staying organized is easy for us.

May 12

Psalm 144

A Prayer for the Nations

I praise you Lord! You are my mighty rock and you teach me. You are my friend my fortress where I am safe. You are my shield and you make me the ruler of your people. Open the heavens like a curtain and come down Lord. Reach down from heavens and set me free. Save me.

The Winds that Scatter

And we have spread out the spacious earth how excellently we do spread out. And of everything we have created pairs that ye may receive instruction. Hasten ye then at once to God I am from him a Warner to you clear and open. Is this the legacy they have transmitted one to another.

You are grateful being organized is easy for you.

You are grateful your ability to organized improves your productivity.

You are grateful staying organized and on top of things makes your life run smoothly and orderly always.

You are grateful you can relax knowing everything is in order.

You are grateful to be highly organized and efficient.

You are grateful to organize your time and maintain control over your life.

You are grateful you enjoy keeping everything tidy and clean.

You are grateful to consistently plan and organize to succeed.

You are grateful to organize your mind and life.

You are grateful to have excellent organizational skills.

May 13

1 John 4:1

God is Love

Dear friends, test them all to find out if they really do come from God. His spirit says that Jesus Christ had a truly human body. Children you belong to God, Gods spirit is in you and is more powerful, everyone who knows God will listen to us.

Hud

The son replied, I will betake the same mountain and it will give me from the water. Noah said this day nothing can save you from the command of Allah. The ark rested on mount Al-Judi and the word went forth. And Noah called upon his Lord and said, "O my Lord! Surely my son is of my family! And thy promise is true and thou art the justest of judges.

We are grateful being organized is easy for me.

We are grateful my ability to organized improves with my productivity.

We are grateful staying organized and on top of things makes our life run smoothly and orderly always.

We are grateful we can relax knowing everything is in order.

We are grateful to be highly organized and efficient.

We are grateful to organize our time and maintain control over our life.

We are grateful we enjoy keeping everything tidy and clean.

We are grateful to consistently plan and organize to succeed.

We are grateful to organize our mind and life.

We are grateful to have excellent organizational skills.

May 14

1 Corinthians 1:18

Christ is Gods Wisdom and Power

The message for those of us who are being saved, it is Gods power at work. God was wise decided to let the people of this world use their wisdom to learn about him.

The Gold Adornments

When Jesus the son of Mary is held up as an example. We granted our favor to him and made him an example to the children of Israel. And it if were our will we could make angels from amongst you succeeding each other on the earth. And Jesus shall be a sign for the coming of the hour of judgment therefore follow ye me. This is a straight way. When Jesus came with clear signs he said, Now have I come to you with wisdom in order to make clear to you. Therefore obey me. For Allah he is my Lord and your Lord. So worship ye him this is a straight way.

I can maintain cleanliness and purity always.

I have good personal hygiene.

I can keep my home, car and where I work neat and clean always.

I balance my body with clean and fresh nutrients.

I get a good daily dose of pure clean fresh air.

Every day I set an intention to experience love, peace cleanliness and purity.

Purity, holiness and cleanliness will exalt the human condition.

I keep myself clean, bright and pure always.

Cleanliness preserves beauty.

Keeping my mind, body and soul clean and tidy is important to me.

May 15

Mark 12:28

The Most Important Commandment

Jesus answered, the most important one says people of Israel, you have only one Lord and God. You must love him with all your heart, soul, mind and strength. The second most important commandment says, Love others as much as you love yourself. The man replied teacher you are certainly right to say there is one God.

Joseph

These are the symbols or verses of the perspicuous book. We have sent it down as an Arabic Quran in order that ye may learn wisdom. We do relate unto thee the most beautiful of stories in that we reveal to thee this portion of the Quran. Behold Joseph said to his father. O my father! I did see eleven stars and the sun and the moon. I saw them prostrate themselves there until you leave me.

You can maintain cleanliness and purity always.

You have good personal hygiene.

You can keep your home, car and where you work neat and clean always.

You balance your body with clean and fresh nutrients.

You get a good daily dose of pure clean fresh air.

Every day you set an intention to experience love, peace cleanliness and purity.

Purity, holiness and cleanliness will exalt the human condition.

You keep myself clean, bright and pure always.

Cleanliness preserves beauty.

Keeping your mind, body and soul clean and tidy is important to you.

May 16

Luke 9

Instructions for the 12 Apostles

Jesus called together his 12 apostles and gave them power over all. Then he sent them to tell about God's kingdom and to heal. Take a walking stick or a traveling bag or food or money or even a change of clothes when you are welcomed into a home stay there until you leave that town.

The Cave

Praise be to Allah who hath sent to his servant the book. He hath made it straight and clear in order that he may warn. He may give glad tidings to the believers who work righteous deeds that they shall have a goodly reward. Wherein they shall remain forever.

I am grateful to keep myself clean and pure always.

I am grateful my environment is neat and clean all the time.

I am grateful to maintain cleanliness and purity always.

I am grateful my home is a clean, heavenly paradise.

I am grateful to maintain and recognize purity and good health.

I am grateful my home, car and workplace are clean and pure always.

I am grateful my soul, heart, body and mind is pure.

I am grateful to love, care and clean for my environment.

I am grateful to have good hygiene and clean eating habits.

I am grateful for purified and clean fresh air and water.

May 17

Hebrews 13:20

Prayers and Greetings

God gives peace and he raised our Lord Jesus Christ. Now Jesus is like a great shepherd was used to make Gods eternal agreement. I pray that God will make you ready to obey him and that you will always be eager to do right. May Jesus help you do what pleases God to Jesus Christ by glory forever and ever. Amen.

Muhammad

Those who believe and work deeds of righteousness and believe in the revelation sent down to Muhammad for it is the truth from their Lord he will improve their condition. Those who believe follow the truth from their Lord, thus does Allah set forth for men their lessons by similitudes.

You are grateful to keep yourself clean and pure always.

You are grateful your environment is neat and clean all the time.

You are grateful to maintain cleanliness and purity always.

You are grateful your home is a clean, heavenly paradise.

You are grateful to maintain and recognize purity and good health.

You are grateful your home, car and workplace are clean and pure always.

You are grateful your soul, heart, body and mind is pure.

You are grateful to love, care and clean for your environment.

You are grateful to have good hygiene and clean eating habits.

You are grateful for purified and clean fresh air and water.

May 18

Romans 7:1

An Example from Marriage

My friends you surely understand enough about law. For example, the law says that a man's wife must remain his wife as long as he lives. That is how it is with you, my friends. You are now part of the body of Christ. You are free to belong to Christ so that we could serve God.

The Criterion

Is that best or the eternal garden promised to the righteous? For them that is a reward as well as a goal of attainment. For them there will be therein all that they wish for and they will dwell there for ages and a promise to be prayed for from thy Lord. The day he will gather them together as well as those whom they worship besides Allah.

We are grateful to keep ourselves clean and pure always.

We are grateful our environment is neat and clean all the time.

We are grateful to maintain cleanliness and purity always.

We are grateful our home is a clean, heavenly paradise.

We are grateful to maintain and recognize purity and good health.

We are grateful our home, car and workplace are clean and pure always.

We are grateful our souls, hearts, bodies and minds are pure.

We are grateful to love, care and clean for our environment.

We are grateful to have good hygiene and clean eating habits.

We are grateful for purified and clean fresh air and water.

May 19

Matthew 5:1

The Sermon on the Mount and Blessings

God blesses those people who are humble. The earth will belong to them. God blesses those people who want to obey him. They will be given what they want. God blesses those people who are merciful. They will be treated with mercy. God blesses those people whose hearts are pure.

The Inner Apartments

O ye who believe! Allah is he who hears and knows all things. O ye who believe. Raise not your voices above the voice of the prophet nor speak aloud to him in talk as ye may speak aloud to one another. Those that lower their voices in the presence of Allah's messenger their hearts has Allah tested for piety and for them is forgiveness and a great reward.

From this moment on I enjoy everything I do.

I am well respected.

My potential is unlimited and it shows.

I am the go to person to get things done right.

I am even tempered and well balanced.

My family, friends, coworkers and the universe think very well of me.

Every day my reputation gets better and better.

I am famous and well known for the good I do and bring.

The universe recognizes and praises our God because of my success and fame.

I have established an excellent reputation in my community now and forever.

May 20

Matthew 5:23

Jesus Teaches, Preaches and Heals

Jesus went all over Galilee teaching in the Jewish meeting places and preaching the good news about God's kingdom. He also healed every kind. News spread about him all over Syria. Jesus healed all of them.

The Prophets

Who can keep you safe by night and by day. We gave the good things of this life to these men and their father.

From this moment on you enjoy everything you do.

You are well respected.

Your potential is unlimited and it shows.

You are the go to person to get things done right.

You are even tempered and well balanced.

Your family, friends, coworkers and the universe think very well of you.

Every day your reputation gets better and better.

You are famous and well known for the good you do and bring.

The universe recognizes and praises our God because of your success and fame.

You have established an excellent reputation in your community now and forever.

May 21

2 Timothy

Please the Lord

When Christ Jesus comes as king he will be the judge of everyone. So with God and Christ as witness I command you to preach. You must correct people. But also cheer them up. The time is coming. You must stay calm. You must work hard to tell the good news and to do your job well. A crown will be given to me for pleasing the Lord.

The Heifer

Allah is full of bounty to mankind but most of them are. Know that Allah heareth and knoweth all thine. Who is he that will loan to Allah a beautiful loan which Allah will double unto his credit and multiply many times. It is Allah that giveth you plenty and to him shall be your return. Hast thou turned thy vision to the chiefs of the children of Israel after the time of Moses?

From this moment on we enjoy everything we do.

We are well respected.

Our potential is unlimited and it shows.

We are the go to people to get things done right.

We are even tempered and well balanced.

Our family, friends, coworkers and the universe think very well of us.

Every day our reputation gets better and better.

We are famous and well known for the good we do and bring.

The universe recognizes and praises our God because of my success and fame.

We have established an excellent reputation in we community now and forever.

May 22

Psalm 107

The Lord is Good to His People

You should celebrate offering sacrifices and singing joyful songs to tell what he has done. You should praise the Lord for his love and for the wonderful things he does for all of us. Honor the Lord when you and your leaders meet for worship. In need he will come to your rescue and your families will grow as fast as a heard of sheep. Be wise and remember this and think about the kindness of the Lord.

Ta Ha

So go ye both to him and say verily we are messengers sent by thy Lord and send forth therefore the children of Israel with us. I am with you. I hear and see everything. And peace to all who follow guidance! Our Lord is he who gave to each created things its form and nature and further gave it guidance.

I am grateful to be well respected in the world.

I am grateful to be honored and respected.

I am grateful for my talents and skills.

I am grateful to enjoy enthusiasm and support for my accomplishment I am grateful for my good, attractive honest, kind, generous, friendly, rich, helpful, trustworthy and compassionate reputation.

I am grateful for fortune, fame and righteousness.

I am grateful to be well known, famous, well liked.

I am grateful I attract and celebrate great success, good fortune, happiness, wisdom and good health with everyone.

I am grateful for all the blessings and opportunities that improve my excellent reputation.

May 23

Proverbs 5

Be Faithful to Your Wife

My son, if you listen closely to my wisdom and good sense you will have sound judgment and you will always know the right thing to say. You should be faithful to your wife just as you take water from your own well. And my son pay close attention and obey me and you will live and let my instructions be your greatest treasure.

Jonah

My work to me and yours to you. Ye are free from responsibility for what I do and I for what ye do. It is he who giveth life. And to him shall all be brought back. O mankind! There hath come to you a direction from your Lord and a healing. For those who believe, a guidance and mercy.

You are grateful to be well respected in the world.

You are grateful to be honored and respected.

You are grateful for your talents and skills.

You are grateful to enjoy enthusiasm and support for your accomplishment.

You are grateful for your good, attractive, honest, kind, generous, friendly, rich, helpful, trustworthy and compassionate reputation.

You are grateful for fortune, fame and righteousness.

You are grateful to be well known, famous, well liked.

You are grateful you attract and celebrate great success, good fortune, happiness, wisdom and good health with everyone.

You are grateful for all the blessings and opportunities that improve your excellent reputation.

May 24

Philippians 4:10

Paul Gives Thanks

The Lord has made me very grateful that at last you have thought about me. Actually you were thinking about me all along. I have learned to be satisfied with whatever I have. I have been paid back everything and with interest. I am completely satisfied with the gifts.

The Cave

Moses said to him, may I follow thee on the footing that thou teach something of the truth which thou hast been taught? The other said verily thou wilt be able to have patience with me. Have patience bout things which thy understanding is complete? Moses said thou wilt find me if Allah so wills truly patient.

We are grateful to be well respected in the world.

We are grateful to be honored and respected.

We are grateful we are well known for our talents and skills.

We are grateful to enjoy enthusiasm and support for our accomplishments.

We are grateful for our good, attractive, honest, kind, generous, friendly, rich, helpful, trustworthy and compassionate reputation.

We are grateful for fortune, fame and righteousness.

We are grateful to be well known, famous, well liked.

We are grateful we attract and celebrate great success, good fortune, happiness, wisdom and good health with everyone.

We are grateful for all the blessings and opportunities that improve our excellent reputation.

May 25

Acts 5:38

Temple

If God is behind it you cannot stop it anyway. The apostles left the council and were happy because God had considered them worthy. Every day they spent time in the temple and in one home after another. They never stopped teaching and telling the good news that Jesus is the messiah.

Hud

The word came too Noah! Come down from the ark with peace from us and blessing on thee and on some of the peoples who with spring from those with thee but there will be other people to whom we shall grant their pleasures for a time in the end. Such are some of the stories of the unseen which we have revealed onto thee before this neither thou nor thy people knew them so persevere patiently for the end for those who are righteous.

I am grateful being organized is easy for me.

I am grateful my ability to organize improves my productivity.

I am grateful staying organized and on top of things makes my life run smoothly and orderly always.

I am grateful I can relax knowing everything is in order.

I am grateful to be highly organized and efficient.

I am grateful to organize my time and maintain control over my life.

I am grateful I enjoy keeping everything tidy and clean.

I am grateful to consistently plan and organize to succeed.

I am grateful to organize my mind and life.

I am grateful to have excellent organizational skills.

May 26

John 13:31

The New Command

Now the son of man will be given glory and he will bring glory to God. Then after God is given glory because of him. God will bring glory to him and God will do it. My children then you will look for me. I tell you just as I told the people you cannot go where I am going. But I am giving you a new command. You must love each other just as I loved you if you love each other everyone will know that you are my disciples.

Hud

And of a surety to all will your Lord pay back in full the recompense of their deeds for he knoweth well all that they do. Therefore stand firm in the straight path as thou art commanded thou and those who with thee turn into Allah. And establish regular prayers at the two ends of the day and at the approaches of the night for those things that are good. And be steadfast in patience.

I am highly creative.

My imagination is always free and active.

I am highly imaginative and naturally creative person.

I am full of inspiration, motivation and creativity.

My creativity flows effortlessly and divinely.

I always come up with amazing brilliant, creative new ideas.

My imagination gets stronger and stronger every day.

I find it easy to be creative.

I enjoy practicing creativity.

I have a good and powerful imagination.

May 27

John 4:34

Jesus and the Samaritan Woman

Jesus said, my food is to do what God wants. He is the one who sent me and I must finish the work that he gave me to do. You may say that there are still four months until harvest time. But I tell you look and you will see that the fields are ripe and ready to harvest. I am sending you to harvest crops in fields where others have done all the hard work.

The Ants

Say praise be to Allah and peace on his servants whom he has chosen. Allah has created the heavens and the earth and who sends you down rain from the sky. Yes with it we cause to grow well planted orchards full of beauty and delight it is in your power to cause the growth of the trees in them.

You are highly creative.

Your imagination is always free and active.

You are highly imaginative and naturally creative person.

You are full of inspiration, motivation and creativity.

My creativity flows effortlessly and divinely.

You always come up with amazing brilliant creative new ideas.

My imagination gets stronger and stronger every day.

You find it easy to be creative.

You enjoy practicing creativity.

You have a good and powerful imagination.

May 28

Luke 8:54

Jesus Heals

Jesus took hold of the girls hand and said child get up. She came back to life and got right up. Jesus told them to give her something to eat. Her parents were surprised.

The Table Spread

O ye who believe! Allah doth but make a trial of you in a little matter of fame well within reach of your hands and your lances that he may test.

We are highly creative.

My imagination is always free and active.

We are highly imaginative and naturally creative person.

We are full of inspiration, motivation and creativity.

Our creativity flows effortlessly and divinely.

We always come up with amazing brilliant creative new ideas.

Our imagination gets stronger and stronger every day.

We find it easy to be creative.

We enjoy practicing creativity.

We have a good and powerful imagination.

May 29

Luke

An Angel Tells About the Birth of Jesus

The angel answered I am Gabriel, Gods servant and I was sent to tell you this good news. You have believed what I have said. But everything will take place when it is supposed to. The angel answered the Holy Spirit will come down to you and God's power will come over you. So your child will be called the holy son of God.

The Gold Adornments

But the mercy of thy Lord is better then the wealth which they a mass. Allah most gracious silver roofs for their houses, and silver stairways on which to go up and silver doors to their houses and thrones of silver on which they should recline and also adornments of gold

I am grateful an endless reservoir of creativity lies within me.

I am grateful to practice bring creative every day.

I am grateful creative, brilliant positive ideas flow to me.

I am grateful creative inspiration flows though me.

I am grateful divine motivation inspiration and creativity are natural and blessings.

I am grateful great joy is expressed by creativity.

I am grateful to be inventive unique creative always.

I am grateful for my powerful intelligent creative imagination.

I am grateful to be a creative genius.

I am grateful to be powerful artistic, resourceful and a visionary.

May 30

Luke 9:48

Child Get Up

And he said to her daughter your faith has made you well go in peace. Jesus answered she will be made well. He did not allow anyone to enter. Child arise. She got up immediately and he gave orders for something to be given her to eat. Her parents were amazed.

The Pilgrimage

Thus have we sent down clear signs and verily Allah doth guide whom he will. Those who believe in the Qur'an those who follow the Jewish scriptures and the Christians. Allah will judge between them on the day of judgment for Allah is witness of all things, To Allah bow down in worship all things that are in the heavens and on earth, the sun, the moon, the stars, the hills, the trees, the animals and a great number among mankind.

You are grateful an endless reservoir of creativity lies within you.

You are grateful to practice bring creative every day.

You are grateful creative, brilliant positive ideas flow to you.

You are grateful creative inspiration flows through you.

You are grateful divine motivation inspiration and creativity are natural and blessings.

You are grateful great joy is expressed by creativity.

You are grateful to be inventive unique creative always.

You are grateful for your powerful intelligent creative imagination.

You are grateful to be a creative genius.

May 31

Psalm 18:16

Lord Praised for Giving Deliverance

He sent from on high. He drew me out of many waters he delivered me. The Lord was my stay, he brought me forth also into a broad place. He rescued me because he delighted in me. The Lord has rewarded me according to my righteousness. According to the cleanness of my hands he has recompensed me. For I have kept the ways of the Lord.

Joseph

Jacob said, never will I send him with you until ye swear a solemn oath to me in Allah's name that ye will be sure to bring him back. And when they had sworn their oath he said, over all that we say be Allah the witness and guardian. For he was by our instruction full of knowledge and experience.

We are grateful an endless reservoir of creativity lies within me.

We are grateful to practice bring creative everyday.

We are grateful creative, brilliant positive ideas flow to us.

We are grateful creative inspiration flows through us.

We are grateful divine motivation inspiration and creativity are natural and blessings.

We are grateful great joy is expressed by creativity.

We are grateful to be inventive unique creative always.

We are grateful for our powerful intelligent creative imagination.

We are grateful to be a creative genius.

We are grateful to be powerful artistic, resourceful and a visionary.

June 1

Colossians 2:9

Christ Brings Real Life

God lives fully in Christ. And you are fully grown because you belong to Christ. Who is over every power and authority. Just as circumcision removes flesh from the body. Then you were raised because you had faith in the power of God who raised Christ. But God let Christ make you alive when he forgave.

The Believers

Further we sent a long line of prophets for your instruction. We sent Noah to his people he said o my people worship Allah. So we inspired him with this message, construct the ark within our sight and under our guidance, then when comes our command and the foundations of the earth gush forth take thou on board pairs of every species male and female and thy family.

I can and will have more than I ever dreamed possible.

I choose happiness, good health, wealth, love and abundance.

I give and receive abundance in all its forms.

I am prosperous, healthy, happy and live in abundance.

Perfect abundance and prosperity and love are my reality.

Feeling joyful attracts more abundance.

I am willing to be more abundant and resourceful now.

All the abundance of the universe already exists within me.

Every action I take moves me towards greater abundance and happiness.

I am an open channel for abundance, love, joy, prosperity and happiness.

June 2

1 Peter 2:11

Live as God's Servants Should

Then on the Day of Judgment they will honor God by telling the good things they saw you do. The Lord wants you to obey all authorities the emperor who rules over everyone. You must obey governors.

The Spider

Recite what is sent of the book by inspiration to thee and establish regular prayers. We believe the revelation which has come down to us and that which came down to you our God and your God is one and it is to him we bow in Islam. And thus it is that we have sent down the book to thee.

You can and will have more than you ever dreamed possible.

You choose happiness, good health, wealth, love and abundance.

You give and receive abundance in all its forms.

You are prosperous, healthy, happy and live in abundance.

Perfect abundance and prosperity and love are your reality.

Feeling joyful attracts more abundance.

You are willing to be more abundant and resourceful now.

All the abundance of the universe already exists within you.

Every action you take moves you towards greater abundance and happiness.

You are an open channel for abundance, love, joy, prosperity and happiness.

June 3

Act 12:7

Rescue

Suddenly an angel from the Lord appeared and light flashed around. The angel poked Peter in the side and woke him up then he said quick get up. The angel said get dressed and put your sandals on. Peter did what he was told. Then the angel said now put on your coat and follow me. Peter left with the angel but he thought everything was only a dream. Peter now realized what had happened.

The Mount

By a decree inscribed in a scroll unfolded. By the much frequented house of worship. By the canopy raised high and by the ocean filled with swell. As to the righteous they will be in gardens and in happiness enjoying the bliss which their Lord hath bestowed on them and their Lord shall deliver them.

We can and will have more than we ever dreamed possible.

We choose happiness, good health, wealth, love and abundance.

We give and receive abundance in all its forms

We are prosperous, healthy, happy and live in abundance.

Perfect abundance and prosperity and love are our reality.

Feeling joyful attracts more abundance.

We are willing to be more abundant and resourceful now.

All the abundance of the universe already exists within us.

Every action we take moves us towards greater abundance and happiness.

We are an open channel for abundance, love, joy, prosperity and happiness.

June 4

Matthew 13:14

A Hidden Treasure

The kingdom of heaven is like what happens when someone finds treasure hidden in a field and buries it again. A person like that is happy and goes and sells everything in order to buy that field. The kingdom of heaven is like what happens when a shop owner is looking for fine pearls. After finding a very valuable one the owner goes and sells everything in order to buy that pearl. The kingdom of heaven is like what happens when a net is thrown into a lake and catches all kinds of fish.

The Rocky Tract

These are the Ayat of revelation of a Qur'an that makes things clear. We send the angels down except for just cause. We have sent down the message and we will assuredly guard it.

I am grateful for abundance and prosperity.

I am grateful to give thanks every day.

I am grateful I allow for greater abundance to come.

I am grateful to be a powerful prosperity, love and abundance magnet.

I am grateful to be entitled to joy, love and abundance.

I am grateful to be surrounded by riches and abundance.

I am grateful to enjoy overflowing abundance into my life.

I am grateful to live in a rich abundant universe.

I am grateful to resonate in harmony with the planets abundance.

I am grateful to welcome and accept success and abundance.

June 5

Matthew 7:7

Ask, Search and Knock

Ask and you will receive. Search and you will find. Knock and the door will be opened to you. Everyone who asks will receive. Everyone who searches will find. And the door will be opened for everyone who knocks. Your heavenly father is even more ready to give good things to people who ask. Treat others as you want them to treat you.

The Elephant

For the covenants of security and safeguard enjoyed by the Quarish. Their covenants covering safe journey by winter and summer. Let them adore the Lord of this house. Who provides them with good and with security.

You are grateful for abundance and prosperity.

You are grateful to give thanks every day.

You are grateful you allow for greater abundance to come.

You are grateful to be a powerful prosperity, love and abundance magnet.

You are grateful to be entitled to joy, love and abundance.

You are grateful to be surrounded by riches and abundance.

You are grateful to enjoy overflowing abundance into your life.

You are grateful to live in a rich abundant universe.

You are grateful to resonate in harmony with the planets abundance.

You are grateful to welcome and accept success and abundance.

June 6

2 Timothy 1:3

Gratitude

I am always grateful for you as I pray to the God my ancestors and I have served with a clear conscience, I remember I want to see you. Because that will make me truly happy. I ask you to make full use of the gift that God gave you when I placed my hands on you. Use it well. God's spirit gives us power, love, and self-control.

The Light

Allah belongs the dominions of the heavens and the earth and to Allah is the final goal of all. Do you see that Allah makes the clouds move gently then joins them together then makes them into a heap. Then will you see rain issue from their midst. And he sends down from the sky mountain masses of clouds wherein is hail.

We are grateful for abundance and prosperity.

We are grateful to give thanks every day.

We are grateful we allow for greater abundance to come.

We are grateful to be a powerful prosperity, love and abundance magnet.

We are grateful to be entitled to joy, love and abundance.

We are grateful to be surrounded by riches and abundance.

We are grateful to enjoy overflowing abundance into your life.

We are grateful to live in a rich abundant universe.

We are grateful to resonate in harmony with the planets abundance.

We are grateful to welcome and accept success and abundance.

June 7

Romans 7:1

An Example of Marriage

You are now part of the body of Christ. You are free to belong to Christ so that we could serve God. We can serve God in a new way by obeying his spirit and in the old way by obeying the written law.

The Crowds

Say it is Allah I serve with my sincere and exclusive devotion. Those who turn to Allah in repentance for them is good news. And so announce the good news to my servants. Those who listen to the word and follow the best meaning in it.

All my desires are committed to memory.

All my goals are carved on my heart.

Daily commitment to my goals makes every day more successful.

Every activity I perform is in accordance with the commitment of my goals.

Every day I am more committed to my goals.

Every day I reassert and reaffirm my commitment to create my perfect reality.

I am committed to being the best I could be.

I am committed to living my life passionately and purposefully.

I am committed in making positive changes.

I am deeply committed to attaining the life of my dreams.

June 8

Psalm 8

The Wonderful Name of the Lord

I think of the heaven your hands have made and the moon and stars you put in place. You put all of it under your power, the sheep, cattle and every wild animal, the birds in the sky, the fish in the sea and all oceans creatures.

The Repentance

The vanguard of Islam the first of those who gave them aid also those who follow them in all good deeds. Well pleased is Allah with them for them hath he prepared gardens under which rivers flow to dwell therein forever, that is the supreme felicity of their goods. Take alms so that mightiest purify and sanctify them and pray on for them and Allah is one source of security for them and Allah is one who heareth and knoweth all.

All your desires are committed to memory.

All your goals are carved on my heart.

Daily commitment to your goals makes every day more successful.

Every activity you perform is in accordance with the commitment of your goals.

Every day you are more committed to your goals.

Every day you reassert and reaffirm your commitment to create your perfect reality.

You are committed to being the best you could be.

You are committed to living your life passionately and purposefully.

You are committed in making positive changes.

You are deeply committed to attaining the life of your dreams.

June 9

Luke 9:29

Sons of God

While he was praying his face changed and his clothes became shining white. Suddenly Moses and Elijah were there speaking with him. They appeared in heavenly glory and talked about all that Jesus would mean. Let us make 3 shelters one for you, one for Moses and one for Elijah. From the cloud a voice spoke, this is my chosen son listen to what he says.

Mary

Relate the book the story of Mary when she withdrew from her family to a place in the east. She placed a screen to screen herself from them then sent her our angel. He said I am a messenger from your Lord to announce to you a gift of a holy son.

All our desires are committed to memory.

All our goals are carved on our heart.

Daily commitment to our goals makes every day more successful.

Every activity we perform is in accordance with the commitment of our goals.

Every day we are more committed to our goals.

Every day we reassert and reaffirm our commitment to create our perfect reality.

We are committed to being the best we could be.

We are committed to living our life passionately and purposefully.

We are committed in making positive changes.

We are deeply committed to attaining the life of our dreams.

June 10

Revelation 2:18

Treat Others As You Want To Be Treated

I know everything about you, including your love, faith, service and how you have endured. I know that you are doing more now than you have ever done before. All the churches will see that I know everyone's thoughts and feelings. I will treat each of you as you deserve.

The Rocky Tract

And the hour is surely coming when this will manifest. Verily it is thy Lord who is the master creator knowing all things. And he bestowed upon thee the seven oft repeated verses and the grand Qur'an. Lower thy wing in gentleness to the believers.

I am grateful to create my ideal life.

I am grateful to be in joyfully committed to attaining the perfect life.

I am grateful to put 100%effort and commitment into my goals.

I am grateful to do my absolute best all the time.

I am grateful to be committed to finishing the work I start.

I am grateful to be successful and live an honorable, purposeful, good life.

I am grateful to be passionately committed to achieving my dreams and goals.

I am grateful to be better than yesterday.

I am grateful to be committed to living a happy, healthy, rich, attractive and successful life through purposeful action and positive intentions and thoughts.

I am grateful to honor and keep my commitments to myself and others.

June 11

Acts 1:1

Holy Spirit

Jesus was taken up to heaven. He gave orders to the apostles he had chosen with the help of the Holy Spirit. Wait here for the father to give you the Holy Spirit just as I told you he has promised to do. John baptized with water but in a few days you will be baptized with the Holy Spirit.

The Prophets

Say what has come to me by inspiration is that your Allah is one Allah you therefore bow to his will in Islam. It is he who knows what is open in speech and what you hide in your hearts.

You are grateful to create my ideal life.

You are grateful to be in joyfully committed to attaining the perfect life.

You are grateful to put 100%effort and commitment into your goals.

You are grateful to do your absolute best all the time.

You are grateful to be committed to finishing the work I start.

You are grateful to be successful and live an honorable purposeful good life.

You are grateful to be passionately committed to achieving your dreams and goals.

You are grateful to be better than yesterday.

You are grateful to be committed to living a happy, healthy, rich, attractive and successful life through purposeful action and positive intentions and thoughts.

You are grateful to honor and keep your commitments to yourself and others.

June 12

Luke 8:32

What Jesus Did

Jesus got back into the boat to start back the man who had been healed begged to go with him. But Jesus sent him off and said go back home and tell everyone how much God has done for you. The man then went all over town telling everything that Jesus had done for him.

The Cave

Praise be to Allah who hath sent his servant the book. He hath made it straight and clear in order that he may warn and that he may give glad tidings to the believers who work righteous deeds that they shall have a goodly reward.

We are grateful to create our ideal life.

We are grateful to be in joyfully committed to attaining the perfect life.

We are grateful to put 100% effort and commitment into our goals.

We are grateful to do our absolute best all the time.

We are grateful to be committed to finishing the work we start.

We are grateful to be successful and live an honorable purposeful good life.

We are grateful to be passionately committed to achieving our dreams and goals.

We are grateful to be better than yesterday.

We are grateful to be committed to living a happy, healthy, rich, attractive and successful life through purposeful action and positive intentions and thoughts.

We are grateful to honor and keep our commitments to ourselves and others.

June 13

James 5:7

Be Patient and Kind

My friends be patient until the Lord returns. Think of farmers who wait patiently for the spring and summer rains to make their valuable crops grow. Be patient like those farmers. The judge is right outside the door. My friends follow the example of the prophets who spoke for the Lord. They were patient. We praise the ones who endured the most.

The Women

And we would then have given them from our presence a great reward. And we would have shown them the straightway. All who obey Allah and the apostle are in the company of those on whom is the grace of Allah of the prophets who teach, the sincere lovers of truth, the witnesses who testify and the righteous who do good. Ah. What a beautiful fellowship.

I am an excellent communicator.

I enjoy talking to people and they enjoy talking to me.

I am assertive, outgoing, and confident when communicating with others.

My communication skills are strong and I can influence easily.

I am a natural leader with great charisma.

I can express my wise opinions easily and well.

I can remain calm when communicating with others

Speaking, listening and understanding others are easy.

My strong communication skills get better and better.

I can express myself easy and listen to what others are saying.

June 14

1 Corinthians 1:18

Christ is God's Power and Wisdom

For those of us who are being saved it is God's power at work. God was wise and decided to let the people of this world use their wisdom to learn about him. Our message is God's power and wisdom for the Jews and Greeks that he has chosen.

The Prostration

This is the revelation of the book from the Lord of the worlds. It is Allah who has created the heavens and the earth and all between them in six days and is firmly established himself on the throne of authority. Ye have none besides him to protect or intercede for you and will ye then receive admonition. He rules all affairs from the heavens to the earth in the end will all affairs go up to him on a day the space whereof will be as a thousand years of your reckoning.

You are an excellent communicator.

You enjoy talking to people and they enjoy talking to you.

You are assertive, outgoing, and confident when communicating with others.

Your communication skills are strong and you can influence easily.

You are a natural leader with great charisma.

You can express your wise opinions easily and well

You can remain calm when communicating with others.

Speaking, listening and understanding others are easy.

Your strong communication skills get better and better.

You can express yourself easy and listen to what others are saying.

June 15

Acts 9:3

Saul Becomes a Follower of the Lord

When Saul had reached Damascus a bright light from heaven suddenly flashed around him. He fell to the ground and heard a voice that said Saul. Saul asked who you are. "I am Jesus, the Lord answered, now get up and go into the city where you will be told what to do." The men stood with Saul. They had heard the voice but they had not seen anyone. Saul got up from the ground.

Joseph

These are the symbols or verses of the perspicuous book. We have sent it down as an Arabic Qur'an in order that you may learn wisdom. We do relate unto you the most beautiful of stories in that we reveal to you this portion of the Qur'an. Joseph said to his father I did see stars and the sun and the moon.

We are an excellent communicator.

We enjoy talking to people and they enjoy talking to us.

We are assertive, outgoing, and confident when communicating with others.

Our communication skills are strong and we can influence easily.

We are a natural leader with great charisma.

We can express my wise opinions easily and well.

We can remain calm when communicating with others.

Our speaking, listening and understanding others is easy.

Our strong communication skills get better and better.

We can express myself easy and listen to what others are saying.

June 16

John 5:31

Witnesses to Jesus

I speak for myself there is way to prove I am telling the truth. There is someone else who speaks for me and I know what he says is true. You sent messengers to John and he told them the truth. I tell you these things so that you may be saved. John was a lamp that gave a lot of light.

Expounded

Say thou I am but a man like you and it is revealed to me by inspiration that your God is one God so stand true to him and ask for his forgiveness. For those who believe and work deeds of righteousness is a reward. So he completed them as seven firmaments in two days and he assigned to each heaven its duty and command. And we adorned the lower heavens with lights and provided it with guard.

I am grateful my communication skills are improving.

I am grateful to be confident when conversing.

I am grateful to enjoy conversations.

I am grateful my communication skills are excellent always.

I am grateful I remain positive and outgoing.

I am grateful to be natural at communicating well and easy to get along with always.

I am grateful to listen to what others say.

I am grateful all forms of my communication are positive, simple, clear, wise and friendly.

I am grateful I always communicate in terms of optimism, success and prosperity.

I am grateful to be friendly, and cheerful in all my communications.

June 17

1 Corinthians 5:12

Honor God with Your Body

Some of you say we can do anything we want to. I stay true. You also say food is meant for our bodies and our bodies are meant for food. We are to use them for the Lord who is in charge of our bodies.

The Table Spread

By its standards have been judged the Jews by the prophets who bowed as in Islam to Allah's will, by the rabbis and the doctors of law; for to them was entrusted the protections of Allah's book and they were witnesses there to. And we ordained therein for them life for life, eye for eye, nose for nose, ear for ear, tooth for tooth and equal for equal. If anyone remits the retaliation by way of charity it is an act of atonement for himself.

You are grateful your communication skills are improving.

You are grateful to be confident when conversing.

You are grateful to enjoy conversations.

You are grateful your communication skills are excellent always.

You are grateful you remain positive and outgoing.

You are grateful to be natural at communicating well and easy to get along with always.

You are grateful to listen to what others say.

You are grateful all forms of your communication are positive, simple, clear, wise and friendly.

You are grateful you always communicate in terms of optimism, success and prosperity.

You are grateful to be friendly, and cheerful in all my communications.

June 18

Psalm 26

The Prayer of an Innocent Person

Show that I am right Lord. I stay true to myself and I have trusted you. Test my thoughts and find out what I am like. I am always faithful to you. I wash my hands Lord to show my innocence and I worship at your altar while gratefully singing about your wonders. I love this temple where you live and where your glory shines.

The Romans

It is Allah who created them after strength gave you. He created as he wills and it is he who has all knowledge and power. Those endued with knowledge and faith will say.

We are grateful our communication skills are improving.

We are grateful to be confident when conversing.

We are grateful to enjoy conversations.

We are grateful our communication skills are excellent always.

We are grateful we remain positive and outgoing.

We are grateful to be natural at communicating well and easy to get along with always.

We are grateful to listen to what others say.

We are grateful all forms of our communication are positive, simple, clear, wise and friendly.

We are grateful we always communicate in terms of optimism, success and prosperity.

We are grateful to be friendly, and cheerful in all our communications.

June 19

Hebrews 2:5

Jesus Leads Us to be Saved

The one who leads us to be saved. We know that God did put the future world under the power of angels. Somewhere in the scriptures someone says to God what makes you care about us humans you have crowned us with glory and honor. Jesus led many of God's children to be saved and to share in his glory. Jesus and the people he makes holy all belong to the same family.

The Ways of Ascent

The angels and the spirit ascend unto him a day the measure whereof is of 50000years. Therefore hold patience a patience of beautiful contentment. They see the day quite near. The day that the sky will be like molten brass and the mountains will be like wool.

I love meeting people and approach them with enthusiasm and confidence.

I live in the present and am confident in the future

My attractive personality exudes a good attitude and confidence.

I am self-reliant, creative and persistent always.

I am energetic, enthusiastic and confident in all my ways.

I am well groomed, healthy and full of confidence.

I always see only the good in others.

I hold a good attitude and am well loved and respected.

My high self-esteem enables me to respect others and receive it.

My mind is full of good attitudes and positive, helpful thoughts always.

June 20

1 Thessalonians 5:12

Final Instructions and Greetings

My friends we ask you to be thoughtful of your leaders who work hard and tell you how to live for the Lord. Show them great respect and love because of their work. Try to get along with each other. My friend we beg you who is living right. Encourage anyone who feels left out, help all, be patient with everyone. Always be joyful and never stop praying. Whatever happens keep thanking God.

Qaf

To be observed and commemorated by every devotee turning to Allah. And we send down from the sky rain charged with blessing and we produce therewith gardens and grains for harvests.

You love meeting people and approach them with enthusiasm and confidence.

You live in the present and you are confident in the future.

Your attractive personality exudes a good attitude and confidence.

You are self-reliant, creative and persistent always.

You are energetic, enthusiastic and confident in all your ways.

You are well groomed, healthy and full of confidence.

Your always see only the good in others.

You hold a good attitude and you are well loved and respected.

Your high self-esteem enables you to respect others and receive it.

Your mind is full of good attitudes and positive helpful thoughts always.

June 21

1 Corinthians 7:17

Obey the Lord

Obeying the Lord at all times. In every church I tell the people to stay as they were when thy Lord Jesus chose them and God called them to be his own. Now I say the same thing to you. The important thing is to obey God's commands. You can win your freedom. When the Lord chooses they become free people.

The Sure Reality

This is the message sent down from the Lord of the worlds. Verily it is truth assured certainly. So glorify the name of your Lord most high.

We love meeting people and approach them with enthusiasm and confidence.

We live in the present and we are confident in the future.

Our attractive personality exudes a good attitude and confidence.

We are self-reliant, creative and persistent always.

We are energetic, enthusiastic and confident in all our ways.

We are well groomed, healthy and full of confidence.

We always see only the good in others.

We hold a good attitude and we are well loved and respected.

Our high self-esteem enables us to respect others and receive it.

Our mind is full of good attitudes and positive helpful thoughts always.

June 22

1 Corinthians 11:13

Rules of Worship

I am proud of you because you always remember me and obey the teachings I gave you. Now I want you to know that Christ is the head over all men. But God is the head over Christ. A woman should wear something on her head. Men were created to be like God and to bring honor to God. Women were created to bring honor to men.

The Cleaving Asunder

When the sky is cleft asunder when the stars are scattered when the oceans burst forth. Then shall each soul know what it hath sent forward and what it hath kept back. Him who created thee fashioned thee in due proportion and gave thee just bias.

I am grateful to be energetic, enthusiastic and confident all the time.

I am grateful to bring out the best in everyone.

I am grateful to be well groomed healthy and confident.

I am grateful to face others with confidence in myself and others.

I am grateful to be self-reliant, creative and attractively good.

I am grateful to encourage a good life by optimism.

I am grateful to see and attract only good positive results.

I am grateful to have a high self-esteem and attractive self-image.

June 23

13:31

Jesus and Herod

Jesus said to them go tell that I am going to heal people today and tomorrow and 3 days later. I am going on my way today and tomorrow and the next day. Blessed is the one who cares in the name of the Lord. When you are invited to be a guest go and sit in the place. Then the one who invited you will come and say my friend take a better seat.

The Heights

I am but a Warner and a bringer of glad tidings to those who have faith. It is he who created you from a single person and made his mate of like nature. In order that he might dwell with her in love. She bears a light burden and comes to it unnoticed. For my protector is Allah who revealed the book from time to time he will choose the righteous.

You are grateful to be energetic, enthusiastic and confident all the time.

You are grateful to bring out the best in everyone.

You are grateful to be well groomed, healthy and confident.

You are grateful to face others with confidence in yourself and others.

You are grateful to be self-reliant, creative and attractively good.

You are grateful to encourage a good life by optimism.

You are grateful to see and attract only good positive results.

You are grateful to have a high self-esteem and attractive self-image.

June 24

John 14:15

The Holy Spirit is Promised

Jesus said to his disciples. If you love me you will do as I command. Then I will ask the father to send you. The Holy Spirit who will help you always, be with you. The spirit what is true. But you know the spirit who is will show you what is true. But you know the spirit who is with you and will keep living with you. Because I live you will live then you will know that I am one with the father.

Those Range in Ranks

Sincere and devoted servants of Allah for them is a sustenance determined. Fruits and delights and they shall enjoy honor and dignity in gardens of felicity. Facing each other on thrones of dignity. Round will be passed to them a cup from a clear flowing fountain crystal white of a taste delicious to those who drink therefore.

We are grateful to be energetic, enthusiastic and confident all the time.

We are grateful to bring out the best in everyone.

We are grateful to be well groomed, healthy and confident.

We are grateful to face others with confidence in ourselves and others.

We are grateful to be self-reliant, creative and attractively good.

We are grateful to encourage a good life by optimism.

We are grateful to see and attract only good positive results.

We are grateful to have a high self-esteem and attractive self-image.

June 25

Psalm 63

God Is Powerful and Kind

God can save me and I calmly wait for him. God is the mighty rock that keeps me safe and the fortress where I am secure. God gives inward peace and I depend on him. God alone is the mighty rock that keeps me safe and he is the fortress where I feel secure. God saves me and honors me. He is that mighty rock where I find safety. Trust God, my friends and always tell him each of your concerns. God is our place of safety.

The Confederates

Verily Allah is full of knowledge and wisdom. But follow that which comes to thee by inspiration from thy Lord for Allah is well acquainted with all that ye do. And put thy trust in Allah and enough is Allah as a disposer of affairs.

I am a person of faith and focus on godly heavenly things always.

I firmly believe in the word of God.

I will remain strong in my faith.

Thought God I have strength, power and authority and everything this world contains.

I gird myself with a shield of faith.

I am grounded in my faith in God.

I please the Lord with my faith and divine lifestyle all the time.

My faith will guard, protect, sustain and deliver you.

My faith is like pure gold.

My body, mind and soul are faithful, loyal, true and peaceful.

June 26

John 12:23

The Son of Man Lifted Up

Jesus said the time came for the son of man to be given his glory. My servants will be with me where I am. If you serve me my father will honor you.

The Thunder

These are the signs or verse of the book that which have been revealed unto you from your Lord is the truth. Allah does know what every female womb does bear. Every single thing is before his sight in due proportion. He knows the unseen and that which is open he is the great the most high. It is the same to him whether any of you conceal his speech or declare it openly.

You are a person of faith and focus on godly heavenly things always.

You firmly believe in the word of God.

You will remain strong in your faith.

Thought God I have strength, power and authority and everything this world contains.

You gird yourself with a shield of faith.

You are grounded in my faith in God.

You please the Lord with your faith and divine lifestyle all the time.

Your faith will guard, protect, sustaining and deliver you.

Your faith is like pure gold.

Your body, mind and soul are faithful, loyal, true and peaceful.

June 27

2 Timothy 2:1

The Last Days

Good solider of Jesus Christ. Timothy my child Christ Jesus is kind and you must let him make you strong. You have often heard me teach. I want you to tell these same things to followers who can be trusted to tell others. As a good soldier of Christ Jesus you must endure. Soldiers on duty try to please their commanding officer. One wins an athletic contest with obeying rules. And farmers who work are the first to eat what grows in their field.

Ya Sin

Their hands will speak to us and their feet bear witness to all that they did. And if it had been our will we could have transformed them to remain in their places. A message and a Quran making things clear. That it may give admonition to any who are alike.

We are a person of faith and focus on godly heavenly things always.

We firmly believe in the word of God.

We will remain strong in our faith.

Thought God I have strength, power and authority and everything this world contains.

We gird ourself with a shield of faith.

We are grounded in our faith in God.

We please the Lord with our faith and divine lifestyle all the time.

Our faith will guard, protect, sustaining and deliver us.

Our faith is like pure gold.

Our body, mind and soul are faithful, loyal, true and peaceful.

June 28

Psalm 91

The Lord is My Fortress

Live under the protection of God most high God all powerful. You are my fortress my place of safety you are my God and I trust you. The Lord will keep you safe. He will spread his wings over you and keep you secure. His faithfulness is like a shield on a city wall.

Hud

He said o my people see you whether I have a clear sign from my Lord and he has given me sustenance pure and good as from himself. I only desire your betterment to the best of my power and my success in my task can only come from Allah. In him I trust and unto him I turn. These are some of the stories of communities which we related unto you. In that is a sign for that day for which mankind will be fathered together that will be a day of testimony.

I am grateful I am completely devoted to God.

I am grateful I have faith God speaks to me.

I am grateful to live a life of faith, hope and love.

I am grateful to be faithful and true to myself and all others.

I am grateful my faith guides my good living.

I am grateful for a faithful, pure soul of infinite powers, love, wisdom and faith.

I am grateful to serve God all the time.

I am grateful to believe in one God and master ruler of the universe.

I am grateful God delivers in every situation all the time.

I am grateful my strong faith makes me invincible, indestructible and eternally divine.

June 29

John 21:20

Jesus and His Favorite People

Peter says Jesus favorite disciple is following them. He was the same one who had sat next to Jesus at the meal. Jesus answered what is it to you if I want him to live until I return? You must follow me.

The Cave

Praise be to Allah who sent to his servant the book and faith He hath made it straight and clear in order that he may give glad tidings to the believers who work righteous deeds that they should have a goodly reward. Wherein they shall remain forever. We relate to them the story of truth they were youths who believed in their Lord and we advanced them in guidance. We gave strength to their hearts.

You are grateful you are completely devoted to God.

You are grateful you have faith God speaks to you.

You are grateful to live a life of faith, hope and love.

You are grateful to be faithful and true to yourself and all others.

You are grateful your faith guides your good living.

You are grateful for a faithful pure soul of infinite powers, love, wisdom and faith.

You are grateful to serve God all the time.

You are grateful to believe in one God and master ruler of the universe.

You are grateful God delivers in every situation all the time.

You are grateful your strong faith makes you invincible, indestructible and eternally divine.

June 30

Luke 3:10

The Preaching of John the Baptist

The crowds asked John what should we do? John told them if you have two coats give one to someone. If you have food share it with someone else. When tax collectors came to be baptized they asked John teacher what should we do? John told them don't make people pay more. Some soldiers asked him and what about us? Be satisfied with your pay.

Al-a-Al

Glorify the name of your guardian Lord most high who has created and further given order and proportion who has ordained laws and granted guidance. And who brings out the green and luscious pasture. By the degrees shall we teach you the message. For he knows what is manifest and what is hidden and we will make it easy for you to follow the simple path.

We are grateful we are completely devoted to God.

We are grateful we have faith God speaks to us.

We are grateful to live a life of faith, hope and love.

We are grateful to be faithful and true to ourselves and all others.

We are grateful our faith guides our good living.

We are grateful for a faithful pure soul of infinite powers, love, wisdom and faith.

We are grateful to serve God all the time.

We are grateful to believe in one God and master ruler of the universe.

We are grateful God delivers in every situation all the time.

We are grateful our strong faith makes me invincible, indestructible and eternally divine.

July 1

Revelation 16:5

Angel Empties a Bowl

Then I heard the angel who has power over water say you have always been and you will always will be the holy God. You had the right to judge in this way. I heard the altar shout. Yes Lord God all powerful your judgments are honest and fair. The fourth angel emptied his power on the sun.

The Prophets

Closer and closer to mankind comes their reckoning. Comes aught to them of a renewed message from their Lord but they listen to it. Is this one more than a man like yourselves. He is the one that heareth and knoweth all things.

I forgive and let go of the past and live only in the present.

I realize my parents gave their best and I forgive them and they forgive me.

I forgive myself and manage to live the best life.

It is easy for me to forgive others.

I follow a path of forgiveness and life has become a clean state.

I move beyond forgiveness to understanding, compassion and kindness to all.

I am forgiving, loving, gentle and kind always.

I forgive everyone from my life and love myself into the future.

I am ready and I am healed. I am willing to forgive all is well.

I return to the basics of life, forgiveness, courage, gratitude, love and humor.

July 2

John 8:11

The Truth Will Set You Free

Jesus told the people who had faith in him. If you keep on obeying what I said you truly are my disciples. You will know the truth and the truth will set you free. They answered we are Abraham's children! Jesus replied, the son will always remain in the family if the son gives you freedom you are free.

Repentance

Say spend for the cause willingly. Let their wealth and their following in sons dazzle you in reality Allah's plan.

You forgive and let go of the past and live only in the present.

You realize your parents gave their best and you forgive them and they forgive you.

You forgive yourself and manage to live the best life.

It is easy for you to forgive others.

You follow a path of forgiveness and life is a clean state.

You move beyond forgiveness to understanding, compassion and kindness to all.

You are forgiving, loving, gentle and kind always.

You forgive everyone from your life and love yourself into the future.

You are ready and you are healed.

You are willing to forgive all is well.

You return to the basics of life, forgiveness, courage, gratitude, love and humor.

July 3

Galatians 2:15

The Law and the Promise

My friends I will use an everyday example to explain what I mean. Once someone agrees to something one can change or cancel the agreement. That is how it is with the promises. God made to Abraham and his descendants.

The Ranks

And remember Jesus the son of Mary said o children of Israel. I am the messenger of Allah sent to you confirming the law which came before me and giving glad tidings of a messenger to come after me whose name shall be Ahmed. But when he came to them with clear signs.

We forgive and let go of the past and live only in the present.

We realize our parents gave their best and we forgive them and they forgive us.

We forgive ourselves and manage to live the best life.

It is easy for us to forgive others.

We follow a path of forgiveness and life has become a clean state.

We move beyond forgiveness to understanding, compassion and kindness to all.

We are forgiving, loving, gentle and kind always.

We forgive everyone from my life and love myself into the future.

We are ready and we are healed.

We are willing to forgive all is well.

We return to the basics of life, forgiveness, courage, gratitude, love and humor.

July 4

Psalm 69

God Can be Trusted

Save our God. Lord God all powerful ruler of Israel, it is for your sake atonement. I pray to you Lord. So when the time is right answer me and help me with your wonderful love. Answer me Lord. You are kind and good. You are truly merciful.

The Victory

Allah's good pleasure was on the believers when they swore fealty to you under the tree. He knew what was in their hearts and he sent down tranquility to them and he rewarded them with a speedy victory. And many gains will they acquire besides and Allah was exalted in power full of wisdom. Allah has promised you many gains that you shall acquire and he has given you these beforehand.

I am grateful to forgive everyone in my past and release them to love.

I am grateful to be healed with forgiveness and compassion.

I am grateful to forgive myself.

I am grateful I set my past free and forgive my participation.

I am grateful to trust my present and future decisions based on good intentions.

I am grateful I forgive others as I forgive myself.

I am grateful to forgive with ease, sincerity, and loving compassion.

I am grateful to achieve inner peace by forgiveness.

I am grateful to live in an ocean of love, kindness and forgiveness.

I am grateful to share the gift of forgiveness.

July 5

Revelation 1:17

A Vision of the Risen Lord

I am the first and the last and the living one. I am alive forever more and I have keys to the world. While what you have seen and what is and what will happen after these things. I will explain the mystery of the seven stars that you saw on my right side and the seven gold lamp stands. The seven stars are the angels of the seven churches and the lamp stands are the seven churches.

The Night Journey

Glory to him. He is high above all that they say and exalted and great beyond measure. The seven heavens and the earth and all beings therein declares his glory but celebrates his praise and yet ye understand.

You are grateful to forgive everyone in your past and release them to love.

You are grateful to be healed with forgiveness and compassion.

You are grateful to forgive yourself.

You are grateful you set your past free and forgive your participation.

You are grateful to trust your present and future decisions based on good intentions.

You are grateful you forgive others as you forgive yourself.

You are grateful to forgive with ease, sincerity, and loving compassion.

You are grateful to achieve inner peace by forgiveness.

You are grateful to live in an ocean of love, kindness and forgiveness.

You are grateful to share the gift of forgiveness.

July 6

Philippians 1:3

Paul's Prayer

I pray that God our father and the Lord of Jesus Christ will be kind to you and will bless you with peace. Everything I think of you. I thank God and whenever I mention you in my prayers it makes me happy. This is because you have taken part with me in spreading the good news from the first day you heard about it.

The Heifer

Their prophets said to them Allah has appointed Talut as king over you. Allah has chosen him above you and has gifted him abundance with knowledge and bodily prowess. Allah grants his authority to whom he pleases. Allah cares for all and he knows all things.

We are grateful to forgive everyone in our past and release them to love.

We are grateful to be healed with forgiveness and compassion.

We are grateful to forgive ourselves.

We are grateful we set our past free and forgive our participation.

We are grateful to trust our present and future decisions based on good intentions.

We are grateful we forgive others as we forgive ourselves.

We are grateful to forgive with ease, sincerity, and loving compassion.

We are grateful to achieve inner peace by forgiveness.

We are grateful to live in an ocean of love, kindness and forgiveness.

We are grateful to share the gift of forgiveness.

July 7

Psalm 20

A Prayer for Victory

I pray that the Lord will listen and the God of Jacob will keep you safe. May the Lord send help from his temple and come to rescue from mount Zion. Remember your gifts and be pleased with what you bring. May God do what you want most and let all go well for you. Then you will win victories and we will celebrate while raising our banners.

The Moon

The hour of judgment is nigh and the moon is cleft asunder. Then he called on his Lord, So we opened the gates of heaven with water pouring forth with springs so the waters met and rose to the extent decreed. We bore him on earth made from broad planks and caulked with palm fiber.

I am attracting a passionate romance.

My mind, body and soul are perfectly attuned to attracting a romantic relationship.

I radiate a loving energy that will draw romantic passionate beings.

My thoughts are effortlessly concentrated on romance and love.

I am full of romantic loving energy.

Passion, romance, love, good health and wealth are my future.

I naturally attract love and romance.

Others notice my passionate, romantic, loving energy.

I find it easy to manifest exciting romance.

I have the power to experience deeply moving and interesting romance always.

July 8

Psalm 107

The Lord is Good

The Lord is good to thy people. Shout praises to the Lord. He is good to us. Everyone the Lord has rescued should praise him everyone he has brought from the east and the west, the north and south. You prayed to the Lord and he rescued you. He brought you to a town. You should praise the Lord for his love and for the wonderful things he does for all of us. To everyone he gives something to drink and to everyone he gives good things to eat.

The Folding Up

When the sun with the spacious light is folded up. When the stars fall losing their luster. When the scrolls are laid open. When the sky is unveiled.

You are attracting a passionate romance.

Your mind, body and soul are perfectly attuned to attracting a romantic relationship.

You radiate a loving energy that will draw romantic passionate beings.

Your thoughts are effortlessly concentrated on romance and love.

You are full of romantic loving energy.

Passion, romance, love, good health and wealth are your future.

You naturally attract love and romance.

Others notice my passionate, romantic, loving energy.

You find it easy to manifest exciting romance.

You have the power to experience deeply moving and interesting romance always.

July 9

Acts 19:34

Great is Artemis

But when the crowd says that he was Jewish they all shouted for two hours. Great is Artemis the goddess of the Ephesians. Finally a town official made the crowd be quiet then he said people of Ephesus who in the world does know that our city is the center for worshiping the great goddess Artemis. Know her image which fell from heaven is right here.

Ta Ha

O my Lord. Expand me my breast ease my task for me. So I may understand what I say. And give me a minister from my family. Aaron my brother add to my strength through him. And make him share my task.

We are attracting a passionate romance.

Our mind, body and soul are perfectly attuned to attracting a romantic relationship.

We radiate a loving energy that will draw romantic passionate beings.

Our thoughts are effortlessly concentrated on romance and love.

We are full of romantic loving energy.

Passion, romance, love, good health and wealth are our future.

We naturally attract love and romance.

Others notice our passionate romantic loving energy.

We find it easy to manifest exciting romance.

We have the power to experience deeply moving and interesting romance always.

July 10

John 1:11

Love Each Other

From the beginning you were told that we must love each other. My friends our love for each other proves that we have life. We know what love is because Jesus gave his life for us. That's why we must give our lives for each other.

The Spider

Those who believe and work righteous deeds from them shall we reward them according to the best of their deeds. We have enjoined on man kindness to parents. You have all to return to me and I will tell you the truth of all that you did.

I am grateful to receive and send romantic love freely and joyfully.

I am grateful I find passionate exciting romantic love everywhere.

I am grateful to love the people who bring out the best in me.

I am grateful to be loving, loved and lovable.

I am grateful to attract an everlasting, kindled, romantic relationship.

I am grateful to be full of exciting passionate romantic sexy loving energy.

I am grateful to enjoy being loved, romanced and pleased all the time.

I am grateful to accept and give perfect divine love.

I am grateful exciting romance fills my life and I fill others' lives.

I am grateful I can romance, pleasure and love easily, joyfully and eternally.

July 11

1 Corinthians 1:18

Christ is God's Power and Wisdom

God was wise and decided to let the people of this world use their wisdom to learn about him.

The Heights

My Lord hath commanded justice and that ye set your whole selves to him at every time and place of prayer. Call upon him making your devotion sincere as in his sight such as he created you in the beginning so shall ye return. Some he hath guided. O children of Adam! Wear your beautiful apparel at every time and place of prayer eat and drink.

You are grateful to receive and send romantic love freely and joyfully.

You are grateful you find passionate exciting romantic love everywhere.

You are grateful to love the people who bring out the best in you.

You are grateful to be loving, loved and lovable.

You are grateful to attract an everlasting kindled romantic relationship.

You are grateful to be full of exciting passionate romantic sexy loving energy.

You are grateful to enjoy being loved, romanced and pleased all the time.

You are grateful to accept and give perfect divine love.

You are grateful exciting romance fills your life and you fill others lives.

You are grateful you can romance, pleasure and love easily, joyfully and eternally.

July 12

Matthew 13:10

Why Jesus Used Stories

Jesus answered I have explained the secrets about the kingdom of heaven to you. Everyone who has something will be given more. I use stories when I speak to them because Gods promise came true.

Ya Sin

They will be brought up before our judgment seat as a troop. Verily we know what they hide as well as what they disclose. Does man see that we created him from sperm? Yet behold he makes comparisons for us. He will give them life who created them for the first time.

We are grateful to receive and send romantic love freely and joyfully.

We are grateful we find passionate exciting romantic love everywhere.

We are grateful to love the people who bring out the best in us.

We are grateful to be loving, loved and lovable.

We are grateful to attract an everlasting kindled romantic relationship.

We are grateful to be full of exciting passionate romantic sexy loving energy.

We are grateful to enjoy being loved, romanced and pleased all the time.

We are grateful to accept and give perfect divine love.

We are grateful exciting romance fills my life and we fill others lives.

We are grateful we can romance, pleasure and love easily, joyfully and eternally.

July 13

Proverbs

The Lord is in Charge

The Lord controls rulers just as he determines the course of rivers. We may think we are doing the right thing but the Lord always knows what is in our hearts. Doing what is right and fair pleases the Lord more than an offering. If you plan and work hard you will have plenty. God is always fair. When justice is done, good citizens are glad. If you try to be kind and good you will be blessed with life and goodness and honor.

The Heifer

Allah grants his authority to whom he pleases. Allah cares for all and he knows all things. And further their prophet said to them a sign of his authority is that there shall come to you the Ark of the Covenant.

I am strong in all of life's circumstances.

I am bold, brave and strong.

I use my inner and outer strength in all situations.

I focus and maintain my extraordinary strength and beauty.

I practice using my inner and outer strength and flexibility always.

I am naturally strong, healthy and attractive.

I can protect myself and others with my strength and power.

I am a strong, independent individual.

I am flexible, energetic, courageous and strong.

I remain strong, physically, mentally, emotionally and spiritually.

July 14

Psalm 40

A Prayer for Help to Restore Health

You Lord God bless everyone who cares and you rescue those people. You protect them and keep them alive. You make them happy here in this land. You always heal them and restore their strength. I pray Lord heal me.

Friday

Whatever is in the heavens and on earth doth declare the praises and glory of Allah the sovereign the holy one the exalted in might, the wise. Such is the bounty of Allah which he bestows on whom he will and Allah is the Lord of the highest bounty. The similitude of those who were charged with obligations of the Mosaic Law. The blessing from the presence of Allah is better. And Allah is best to provide for all needs.

You are strong in all of life's circumstances.

You are bold, brave and strong.

You use your inner and outer strength in all situations.

You focus and maintain my extraordinary strength and beauty.

You practice using your inner and outer strength and flexibility always.

You are naturally strong, healthy and attractive.

You can protect yourself and others with your strength and power.

You are a strong, independent individual.

You are flexible, energetic, courageous and strong.

You remain strong, physically, mentally, emotionally and spiritually.

July 15

Matthew 13:24

Good Seed

Jesus then told this story the kingdom of heaven is like what happened when a farmer scattered good seed in a field. The plant came up and began to ripen good seed.

Folded in Garments

O you folded in garments and stand to prayer but not all night. Or a little more and recite the Quran in slow, measure and rhythmic tones. Soon shall we send down to you a weighted message. Truly the rising by night is most potent for governing the soul and most suitable for forming the word of prayer and praise. True there is for you by day prolonged occupation with ordinary duties. But keep in remembrance the name of your Lord and devote yourself to him whole heartedly.

We are strong in all of life's circumstances.

We are bold, brave and strong.

We use our inner and outer strength in all situations.

We focus and maintain our extraordinary strength and beauty.

We practice using our inner and outer strength and flexibility always.

We are naturally strong, healthy and attractive.

We can protect ourselves and others with our strength and power.

We are strong, independent individuals.

We are flexible, energetic, courageous and strong.

We remain strong, physically, mentally, emotionally and spiritually.

July 16

John 6:20

The Words of Eternal Life

See the son of man go up to heaven where he came from. The spirit is the one who gives life. The words I have spoken to you are from that life giving spirit. Jesus said this because from the beginning he knew he would have faith in him.

The Wise

These are verses of the wise book. A guide and mercy to the doers of good. Those who establish regular prayer and give regular charity and have in their hearts the assurance of the hereafter. These are on true guidance from their Lord and these are the ones who will prosper. There are among men those who work righteous deeds. There will be gardens of bliss to dwell therein. The promise of Allah is true and he is exalted in power, wise.

I am grateful my body, mind and soul are healthier and stronger every day.

I am grateful to be strong, confident and kind.

I am grateful to manifest perfect health, strength and beauty.

I am grateful to have inner and outer strength and power.

I am grateful to enjoy exercising and staying fit.

I am grateful to be whole, perfect, strong, powerful, loving and happy always.

I am grateful to practice on strength building and flexibility.

I am grateful to have super strength, power, endurance and stamina all the time.

I am grateful to get power from Gods divine source.

July 17

Mark 16:9

Jesus Appears to Mary Magdalene

Very early on the first day of the week after Jesus had risen, he appeared to Mary Magdalene. They heard that Jesus was alive and that Mary had seen him. Go and preach the good news to everyone in the world. Anyone who of them believes me and is baptized will be saved.

Al Inram

Of the good that they do for Allah knows well those that do right. Say Allah knows well all the secrets of the heart. Allah made it but a message of hope for you and an assurance to your hearts in any case there is help except from Allah the exalted the wise.

You are grateful your body, mind and soul are healthier and stronger every day.

You are grateful to be strong, confident and kind.

You are grateful to manifest perfect health, strength and beauty.

You are grateful to have inner and outer strength and power.

You are grateful to enjoy exercising and staying fit.

You are grateful to be whole, perfect, strong, powerful, loving and happy always.

You are grateful to practice on strength building and flexibility.

You are grateful to have super strength, power, endurance and stamina all the time.

You are grateful to get power from Gods divine source.

July 18

Psalm 78

What God Has Done for His People

My friends I beg you to listen as I teach. I will give instructions and explain the mystery of what happened long ago. God gave a command to the clouds and he opened the doors in the skies from heaven he sent grain that they called manna. He gave them more then enough.

The Table Spread

O people of the book you have ground to stand upon stand fast by the law, the gospel and all the revelations that has come to you from your Lord. It is the revelation that comes to you from your Lord. Turn they to Allah and seek his forgiveness. For Allah is oft forgiving most merciful. Christ is the son of Mary was an apostle. His mother was a woman of truth. They both eat their daily food.

We are grateful our body, mind and soul are healthier and stronger every day.

We are grateful to be strong, confident and kind.

We are grateful to manifest perfect health, strength and beauty.

We are grateful to have inner and outer strength and power.

We are grateful to enjoy exercising and staying fit.

We are grateful to be whole, perfect, strong, powerful, loving and happy always.

We are grateful to practice on strength building and flexibility.

We are grateful to have super strength, power, endurance and stamina all the time.

We are grateful to get power from Gods divine source.

July 19

John 8:31

The Truth Will Set You Free

Jesus told the people who had faith in him. If you keep on obeying what I have said you truly are my disciples. You will know the truth and the truth will set you free. They answered we are Abraham's children. The son gives you freedom you are free. I know you are born from Abraham's family.

Ibrahim

Our Lord! Truly you do know what we conceal and what we reveal. Praise be to Allah who has granted unto me in old age Ismail and Isaac for truly my Lord is he the hearer of prayer. O my Lord. Make me one who establishes regular prayer. O our Lord and accept you my prayer. O our Lord covers us with your forgiveness, me and my parents and all believers on the day that the reckoning will be established.

I trust the process of life.

I trust in the power of love to heal and guide me.

I am respected, trusted and professional.

I believe in the power of love to heal my body, mind and soul.

I am fearless, and trust it's all happening perfectly.

I trust myself and my intuitive insights.

All my relationships are filled with love, respect and trust.

I trust myself to deal in life with wisdom, grace and beauty.

I trust the universe to bring the right people and circumstances always.

I am blessed with security and trust everything will be okay.

July 20

Luke 4:31

A Man Cleansed

Jesus went to the town of Copperhaun in Galilee and taught the people on the Sabbath. His teaching amazed them because he spoke with power. You are God's holy one. Jesus ordered quiet. They were amazed.

The Cattle

Say be good to your parents. Provide sustenance for you and for them. Whether open or secret take not life which Allah hath made sacred.

You trust the process of life.

You trust in the power of love to heal and guide you.

You are respected, trusted and professional.

You believe in the power of love to heal your body, mind and soul.

You are fearless, and trust it's all happening perfectly.

You trust yourself and your intuitive insights.

All your relationships are filled with love, respect and trust.

You trust myself to deal with life with wisdom, grace and beauty.

You trust the universe to bring the right people and circumstances always.

You are blessed with security and trust everything will be okay.

July 21

Psalm 50

What Pleases God

From east to west powerful Lord God has been calling together everyone on earth. God shines brightly from Zion the most beautiful city. Our God approaches. God comes to judge his people. He shouts to the heavens and the earth call my followers together. We made an agreement. The heavens announce God is the judge and He is always honest. I am your God.

Al Imran

These are the signs of Allah. We rehearse them to you in truth. Allah belongs all that is in the heavens and on earth. To him do all questions go back for decision. You are the best of peoples evolved for mankind, enjoining what is right and believing in Allah. If only the people of the book had faith it were best for them.

We trust the process of life.

We trust in the power of love to heal and guide us.

We are respected, trusted and professional.

We believe in the power of love to heal our body, mind and soul.

We are fearless, and trust it's all happening perfectly.

We trust ourselves and our intuitive insights.

All our relationships are filled with love, respect and trust.

We trust ourselves to deal with life with wisdom, grace and beauty.

We trust the universe to bring the right people and circumstances always.

We are blessed with security and trust everything will be okay.

July 22

Psalm 112

Living by the Power of God's Spirit

The Holy Spirit will give you life that comes from Christ Jesus and will set you free. God set you free when he sent his own son to be like us. God used Christ's body. He did this so that we would do what the law commands by obeying the Spirit.

Joseph

So the king said bring him unto me I will take him specially to serve about my own person. Therefore when he had spoken to him he said be assured this day thou art before our own. Presence with rank firmly established and fidelity fully proved. Joseph said set me over the storehouses of the land and I will indeed guard them as one that knows their importance. Thus did we give established power to Joseph in the land to take possession therein as when or where he pleased. We bestow our mercy on whom we please and the reward of those who do good.

I am grateful to be trustworthy, honest and sincere.

I am grateful to be faithful, humble and loyal.

I am grateful I am always truthful to myself and others.

I am grateful to be good and faithful to my word.

I am grateful to be responsible and reliable always.

I am grateful to attract honest and loyal people.

I am grateful to conduct my life with integrity, humor and honesty.

I am grateful to be respected as faithful and reliable.

July 23

Romans 13:1

Obey Rulers

Obey the rulers who have authority over you. Only God can give authority to anyone and he puts these rulers in their places of power. There is need of the authorities just do right and they will praise you for it. After all they are God's servants and it is their duty to help you.

The Ways of Ascent

The angels and the spirit ascend unto him in a day the measure whereof is as 50 000 years. Hold patience a patience of beautiful contentment. They see the day indeed as far off event. It quite near. The day that the sky will be like molten brass and the mountains will be like wool.

You are grateful to be trustworthy, honest and sincere.

You are grateful to be faithful, humble and loyal.

You are grateful you are always truthful to yourself and others.

You are grateful to be good and faithful to your word.

You are grateful to be responsible and reliable always.

You are grateful to attract honest and loyal people.

You are grateful to conduct your life with integrity, humor and honesty.

You are grateful to be respected as faithful and reliable.

July 24

Mark 6:49

Jesus Walks

When the disciples saw Jesus walking on the water they thought he was a ghost. I am Jesus. He then got in the boat with them and the wind died down. Jesus and his disciples crossed the lake and brought the boat to shore near the town of Gennesaret. As soon as they got out of the boat the people recognized Jesus in every village or farm or marketplace. Where Jesus went everyone was healed.

The Ants

These are verses of the Quran a book that makes things clear. A guide and glad tidings for the believers. Those who establish regular prayers and give in regular charity and also have full assurance of the hereafter.

We are grateful to be trustworthy, honest and sincere.

We are grateful to be faithful, humble and loyal.

We are grateful we are always truthful to ourselves and others.

We are grateful to be good and faithful to our word.

We are grateful to be responsible and reliable always.

We are grateful to attract honest and loyal people.

We are grateful to conduct our life with integrity, humor and honesty.

We are grateful to be respected as faithful and reliable.

July 25

Matthew 1:18

The Birth of Jesus

This is how Jesus Christ was born. A young woman named Mary was engaged to Joseph from King David's family. But before they were married she learned that she was going to have a baby by God's Holy Spirit. Joseph was a good man. The angel said Joseph the baby that Mary will have is from the Holy Spirit. Then after her baby is born name him Jesus.

Qaf

And we send down from the sky rain charted with blessing and we produced therewith gardens and grains for harvests and fall and stately palm trees with sheets of fruit stalks piled one over another. As sustenance for Allah's servants and we give new life therewith to land.

I am a success magnet and I attract success in everything I do.

I always spot opportunities and utilize them to find and meet success.

The power of success is within me. I learn from the past and plan for the future.

I focus on success, right thinking and hard work and excel at all of these.

I embrace only positive thoughts and success is ongoing.

I have action plus vision equals success.

I am inspired, enthusiastic and success bound.

I deserve to be successful with a good fortune and good life.

Success is my birthright and I have achieved it.

I am successful in everything I do with everyone.

July 26

Psalm 7

The Lord Always Does Right

You Lord God are my protector. Keep me safe. I am innocent Lord God. See that justice is done. Make the nations come to you as you sit on your throne above them all. Our Lord judges the nations. Judge me and show that I am honest and innocent. You know every heart and mind and you always do right. You God are my shield the protector of everyone whose heart is right.

The Believers

Then the blast overtook them with justice. Then we raised after them other generations. Then sent we our messengers in succession. And we made the son of Mary and his mother as a sign. We gave them both shelter on high ground affording rest and security furnished with springs.

You are a success magnet and you attract success in everything you do.

You always spot opportunities and utilize them to find and meet success.

The power of success is within you. You learn from the past and plan for the future.

You focus on success, right thinking and hard work and excel at all of these.

You embrace only positive thoughts and successes ongoing.

You have action plus vision equals success.

You are inspired, enthusiastic and success bound.

You deserve to be successful with a good fortune and good life.

Success is your birthright and you have achieved it.

July 27

Psalm 72

A Prayer for God to Guide and Help the King

Please help the king to be honest and fair just like you our God let him be honest and fair. Let peace and justice rule every mountain and hill. Let the king defend and rescue. Let the king live forever like the sun and the moon. Let the king be fair with everyone and let there be peace until the moon falls from the sky. Let his kingdom reach from sea to sea. Long live the king! The heavens and the earth and made the light.

The Cattle

Praise to be Allah who created the heavens and the earth and made the light. I tell you that with me are the treasures of Allah, do I know what is hidden, do I tell you that I am an angel. I follow what is revealed to me.

We are a success magnet and we attract success in everything we do.

We always spot opportunities and utilize them to find and meet success.

The power of success is within us. We learn from the past and plan for the future.

We focus on success, right thinking and hard work and excel at all of these.

We embrace only positive thoughts and success is ongoing.

We have action plus vision equals success.

We are inspired, enthusiastic and success bound.

We deserve to be successful with a good fortune and good life.

Success is our birthright and we have achieved it.

We are successful in everything we do with everyone.

July 28

2 Timothy 3

Listen to Good

The time is coming when people listen to good teachers. You must stay calm. You must work to tell the good news to do your job well. I encourage Gods own people to understand the truth about religion. Then they will have the hope of eternal life that God promised long ago. At the proper time God our savior gave this message and told me to announce what he said.

The Family of Imran

O ye who believe. Hold fast altogether by the rope which Allah stretches out to you and be not divided among yourselves and remember with gratitude Allah's favor on you. He saved you. Thus doth Allah make his signs clear to you that ye maybe guided. For Allah has power over all things.

I am grateful to succeed at everything always.

I am grateful to attract success in all areas of my life.

I am grateful I am motivated and action oriented to succeed.

I am grateful to be highly focused on success.

I am grateful to only think positively and am a success magnet.

I am grateful success is easy and natural for me.

I am grateful success, achievement and abundance flow in my life.

I am grateful to believe in myself and strive for success.

I am grateful to use the law of attraction to manifest success.

I am grateful and thankful for all my ongoing successes.

July 29

Psalm 92

Sing Praises to the Lord

It is wonderful to be grateful and to sing your praises Lord most high! It is wonderful every morning to tell about your love and at night to announce how faithful you are. I enjoy praising your name to the music of harps, because everything you do makes me happy and I sing joyful songs. You do great things Lord. Your thoughts are too deep. You will rule forever. Good people will prosper like palm trees and they will grow strong like the cedars of Lebanon.

The Spider

Travel through the earth and see how Allah did originate creation so will Allah produce a later creation for Allah has power over all things. He pleases and he grants mercy to whom he pleases. The meeting with him in the hereafter.

You are grateful to succeed at everything always.

You are grateful to attract success in all areas of your life.

You are grateful you are motivated and action oriented to succeed.

You are grateful to be highly focused on success.

You are grateful to only think positively and are a success magnet.

You are grateful success is easy and natural for you.

You are grateful success, achievement and abundance flow in your life.

You are grateful to believe in myself and strive for success.

You are grateful to use the law of attraction to manifest success.

You are grateful and thankful for all your ongoing successes.

July 30

Acts 20:22

Paul Says Goodbye

I must obey God's spirit. As long as I finish the work that the Lord Jesus gave me to do. And that work is to tell the good news about God's great kindness. I have told you everything God wants you to know. Look after yourselves and everyone that Holy Spirit has placed in your care. Be like a shepherd to God's church. Be on your guard. I now place you in Gods care.

Pilgrimage

Then let them complete the rites prescribed for them perform their vows and again circumnavigate the ancient house. Such is pilgrimage whoever honors the sacred rites of Allah for him it is in the sight of his Lord lawful to you for food in pilgrimage are cattle.

We are grateful to succeed at everything always.

We are grateful to attract success in all areas of our life.

We are grateful we are motivated and action oriented to succeed.

We are grateful to be highly focused on success.

We are grateful to only think positively and are a success magnet.

We are grateful success is easy and natural for us.

We are grateful success, achievement and abundance flow in our life.

We are grateful to believe in ourselves and strive for success.

We are grateful to use the law of attraction to manifest success.

We are grateful and thankful for all our ongoing successes.

July 31

Hebrews 8

A Better Promise

God's promise which came better than the law, appoints his son. And he is the perfect high priest forever. We have a high priest who sits at the right side of God's great throne in heaven. He also serves as the priest in the most holy place inside the real tent there in heaven. This tent of worship was set up by the Lord. I tell the people of Israel this is my new agreement. The time will come when I the Lord will write my laws on their minds and hearts.

The Cattle

If it were Allah's will he could gather them together unto true guidance. Those who listen to the truth be sure will accept so Allah will raise them up then will they be turned unto him.

I am with God and God is with me always.

The divine spirit is omnipresent all around me.

God's love is working through me now and forever.

All my thoughts, words, and actions are divinely guided.

I am a spiritual being and everything is happening for my highest good.

I patiently and respectfully ask for divine guidance.

The universe naturally and respectfully provides for all my needs.

My mind and body and soul are completely aligned with the universe.

I am responsible for my own spiritual growth and development.

I trust everything is working for my highest good all the time.

August 1

Psalm 33

Sing Praises to the Lord

The Lord is truthful he can be trusted. He loves justice and fairness and he is kind to everyone everywhere on earth. The Lord made the heavens and everything in them by his word. As soon as he spoke the world was created at his command, the earth was formed. What the Lord has planned will stand forever. His thoughts never change. Make our hearts glad because we trust you.

The Elephant

Do you see how your Lord dealt with the people of the elephant. For the covenants of security and safeguard enjoyed by the quaraut. Their covenants covering safe journeys by winter and summer. Let them adore the Lord of the house.

You are with God and God is with you always.

The divine spirit is omnipresent all around you.

God's love is working through you now and forever.

All your thoughts, words, and actions are divinely guided.

You are a spiritual being and everything is happening for your highest good.

You patiently and respectfully ask for divine guidance.

The universe naturally and respectfully provides for all your needs.

Your mind and body and soul are completely aligned with the universe.

You are responsible for your own spiritual growth and development.

You trust everything is working for your highest good all the time.

August 2

Psalm 40

A Prayer for Help

I patiently waited Lord for you to hear my prayer. You listened. You let me stand on my feet firm you gave me a new song. A song of praise to you. Many will see this and they will honor and trust you the Lord. God you bless all of those who trust you Lord.

The Spider

Only know do men think that they will be left saying we believe. We did test those before them and Allah will certainly know who are true. We have enjoined on man kindness to parents.

We are with God and God is with us always.

The divine spirit is omnipresent all around us.

God's love is working through us now and forever.

All our thoughts, words, and actions are divinely guided.

We are spiritual beings and everything is happening for our highest good.

We patiently and respectfully ask for divine guidance.

The universe naturally and respectfully provides for all our needs.

My mind and body and soul are completely aligned with the universe.

We are responsible for our own spiritual growth and development.

We trust everything is working for our highest good all the time.

August 3

Mark 12:29

The Most Important Commandment

You must love him with all your heart, soul, mind and strength. The second most important commandment says love others as much as you love yourself. The man replied teacher you are certainly right to say there is only one God.

Ar Rahman

It is he who has taught me the Quran he has created me. He has taught him speech and intelligence. The sun and moon follow courses exactly computed. And the herbs and the trees both alike bow in adoration. And the firmament has he raised high and he set up the balance of justice. So establish weight with justice and in the balance it is he who has spread out the earth for his creatures.

I am grateful to trust everything is working for my highest good all the time.

I am grateful to love others and receive love.

I am grateful to be a divine expression of a loving God.

I am grateful I live in love with God.

I am grateful to be a loving, kind, and forgiving person.

I am grateful the love of God flows through me and works through me.

I am grateful to surrender to Gods will and his all-knowing plan.

I am grateful God is good.

I am grateful all my thoughts, words and actions are good and divinely guided by the heavenly realms.

I am grateful the Lords favor is upon me always and has blessed me.

August 4

Mark 10:14

What Jesus Should Do

Go and preach the good news to everyone in the world. Anyone who believes me and is baptized will be saved. Everyone who believes me will be able to do wonderful things. By using my name they will speak new languages. They will also heal people by placing their hands on them.

The Bee

Verily in this are signs for men who are wise. And the things on this earth which he has multiplied in varying colors and qualities. Verily in this is a sign for men who celebrate the praises of Allah in gratitude. It is he who made the sea subject and marks and sign posts and by the stars men guide themselves.

You are grateful to trust everything is working for your highest good all the time.

You are grateful to love others and receive love.

You are grateful to be a divine expression of a loving God.

You are grateful you live in love with God.

You are grateful to be a loving, kind, and forgiving person.

You are grateful the love of God flows through you and works through you.

You are grateful to surrender to Gods will and his all-knowing plan.

You are grateful God is good.

You are grateful all your thoughts, words and actions are good and divinely guided by the heavenly realms.

You are grateful the Lords favor is upon you always and has blessed you.

August 5

Proverbs 7:1

Pay Attention

My son pay close attention what I tell you to do. Obey me. Let my instructions be your greatest treasure. Keep them at your fingertips and write them in your mind. Let wisdom be your sister and make common sense your closest friend.

Al Rathiyah

The revelation of the book is from Allah the exalted in power full of wisdom. Verily in the heavens and the earth are signs for these who believe. And in the creation the fact that animals are scattered through the earth are signs for those of assured faith. And in the alternation of night and day and the fact that Allah sends down sustenance from the sky revives the earth.

We are grateful to trust everything is working for our highest good all the time.

We are grateful to love others and receive love.

We are grateful to be a divine expression of a loving God.

We are grateful we live in love with God.

We are grateful to be a loving, kind, and forgiving person.

We are grateful the love of God flows through us and works through us.

We are grateful to surrender to Gods will and his all-knowing plan.

We are grateful God is good.

We are grateful all our thoughts, words and actions are good and divinely guided by the heavenly realms.

We are grateful the Lords favor is upon us always and has blessed us.

August 6

Luke 2

Parents are Amazed

Three days later they found Jesus sitting in the temple, listening to the teachers and asking them questions. Everyone who hears him was surprised at how much he knew and at the answers he gave. When his parents found him they were amazed his mother said son why have you done this to us? Your father and I have been searching for you.

Qaf

A voice will say this is what was promised for you for everyone who turned to Allah in sincere repentance who kept his law. Allah most gracious unseen and brought a heart turned in devotion to him. Enter you therein in peace and security and this is a day of eternal life. There will be for them therein all that they wish and more besides in our presence.

I maintain positive changes in all areas of my life.

I have unlimited potential and only good lies before me and after me.

I have the power to improve myself.

I am confident and happy with myself.

I believe in myself.

I have a desire to be loved, loving, healthy, happy, rich, and successful.

It is easy for me to make lasting positive changes.

I am enthusiastic, energetic and strong and healthy always.

I set and achieve all my goals easily and effortlessly.

I choose to be a go getter and a go giver and the more I give the more I get.

August 7

John 4:21

Know God

Jesus said to her believe me the time is coming when you want to worship the father either on this mountain or in Jerusalem. The Jews do know God. Even now the true worshipers are being led by the spirit to worship the father according to the truth. These are the ones the father is seeking to worship him. God is spirit and those who worship God is spirit.

The Table Spread

Both Jews and the Christians say we are sons of Allah and his beloved. He forgives whom he pleaseth and to Allah belongeth the dominion of the heavens and the earth and all that is between unto him is the final goal of all. O people of the book. Now hath come to you making things clear unto you our messenger.

You maintain positive changes in all areas of your life.

You have unlimited potential and only good lies before and after you.

You have the power to improve yourself.

You are confident and happy with yourself.

You believe in yourself.

You have a desire to be loved, loving , healthy, happy, rich, and successful.

It is easy for you to make lasting positive changes.

You are enthusiastic, energetic and strong and healthy always.

You set and achieve all your goals easily and effortlessly.

You choose to be a go getter and a go giver and the more you give the more you get.

August 8

Psalm 110

The Lord Gives Victory

The Lord said to my Lord sit at my right side. The Lord will let your power react out from Zion and you will rule. Your glorious power will be soon on the day you begin to rule. You will wear the sacred robes and shine like the morning sun in all your strength. The Lord has made a promise. The Lord is at your right side.

The Victory

Allah's good pleasure was on the believers when they swore fealty to you under the tree. He knows what was in their hearts and he sent down tranquility to them and he rewarded them with a speedy victory. And many gains will they acquire besides and Allah is exalted in power full of wisdom Allah has promised you many gains that you shall acquire and he has given you these beforehand.

We maintain positive changes in all areas of our life.

We have unlimited potential and only good lies before and after us.

We have the power to improve ourselves.

We are confident and happy with ourselves.

We believe in ourselves.

We have a desire to be loved, loving, healthy, happy, rich, and successful.

It is easy for us to make lasting positive changes.

We are enthusiastic, energetic and strong and healthy always.

We set and achieve all our goals easily and effortlessly.

We choose to be a go getter and a go giver and the more we give the more we get.

August 9

1 Corinthians 1:11

Taking Sides

My dear friends as a follower of Lord Jesus Christ. I beg you to get along with each other. Don't take sides. They said that some of you claim to follow me while others claim to follow Apollos or Peter or Christ. I thank God. I did baptize the family of Stephanas. Christ did not send me to baptize. He sent me to tell the good news.

Ibrahim

O our Lord. I have made some of my offspring to dwell in a valley with cultivation by thy sacred house. O our Lord cover us with thy forgiveness, me, my parents and all believers on the day that the reckoning will be established in Allah's name.

I am grateful financial success comes to me easily.

I am grateful abundance is my true state of being.

I am grateful to be a competent, capable and deserving individual.

I am grateful to think positively and take responsibility.

I am grateful to be motivated, optimistic and solution oriented.

I am grateful to be assertive and in control of myself.

I am grateful to be a winner and attract successful winners.

I am grateful to be beautiful inside and out and am attractive, sexy, funny and irresistible to all.

I am grateful others recognize me because of my beauty, wisdom and good heart.

I am grateful to keep my smile, very pretty and attractive.

August 10

Psalm 9

Sing Praises to the Lord

I will praise you Lord with all my heart and tell about the wonders you have worked. God most high I will rejoice I will celebrate and sing because of you. You take your seat as judge and your fair decisions prove that I was in the right.

Yusuf

Ask at the town where we have been and the caravan in which we returned and you will find we are indeed telling the truth. Jacob said no but you have yourselves contrived a story good enough for you. So patience is most fitting for me. May be Allah will bring them back all to me in the end. For he is indeed full of knowledge and wisdom.

You are grateful financial success comes to you easily.

You are grateful abundance is your true state of being.

You are grateful to be a competent, capable and deserving individual.

You are grateful to think positively and take responsibility.

You are grateful to be motivated, optimistic and solution oriented.

You are grateful to be assertive and in control of yourself.

You are grateful to be a winner and attract successful winners.

You are grateful to be beautiful inside and out and are attractive, sexy, funny and irresistible to all.

You are grateful others recognize you because of your beauty, wisdom and good heart.

You are grateful to keep your smile, very pretty and attractive.

August 11

Proverbs 8

Wisdom Speaks

I am wisdom common sense is my closest friend. I possess knowledge and sound judgment. Every honest leader rules with help from me. I love everyone how loves me and I will be found by all how honestly search. What you receive from me is more valuable than even the finest gold or the purest silver.

The Examined One

It may be that Allah will grant love and friendship between you and those. And Allah is oft forgiving most merciful. Those dealing kindly and justly with them for Allah loveth those who are just.

We are grateful financial success comes to us easily.

We are grateful abundance is our true state of being.

We are grateful to be a competent, capable and deserving individual.

We are grateful to think positively and take responsibility.

We are grateful to be motivated, optimistic and solution oriented.

We are grateful to be assertive and in control of ourselves.

We are grateful to be a winner and attract successful winners.

We are grateful to be beautiful inside and out and be attractive, sexy, funny and irresistible to all.

We are grateful others recognize us because of our beauty, wisdom and good heart.

We are grateful to keep our smile, very pretty and attractive.

August 12

Matthew 2:39

The Most Important Commandment

One of them was an expert in the Jewish law so he tried to test Jesus by asking teacher what is the most important commandment in the law. Jesus answered love the Lord your God with all your heart, soul and mind. This is the first most important commandment. The second most important commandment is like this one. And love others as much as you love yourself. All the Law of Moses and the book of the prophets are based on these two commandments.

The Repentance

Say my Lord knoweth every word spoken in the heavens and on earth. He is the one that heareth and knoweth all things. In the end we fulfilled to them our promise and we saved them and those whom we pleased.

I am content and safe during all my travels and so are my loved ones.

Me and my loved ones safety comes first.

God has given me guardian angels to protect me.

We are divinely protected by God himself at all times.

My mature and responsible actions and reactions keep me safe at all times.

My living environment is safe, secure and divinely protected always.

I am confident my environment is safe and divinely guarded.

My security is guarded by guardian angels always.

I am grounded, safe and secure always.

Earth is a safe place to live and our safety is assured.

August 13

Psalm 116

When the Lord Saves You

I love you Lord, you answered my prayers. You paid attention to me and so I will pray to you as long as I live. You are kind Lord so good and merciful. You protect ordinary people and you saved me and treated me so kindly. You Lord saved my life.

The Thunder

These are the signs or verses of the book and that which have been revealed unto you from your Lord is the truth. Allah is he who raised the heavens without any pillars that you can see, is firmly established on the throne of authority. He has subjected the sun and the moon to his law. Each one runs its course for a term appointed. He does regulate all affairs.

You're content and safe during all your travels and so are your loved ones.

You and your loved ones safety comes first.

God has given you guardian angels to protect you.

You are divinely protected by God himself at all times.

Your mature and responsible actions and reactions keep you safe at all times.

Your living environment is safe, secure and divinely protected always.

You are confident your environment is safe and divinely guarded.

Your security is guarded by guardian angels always.

You are grounded, safe and secure always.

Earth is a safe place to live and your safety is assured.

August 14

Psalm 78

What God has Done for His People

My friends I beg you to listen as I teach. I will give you instructions and explain the mystery of what happened long ago. These are things we learned from our ancestors. God gave his law to Jacob's descendants the people of Israel. And he told our ancestors to teach their children so that each new generation would know his law and tell it. They would trust God and obey his teachings.

Hud

They will dwell therein for all the time that the heavens and the earth endure except as thy Lord willeth for thy Lord is the sure accomplisher of what he planneth. And those who are blessed shall be in the garden and they will dwell therein for all the time that the heavens and the earth endure except as thy Lord willeth.

We are content and safe during all our travels and so are our loved ones.

Us and our loved ones safety comes first.

God has given us guardian angels to protect us.

We are divinely protected by God himself at all times.

Our mature and responsible actions and reactions keep us safe at all times.

Our living environment is safe, secure and divinely protected always.

We are confident our environment is safe and divinely guarded.

Our security is guarded by guardian angels always.

We are grounded, safe and secure always.

Earth is a safe place to live and our safety is assured.

August 15

Psalm 90

God is Eternal

Our Lord in all generations you have been our home. You have always been God long before the birth of the mountains even before you created the earth and the world. To use wisely all the time we have. Help us Lord. When morning comes let your love satisfy all our needs.

The City

I do call to witness this city and you are free inhabitations of this city and of the ties of parent and child. Then will he be of those who believe and enjoin patience, constance and self-restraint and enjoin deeds of kindness and compassion. Such are the companions of the right hand.

I am grateful my family, loved ones and God and I are always safe and secure.

I am grateful I am grounded, safe and secure.

I am grateful I am safe and protected always.

I am grateful God keeps me well protected and I feel safe always.

I am grateful me and my loved ones travel safely.

I am grateful to be in a safe environment all the time.

I am grateful to be free protected in all ways always.

I am grateful earth is a safe place to live.

I am grateful it's safe for me to openly express all my brilliant ideas.

I am grateful guardian angels protect and guard me always.

August 16

Psalm 40

A Prayer for Help

You let me stand on a rock with my feet firm and you gave me a new song, a song of praise to you. Many will see this and they will honor and trust the Lord God. You bless all those who trust you, you Lord God have done many wonderful things and you have planned marvelous things for us. No one is like you.

The Repentance

Perhaps Allah will turn unto them in mercy for Allah is oft forgiving most merciful. Of their goods take away that so thou might purify, sanctify them and pray on their behalf. Verily thy process are a source of security for them. Allah is one who heareth and knoweth. Know they that Allah doth accept repentance from his and receives their gifts of charity.

You are grateful your family, loved ones and God and you are always safe and secure.

You are grateful you are grounded, safe and secure.

You are grateful you are safe and protected always.

You are grateful God keeps you well protected and you feel safe always.

You are grateful you and your loved ones travel safely.

You are grateful to be in a safe environment all the time.

You are grateful to be free protected in all ways always.

You are grateful earth is a safe place to live.

You are grateful it's safe for you to openly express all your brilliant ideas.

You are grateful guardian angels protect and guard you always.

August 17

Psalm 141

A Prayer for the Lord's Protection

I pray to you Lord. Please listen when I pray and hurry to help me. Think of my prayer as sweet smelling incense and think of my hands as an evening sacrifice. Help me to guard my words whenever I say something. Everyone will admit that I was right. You are my Lord and God. I look to you for safety.

The Women to be Examined

O you who believe. Simply because you believe in Allah your Lord. There was indeed in them an excellent example for you to follow and for those whose hope is in Allah and in the last day, truly Allah is free of all wants worthy of all praise.

We are grateful our family, loved ones and God and us are always safe and secure.

We are grateful we are grounded, safe and secure.

We are grateful we are safe and protected always.

We are grateful God keeps us well protected and we feel safe always.

We are grateful us and our loved ones travel safely.

We are grateful to be in a safe environment all the time.

We are grateful to be free protected in all ways always.

We are grateful earth is a safe place to live.

We are grateful it's safe for us to openly express all our brilliant ideas.

We are grateful guardian angels protect and guard us always.

August 18

Luke 22:39

Jesus Prays

Jesus went out to the Mount of Olives as he often did as his disciples went with him. When they got there he told them pray that you won't be tested. Jesus walked on a little way before he knelt down and prayed father if you will please don't make me drink from this cup. Then an angel from heaven came to help him. Jesus prayed sincerely.

The Cattle

Be good to your parents. We provide sustenance for you and for them. Take not life which Allah has made sacred except by way of justice and law thus doth he command you that ye may learn wisdom.

Building a healthy relationship is worthy of all effort, love and care.

Listening and expressing feelings is important to me.

I have many healthy, loving and respectful relationships in my life.

Honest and open communication is my natural strength.

All my relationships are improving everyday as we get closer.

I will act with respect, love and care in all my relationships always.

I put in time, care and attention to make my relationships happy.

I am constantly growing in love with my partner every day.

Me and my partner can communicate and respond positively to each other's needs and wants.

August 19

Mark 2:18

People Ask About Eating

The followers of John the Baptist and the Pharisees often went without eating. Some people came and asked Jesus why the followers of John and those of the Pharisees often go without eating while your disciples never do. Jesus answered the friends of a bridegroom don't go without eating while he is still with them.

The Roman Empire

Within a few years with Allah is the command in the past and in the future on that day shall the believers rejoice. With the help of Allah. Never does Allah depart from his promise. They know but the outer things in the life of this world. It is Allah who begins the process of creation then repeats it then shall you be brought back to him.

Building a healthy relationship is worthy of all effort, love and care.

Listening and expressing feelings is important to you.

I have many healthy, loving and respectful relationships.

Honest and open communication is your natural strength.

All your relationships are improving everyday as you get closer.

You will act with respect, love and care in your relationships always.

You put in time, care and attention to make your relationships happy.

You are constantly growing in love with your partner every day.

You are your partner can communicate and respond positively to each other's needs and wants.

August 20

Psalm 17

The Prayer of an Innocent Person

I am innocent Lord and you listen as I pray and beg for help. I am honest. Only you can say that I am innocent because only eyes can see the truth. You know my heart and even during the night you have tested me and found me innocent. I have made up my mind.

The Night Journey

Establish regular prayers. And pray in the small watches of the morning it would be an additional prayer or spiritual profit for thee soon will thy Lord raise thee to a station of praise and glory. O my Lord. Let my entry be by the gate of truth and honor and likewise my exit by the gate of truth and honor and grant me from thy presence an authority to aid me.

Building a healthy relationship is worthy of all effort, love and care.

Listening and expressing feelings is important to us.

We have many healthy, loving and respectful relationships.

Honest and open communication is our natural strength.

All our relationships are improving everyday as we get closer.

We will act with respect, love and care in all our relationships always.

We put in time, care and attention to make our relationships happy.

We are constantly growing in love with our partner every day.

Us and our partner can communicate and respond positively to each other's needs and wants.

August 21

Psalm 65

God Answers Prayers

Our God you deserve praise in Zion where we keep our promises to you. Everyone will come to you because you answer prayer. You forgave us. You bless your chosen ones and you invite them to live near you in your temple. We will enjoy your house the sacred temple. Our God you save us our prayers for justice.

The Great

Verily the day of sorting out is a thing appointed. The day that the trumpet shall be sounded and you will come forth in crowds. And the heavens shall be opened as if there were doors.

I am grateful me and my partner respect and love.

I am grateful I can communicate my wants and needs clearly and easily.

I am grateful to take into consideration the perspective of my loved ones easily and always.

I am grateful to develop healthy, mutually satisfying and fun loving relationships.

I am grateful to feel more in love in my relationships.

I am grateful to be able to communicate clearly and effectively in all my relationships always.

I am grateful I can listen and express myself easily.

I am grateful to build mutually beneficial and healthy relationships easily and quickly.

I am grateful all my relationships foster respect, love and patience.

August 22

John 3:27

Jesus is Important

At a wedding the groom is the one who gets married. The best man is glad just to be there and to hear the groom. That's why I am glad. Jesus must become more important. God's son comes from heaven and is above all others. Everyone who comes from the earth belongs to the Earth and speaks about earthly things. The one who comes from heaven is above all others.

The Narration

That name of the hereafter we shall give to those who intend high handedness on earth and the end is best for the righteous. If any does good the reward to him is better than his deed.

You are grateful you and your partner respect and love.

You are grateful you can communicate your wants and needs clearly and easily.

You are grateful to take into consideration the perspective of your loved ones easily and always.

You are grateful to develop healthy, mutually satisfying and fun loving relationships.

You are grateful to feel more in love in your relationships.

You are grateful to be able to communicate clearly and effectively in all your relationships always.

You are grateful you can listen and express yourself easily.

You are grateful to build mutually beneficial and healthy relationships easily and quickly.

You are grateful all your relationships foster respect, love and patience.

August 23

Psalm 56

A Prayer of Trust in God

God most high I keep on trusting you. I praise your promises. I trust you. Good people will be glad when they see they get what they deserve and they will wash their feet. Everyone will say it's true. Good people are rewarded. God does indeed rule the earth with justice. Save me God. Protect me. Keep me safe.

The Crowds

On the Day of Judgment the whole of the earth will be but his handful and the heavens will be rolled up in his right hand. Glory to him. High is he. The trumpet will just be sounded when behold they will be standing and looking on. And the earth will shine with the glory of its Lord the record of deeds will be placed open.

We are grateful us and our partner respect and love.

We are grateful we can communicate our wants and needs clearly and easily.

We are grateful to take into consideration the perspective of our loved ones easily and always.

We are grateful to develop healthy, mutually satisfying and fun loving relationships.

We are grateful to feel more in love in our relationships.

We are grateful to be able to communicate clearly and effectively in all our relationships always.

We are grateful we can listen and express ourselves easily.

We are grateful to build mutually beneficial and healthy relationships easily and quickly.

We are grateful all our' relationships foster respect, love and patience.

August 24

Mark 16

Jesus is Alive

But when they looked they saw that the stone had already been rolled away and it was a huge stone. The woman went into the tomb on the right side they saw a young man in a white robe sitting there.

The Inevitable

Many will it bring law many will it exalt and when the earth shall be shaken to its depths and the mountains shall be crumbled to atoms, becoming dust scattered abroad and he shall be sorted out into three classes. Then there will be companions of the right hand and the companions of the left hand. And those foremost in faith will be foremost in the hereafter.

Beautiful people love me and are attracted to me.

Romance, sensuality and intimacy are natural feelings in my relationships.

Romance finds me everywhere I go.

I am needed, accepted, appreciated and treasured.

I am in a joyous intimate relationship with a person who truly loves me.

I am sexually confident and the best lover.

I can always please my partner and am a powerful, sexual, romantic being.

I can attract romance into my life naturally and easily.

I give off romantic intimate energy always.

My mind, body and soul are perfectly attuned to attracting a romantic fun and long lasting relationships.

August 25

Psalm 85

A Prayer for Peace

Our Lord you have blessed your land and made all go well for Jacobs descendants. You have forgiven your people. Our Lord and our God you save us. Please bring us back home. I will listen to you Lord God because you promise peace to those who are faithful. You are ready to rescue everyone who worships you.

The Prophets

Say I do but warn you according to revelation. We shall set up scales of justice for the Day of Judgment so that a soul will be dealt with justly and if there be no more than the weight of a mustard seed. We will bring it to account and enough are we to take account.

Beautiful people love you and are attracted to you.

Romance, sensuality and intimacy are natural feelings in your relationships.

Romance finds you everywhere you go.

You are needed, accepted, appreciated and treasured.

You are in a joyous intimate relationship with a person who truly loves you.

You are sexually confident and the best lover.

You can always please your partner and you are a powerful, sexual, romantic being.

You can attract romance into your life naturally and easily.

You give off romantic intimate energy always.

Your mind, body and soul are perfectly attuned to attracting a romantic fun and long lasting relationships.

August 26

1 Corinthians 2

God's Spirit will Show You

It is as the scriptures say what God has planned for people who love him is more than eyes have seen or ears have heard. God's spirit has shown you everything. His spirit finds out everything what is deep in the mind of God. You are the only one who knows what is in your own mind and God's spirit is the only one who knows what is in God's mind.

The Victory

And that Allah may help thee with powerful help. It is he who sent down tranquility into the hearts of the believers that they might add faith to their faith. For to Allah belong the forces of the heavens and the earth and Allah is full of knowledge and wisdom.

Beautiful people love us and are attracted to us.

Romance, sensuality and intimacy are natural feelings in our relationships.

Romance finds me everywhere we go.

We are needed, accepted, appreciated and treasured.

We are in a joyous intimate relationship with a person who truly loves us.

We are sexually confident and the best lovers.

We can always please our partner and we are powerful, sexual, romantic beings.

We can attract romance into our life naturally and easily.

We give off romantic intimate energy always.

My mind, body and soul are perfectly attuned to attracting a romantic fun and long lasting relationship.

August 27

Romans 5:18

Adam and Christ

Because of the good thing that Christ has done God accepts us and gives us the gift of life. Jesus obeyed him and will make people acceptable to God. God's kindness now rules and God has accepted us because of Jesus Christ our Lord.

The Ways of Ascent

And those in whose wealth are a recognized right. For the needy who asks and him who is prevented for some reason from asking. And those who hold to the truth of the Day of Judgment. For their Lords peace and tranquility and those who guard against their chastity.

I am grateful to be ready and willing to allow deep fulfilling love into my life.

I am grateful I accept romantic love with open arms.

I am grateful to have a wonderful romantic partner and we both please and stimulate each other well.

I am grateful to attract friendship, love, affection and romance in my life.

I am grateful the perfect partner has found me and I am ready for true love.

I am grateful to attract romance.

I am grateful to be brilliant, sexy, attractive, independent and helpful.

I am grateful to be easy to communicate and flirt with.

I am grateful to be in my intimate relationship.

I am grateful to love myself and am irresistible to everyone always.

August 28

Colossians 3

Christ Brings New Life

Now set your heart on what is in heaven. Where Christ rules as Gods creator, Gods right side. Christ is all that matters and he lives in all of us. God loves you and has chosen you as his own special people. So be gentle, kind, humble, meek, and patient.

Yusuf

We have sent it down as an Arabic Quran in order that ye may learn wisdom. We do relate thee the most beautiful of stories in that we reveal to thee this portion of the Quran. Behold Joseph said to his father o my father I did see eleven stars and the sun and the moon and I saw them prostrate themselves to me.

You are grateful to be ready and willing to allow deep fulfilling love into your life.

You are grateful you accept romantic love with open arms.

You are grateful to have a wonderful romantic partner and you both please and stimulate each other well.

You are grateful to attract friendship, love, affection and romance in your life.

You are grateful the perfect partner has found you and you are ready for true love.

You are grateful to attract romance.

You are grateful to be brilliant, sexy, attractive, independent and helpful.

You are grateful to be easy to communicate and flirt with.

You are grateful to be in your intimate relationship.

You are grateful to love yourself and you are irresistible to everyone always.

August 29

Colossians 1:3

A Prayer of Thanks

We have heard your faith in Christ and of your love. In all of Gods people because what you hope for is kept safe for you in heaven. You first heard about this hope when you believed the true message which is the good news. The good news is spreading all over the world with great success.

The Ants

Praise be to Allah and peace on his servants who he has chosen for this message who is better? Yes with it we cause to grow well planted orchards full of beauty of delight. Allah knows what is hidden can they perceive when they shall be raised up for judgment.

We are grateful to be ready and willing to allow deep fulfilling love into our life.

We are grateful we accept romantic love with open arms.

We are grateful to have a wonderful romantic partner and we both please and stimulate each other well.

We are grateful to attract friendship, love, affection and romance in our life.

We are grateful the perfect partner has found us and we are ready for true love.

We are grateful to attract romance.

We are grateful to be brilliant, sexy, attractive, independent and helpful.

We are grateful to be easy to communicate and flirt with.

We are grateful to be in our intimate relationship.

We are grateful to love our self and are irresistible to everyone always.

August 30

Hebrews 8

A Better Promise

What I mean is that we have a high priest who sits at the right side of God's great throne in heaven. He also serves as the priest in the most holy place inside the real tent there in heaven. This tent of worship was set up by the Lord. But now I tell the people of Israel this is my new agreement. The time will come when I the Lord will write my laws on their minds and hearts. I will be there God and they will be my people.

The Repentance

Be with those who are true in word and deed. For Allah to reward those who do good.

I always know how to have a good time.

I am a social butterfly and enjoy playing with others always.

My social calendar is always completely filled and I always have fun.

I have a good sense of humor and enjoy being silly.

I attract fun and amusing experiences always.

My social life is fun, youthful, entertaining and adventurous.

I love to laugh, have fun and play always.

My sense of humor is attractive.

I make and maintain good friends easily now and always.

Joy is a healing choice and I choose it for myself and others.

August 31

Mark 2:5

Jesus Heals

Only God can forgive. Right away Jesus knew what they were thinking I will show you that the son of man has the right to forgive here on earth. So Jesus said to the man get up! Pick up your mat and go on home. The man got right up.

Hud

All that we relate to thee of the stories of the prophets with it we make firm thy heart in them there cometh to thee the truth as well as an exhortation and a message of remembrance to those who believe. Do whatever ye can we shall do our part and wait ye we too shall wait. To Allah do belong the unseen secrets of the heavens and the earth and to him goeth back every affair for decision then worship him and put thy trust in him.

You always know how to have a good time.

You are a social butterfly and enjoy playing with others always.

Your social calendar is always completely filled and you always have fun.

You have a good sense of humor and enjoy being silly.

You attract fun and amusing experiences always.

Your social life is fun, youthful, entertaining, productive and adventurous.

You love to laugh, have fun and play always.

Your sense of humor is attractive.

You make and maintain good friends easily now and always.

Joy is a healing choice and you choose it for yourself and others.

September 1

Psalm 150

The Lord is Good to His People

Shout praises to the Lord. Praise God in his temple. Praise him in heaven his mighty fortress. Praise our God! His deeds are wonderful too marvelous to describe. Praise God with trumpets and all kinds of harps, dancing with stringed instruments, cymbals and clashing cymbals.

The Heights

And if there is among you who believes in the message with which I have been sent and hold yourselves in patience until Allah does decide between us. He is the best to decide if the people of the towns believed Allah. We should indeed have opened out to them all gracious kinds of blessings from heaven and earth.

We always know how to have a good time.

We are social butterflies and enjoy playing with others always.

Our social calendar is always completely filled and we always have fun.

We have a good sense of humor and enjoy being silly.

We attract fun and amusing experiences always.

Our social life is fun, youthful, entertaining, productive and adventurous.

We love to laugh, have fun and play always.

Our sense of humor is attractive.

We make and maintain good friends easily now and always.

Joy is a healing choice and we choose it for ourselves and others.

September 2

Luke 12:3

Your Worth

Five sparrows are sold for just two pennies but God doesn't forget one of them. Even the hairs on your head are counted. You are worth much more than many sparrows.

The Man

Verily we created man from a drop of mingled sperm in order to try him so we gave him the gifts of hearing and sight. We showed him the way to be grateful rests on his will. As to the righteous they shall drink of a cup of wine mixed kafuf fountain where the devotees of Allah do drink making it flow in abundance.

I am grateful to have more fun and enjoy life.

I am grateful I take time each day to laugh and have fun.

I am grateful to attract more fun and amusing experiences.

I am grateful to live, work and play and really enjoy it.

I am grateful to succeed daily at having fun and creating entertaining experiences.

I am grateful to live life fully experiencing everything with joy.

I am grateful others value and enjoy playing with me.

I am grateful to be free to have fun and play all the time.

I am grateful to always have interesting amazing fun experiences to do.

I am grateful to socialize and celebrate life daily.

September 3

Psalm 141

A Prayer for the Lord's Protection

I pray to you Lord. Please listen when I pray and hurry to help me. Think of my prayer as sweet smelling incense and think of my lifted hands as an evening sacrifice. Help me to guard my words. Everyone will admit that I was right. You Lord God and I look to you for safety.

The Inner Apartments

Put not yourselves forward before Allah and his apostle for Allah is he who hears and knows all things. O you who believe. Raise not your voices above the voice of the prophet nor speak aloud to him in talk as you may speak aloud to one another. Those that lower their voices in the presence of Allah's apostle their hearts has Allah tested for piety and for them is forgiveness and a great reward.

You are grateful to have more fun and enjoy life.

You are grateful you take time each day to laugh and have fun.

You are grateful to attract more fun and amusing experiences.

You are grateful to live, work and play and really enjoy it.

You are grateful to succeed daily at having fun and creating entertaining experiences.

You are grateful to live life fully experiencing everything with joy.

You are grateful others value and enjoy playing with me.

You are grateful to be free to have fun and play all the time.

You are grateful to always have interesting amazing fun experiences to do.

You are grateful to socialize and celebrate life daily.

September 4

Acts 20:17

God Wants You to Know

I care what happens to me as long as I finish the work that the Lord Jesus gave me to do. And that work is to tell the good news about God's great kindness. I have gone from place to place preaching to you about God's kingdom but now I know that none of you will see me again.

The Kneeling Down

Say it is Allah who gives you life then he will gather you together for the Day of Judgment. To Allah belongs the dominions of the heavens, the earth and the day that the hour of judgment is established. And you will see every nation bowing. Every nation will be called to its record and this day shall you be recompensed for all that you did. This our record speaks about you with truth.

We are grateful to have more fun and enjoy life.

We are grateful we take time each day to laugh and have fun.

We are grateful to attract more fun and amusing experiences.

We are grateful to live, work and play and really enjoy it.

We are grateful to succeed daily at having fun and creating entertaining experiences.

We are grateful to live life fully experiencing everything with joy.

We are grateful others value and enjoy playing with us.

We are grateful to be free to have fun and play all the time.

We are grateful to always have interesting amazing fun experiences to do.

We are grateful to socialize and celebrate life daily.

September 5

2 Timothy 1

Pray

Night and day I mention you in my prayers. I am always grateful for you and chose us to be as I pray to the God my ancestors and I have served with a clear conscience. So I ask you to make full use of the gift that God gave you when I placed my hands on you. Use it well. The spirit gives us power, love and self-control.

The Narrations

Any that in this life had repented, believed and worked righteousness happily he shall be one of the successful. Your Lord does create and choose as he pleases. Glory to Allah! But those who had been granted true knowledge said alas for you the reward of Allah in the hereafter is best for those who believe and work righteousness save those who steadfastly preserve in good. If any does good the reward to him is better.

I have beautiful and peaceful home, job and relationship channels.

I am at peace with my past, present and future.

I am divine presence expressing as compassion, sincerity and peace.

My mind, body and soul are at peace.

I am peaceful and calm in every situation.

People feel peaceful and comfortable around me.

I give and receive peace and love gracefully and easily.

I feel centered and grounded in the peaceful loving energy of myself.

I am a clear channel of peace, love, beauty, wisdom and well-being.

September 6

Psalm 87

The Glory of Mount Zion

Zion was built by the Lord on the holy mountain and he loves that city more than any other place in all of Israel. Zion you are the city of God and wonderful things are told about you. God most high will strengthen the city of Zion. The Lord will make a list of his people and all who were born here will be included. All who sing and dance will say I too am from Zion.

The Roman Empire

Have we sent down authority to them which points out to them the things to which they worship and when we give them a taste of mercy. See they that Allah enlarges the provision and restricts it to whomsoever he pleases. That which you lay out for charity seeking the countenance of Allah will increase.

You have beautiful and peaceful home, job and relationship channels.

You are at peace with your past, present and future.

You are divine presence expressing as compassion, sincerity and peace.

Your mind, body and soul are at peace.

You are peaceful and calm in every situation.

People feel peaceful and comfortable around you.

You give and receive peace and love gracefully and easily.

You feel centered and grounded in the peaceful loving energy of yourself.

You are a clear channel of peace, love, beauty, wisdom and wellbeing.

September 7

Matthew 25:31

Final Judgment

When the son of man comes in his glory with all his angels. He will sit on his royal throne. The people of all nations will be brought before him and he will separate them as shepherds separate their sheep from their goats. He will place the sheep on his right and the goats on his left. Then the king will say father has blessed you come and receive the kingdom that was prepared for you before the world was created.

The Heifer

O children of Israel! Call to mind the special favor which I bestowed upon you and fulfill your covenant with me as I fulfill a covenant with you. And believe in what I reveal confirming the revelation which is with you. Steadfast in prayer practice, regular charity and bow down your heads and those who bow down in worship.

We have beautiful and peaceful home, job and relationship channels.

We are at peace with our past, present and future.

We are divine presence expressing as compassion, sincerity and peace.

Our mind, body and soul are at peace.

We are peaceful and calm in every situation.

People feel peaceful and comfortable around us.

We give and receive peace and love gracefully and easily.

We feel centered and grounded in the peaceful loving energy of ourselves.

We are a clear channel of peace, love, beauty, wisdom and wellbeing.

September 8

1 Thessalonians 1:4

The Thessalonians Faith and Example

My dear friends God loves you we know he has chosen you to be his people. When we told you the good news it was with the power and assurance that comes from the Holy Spirit. You knew what kind of people we were and how we helped you. So when you accepted the message you followed our example and the example of the Lord.

The Iron

For those who give in charity men and women and loan to Allah a beautiful loan it shall be increased manifold to their credit and they shall have besides a liberal award. And those who believe in Allah and his apostles they are the sincere lovers of truth and the witnesses who testify in the eyes of their Lord.

I am grateful a warm peaceful loving energy surrounds me and those I love always.

I am grateful to connect with what is peaceful and good around me.

I am grateful inside me lies a great reservoir of peace, love and divinity.

I am grateful to discover peace in those around me and they find peace in me.

I am grateful my heart feels peace always.

I am grateful my need of peace and calm is met.

I am grateful to create a home full of joy and peace

I am grateful to be filled with peace of mind.

I am grateful I experience joy, peace, love, serenity, kindness, truth, beauty, generosity and freedom.

I am grateful I accept the blessed flow of the divine.

September 9

Psalm 86

The Lord Will Help

I am your faithful servant and I trust you. Be kind to me. I pray to you all day. Make my heart glad and I serve you and my prayer is sincere. You willingly forgive and your love is always there for those who pray to you. Please listen Lord and answer my prayer for help.

The Confederates

He it is who sends blessings on you as do his angels that he may bring you into light and he is full of mercy to the believers. Their salvation on that day they meet him will be peace and he has prepared for them a generous reward. Truly we have sent you as a witness a bearer of glad tidings and Warner. And as one who invites to Allah grace by his leave and as a lamp spreading light.

You are grateful a warm peaceful loving energy surrounds you and those you love always.

You are grateful to connect with what is peaceful and good around you.

You are grateful inside you lies a great reservoir of peace, love and divinity.

You are grateful to discover peace in those around you and they find peace in you.

You are grateful your heart feels peace always.

You are grateful your need of peace and calm is met.

You are grateful to create a home full of joy and peace.

You are grateful to be filled with peace of mind.

You are grateful you experience joy, peace, love, serenity, kindness, truth, beauty, generosity and freedom.

You are grateful you accept the blessed flow of the divine.

September 10

Revelation 12:10

God's Authority

Then I heard a voice from heaven shout our God has shown his saving power and his kingdom has come. Gods own chosen one has shown his authority. The heavens shout rejoice together with everyone who lives there.

The Sure Reality

And the angels will be on its sides and will that day bear the throne of your Lord above them. That day you will be brought to judgment. Then he that will be given his record in his right hand will say ah here read you my record. I did really understand that my account would one day reach me. And he will be in a life of bliss in a garden on high, eat and drink you with satisfaction because of the good that you sent before them.

We are grateful a warm peaceful loving energy surrounds us and those we love always.

We are grateful to connect with what is peaceful and good around and within us.

We are grateful inside us lies a great reservoir of peace, love and divinity.

We are grateful to discover peace in those around us and they find peace in us.

We are grateful our heart feels peace always.

We are grateful our need of peace and calm is met.

We are grateful to create a home full of joy and peace.

We are grateful to be relaxed and filled with peace of mind.

We are grateful we experience joy, peace, love, serenity, kindness, truth, beauty, generosity and freedom.

We are grateful we accept the blessed flow of the divine.

September 11

Luke 9

Jesus is the Messiah

When Jesus was alone praying his disciples came to him and he asked them what do people say about me they answered some say that you are John the Baptist or Elijah or a prophet from long ago who has come back to life. Jesus then asked them but who do you say I am. Peter answered you are the messiah sent from God. Jesus said to all the people. You must follow me.

The Originator of Creation

Verily we have sent you in truth as a bearer of glad tidings and as a Warner we then bring out a produce of various colors. And in the mountains are tracts white and red of various shades of color and black intense in hue. And so amongst men are crawling creatures and cattle of various colors.

I am extroverted, outgoing, open and friendly.

I will let my positive personality shine always.

I have a full and enjoyable social life.

Being kind, friendly, caring, charismatic, and outgoing is natural for me.

I am a good conversationalist.

I attract excellent relationships because of my fun, friendly and productive lifestyle.

I have a precious, unique and charming personality.

I am great fun to be around.

I am inquisitive, fun, loving, spontaneous and very witty.

I can be my true self with everyone and they love me for that.

September 12

John 4:16

Jesus and the Samaritan Woman

Jesus told her go and bring your husband. The woman answered. I don't have a husband. Jesus replied you're telling the truth. The woman said sir I can see that you are a prophet. My ancestors worshiped on this mountain. Jesus said to her. Believe me the time is coming God will save the world. God is spirit and those who worship God must be led by the spirit to worship him according to the truth.

The Poets

If such were our will we could send down to them from the sky a sign. There comes to them a newly revealed message from Allah most gracious. Verily your Lord is he the exalted in might most merciful. Behold your Lord.

You are extroverted, outgoing, open and friendly.

You will let your positive personality shine always.

You have a full and enjoyable social life.

Being kind, friendly, caring, charismatic, and outgoing is natural for you.

You are a good conversationalist.

You attract excellent relationships because of your fun, friendly and productive lifestyle.

You have a precious, unique and charming personality.

You are great fun to be around.

You are inquisitive, fun, loving, spontaneous and very witty.

You can be your true self with everyone and they love you for that.

September 13

Matthew 18:18

Allowing

I promise you that God in heaven will allow whatever you allow on earth but he will not allow anything you don't allow. I promise that when any two of you on earth agree about something you are praying for my father in heaven will do it for you.

Al-Imran

And hold fast all together by the rope which Allah stretches out for you and remember with gratitude Allah's favor on you. He joined your hearts in love so that by his grace. He saved you. Let them arise out of you a bond of people inviting to all that is good enjoining what is right. They are the ones to attain felicity. On the day when some faces will be lifted up with white. Those faces will be lit with white they will be in the light of Allah's mercy therein to dwell forever.

We are extroverted, outgoing, open and friendly.

We will let our positive personality shine always.

We have a full and enjoyable social life.

Being kind, friendly, caring, charismatic, and outgoing is natural for us.

We are good conversationalists.

We attract excellent relationships because of our fun, friendly and productive lifestyle.

We have a precious, unique and charming personality.

We are great fun to be around.

We are inquisitive, fun, loving, spontaneous and very witty.

We can be our true self with everyone and they love us for that.

September 14

Colossians 6

Christ Brings Life

Be strong in your faith, just as you were taught. And be grateful God lives fully in Christ. And you are fully grown because you belong to Christ who is over every powers authority. When you were baptized it was the same as Christ. Then you were raised to life because you had faith in the power of God who raised Christ.

The Originator of Creation

And Allah did create you from dust then from a sperm drop then he made you in pairs. And no female conceives or lays down her load but with his knowledge. All this is easy to Allah. Not are the two bodies of flowing water alike the one palatable sweet and pleasant to drink and the other is salty and bitter.

I am grateful to be charismatic, positive and outgoing.

I am grateful others are attracted to my charisma and positive energy.

I am grateful I can lead and start conversations with anyone.

I am grateful others love to be around me.

I am grateful to confidently express my amazing friendly personality always.

I am grateful to feel more outgoing, charismatic and social.

I am grateful to have a magnetic personality.

I am grateful being happy, positive and charismatic comes easily and naturally.

I am grateful my true self makes new friends and keeps old friends easily.

I am grateful to enjoy socializing and sharing my divine self with others.

September 15

Luke 10:21

Jesus Thanks the Father

My father has given me everything and he is the only one who really knows the father is the son. But the son wants to tell others about the father so they can know him. Jesus then turned to his disciples and said to them in private you are blessed to see what you see.

The Opener

This is the book about which there is guidance for those conscious of Allah. Who believe in the unseen establishes prayer and spends out of what we have provided for them. Those are upon right guidance from their Lord and it is those who are the successful.

You are grateful to be charismatic, positive and outgoing.

You are grateful others are attracted to your charisma and positive energy.

You are grateful you can lead and start conversations with anyone.

You are grateful others love to be around you.

You are grateful to confidently express your amazing friendly personality always.

You are grateful to feel more outgoing, charismatic and social.

You are grateful to have a magnetic personality.

You are grateful being happy, positive and charismatic comes easily and naturally.

You are grateful your true self makes new friends and keeps old friends easily.

You are grateful to enjoy socializing and sharing your divine self with others.

September 16

Romans 5:1

What it Means to be Acceptable

By faith we have been made acceptable to God. And now because of our Lord Jesus Christ we live at peace with God. Christ has also introduced us to Gods kindness on which we take our stand. So we are happy as we look forward to sharing in the glory of God. And endurance builds character which gives us a hope.

The Woman to be Examined

There was indeed an excellent example for you to follow for those whose hope is in Allah and in the last day. Truly Allah is free of all wants worthy of all praise. It may be that Allah will grant love and friendship between you.

We are grateful to be charismatic, positive and outgoing.

We are grateful others are attracted to our charisma and positive energy.

We are grateful we can lead and start conversations with anyone easily.

We are grateful others love to be around us.

We are grateful to confidently express our amazing friendly personality always.

We are grateful to feel more outgoing, charismatic and social.

We are grateful to have a magnetic personality.

We are grateful being happy, positive and charismatic comes easily and naturally.

We are grateful our true self makes new friends and keeps old friends easily.

We are grateful to enjoy socializing and sharing my divine self with others.

September 17

Psalm 32

The Joy of Forgiveness

Our Lord you bless everyone you forgive. You bless them. I forgive you. We worship you Lord and we should always pray. You are my hiding place. You protect me. You put songs in my heart because you have saved me. Your kindness shields those who trust you Lord.

The Pen

Ask you of them which of them will stand surety for that. They shall be summoned to bow in adoration. A long respite will I grant them truly powerful is my plan. The unseen is in their hands so that they can write it down. So wait with patience for my command of your Lord. This is a message to all the worlds.

I feel safe in my neighborhood.

I choose to love my neighbors.

I am invited to all the neighborhood events.

My neighborhood is filled with kind, generous and lovely people.

I deserve to have the best neighbors.

I treat my neighbors with kindness and respect.

I treat my neighbors the way they like to be treated.

I am able to communicate well with my neighbors.

I am grateful to have super, kind, friendly neighbors.

My neighborhood is fun, safe and clean place to be always.

September 18

John 7:10

Jesus at the Festival of Shelters

After Jesus brothers had gone to the festival he went secretly without telling anyone. During the festival the leaders looked for Jesus and asked where is he? Some were saying Jesus is a good man.

Yusuf

So they concealed him as a treasure. But Allah knows well all that they do. The man in Egypt who bought him said to his wife make his stay among us honorable may be he will bring us much good or we shall adopt him as a son. Thus did we establish Joseph in the land that we might teach him the interpretation of stories and events. And Allah has full power and control over his affairs but most among mankind know it not. When Joseph attained his full manhood. We gave him power and knowledge thus do we reward those who do right.

You feel safe in your neighborhood.

You choose to love your neighbors.

You are invited to all the neighborhood events.

Your neighborhood is filled with kind, generous and lovely people.

You deserve to have the best neighbors.

You treat your neighbors with kindness and respect.

You treat your neighbors the way they like to be treated.

You are able to communicate well with your neighbors.

You are grateful to have super, kind, friendly neighbors.

Your neighborhood is a fun, safe and clean place to be always.

September 19

1 Thessalonians 3:12

Final instructions and Greetings

My friends we ask you to be thoughtful of your leaders who work hard and tell you how to live for the Lord. Show them great respect and love because of their work. Try to get along with each other. My friends we beg you to warn people to live right. Encourage anyone and be patient with everyone. Be good to each other and to everyone else. Always be joyful and never stop praying.

The Range

Now ask them their opinion is it that you Lord have only daughters and they have sons. Or that we created the angels female and they are witnesses thereto. Behold that they say from their own invention Allah has begotten children. Did he choose daughters rather than sons? What is the matter with you? How judge your will you then receive admonition? Or have you manifest authority.

We feel safe in our neighborhood.

We choose to love our neighbors.

We are invited to all the neighborhood events.

Our neighborhood is filled with kind, generous and lovely people.

We deserve to have the best neighbors.

We treat our neighbors with kindness and respect.

We treat our neighbors the way they like to be treated.

We are able to communicate well with our neighbors.

We are grateful to have super, kind, friendly neighbors.

Our neighborhood is a fun, safe and clean place to be always.

September 20

Revelations 3:7

The Letter to Philadelphia

I am the one who is holy and true. I have the keys that belonged to David. When I open a door no one can close it. And when I close a door no one can open it. Listen to what I say I know everything you have done. You obeyed my message and endured. So I will protect you from the time of testing that everyone in all the world must go through. Hold firmly to the crown that you will be given as your reward. Everyone who wins the victory.

Fussilat

In the case of those who say our Lord is Allah and further stand straight and steadfast the angels descend on them from time to time. Receive the glad tidings of the garden of bliss the which you were promised. We are your protectors in this life and in the hereafter therein you shall have all that your souls ask for.

I am grateful to have the most helpful neighbors.

I am grateful my neighbors and I have an active social life.

I am grateful for the good neighborhood I live in.

I am grateful I have a caring and protective relationship with my neighbors.

I am grateful my neighborhood is clean, friendly and safe.

I am grateful my neighbors and I are always helpful.

I am grateful my neighbors are safe, happy, clean and healthy always.

I am grateful me and my neighbors feel good about how we treat each other.

I am grateful to trust my kind, generous neighbors.

September 21

Revelations 20:11

The Judgment at the Great White Throne

I saw a great white throne with someone sitting on it. Books were opened. Then the book of life was opened. Then everyone was judged by what they had done.

The Believer

We did aforetime give Moses the book of guidance and we gave the book in inheritance of the children of Israel. A guide and a message to men of understanding. Patiently then persevere for the promise of Allah is true and ask forgiveness and celebrate the praises of your Lord in the evening and in the morning. Assuredly the creation of the heavens and the earth is greater matter than the creation of men.

You are grateful to have the most helpful neighbors.

You are grateful your neighbors and you have an active social life.

You are grateful for the good neighborhood you live in.

You are grateful you have a caring and protective relationship with your neighbors.

You are grateful m your neighborhood is clean, friendly and safe.

You are grateful your neighbors and you are always helpful.

You are grateful your neighbors are safe, happy, clean and healthy always.

You are grateful you and your neighbors feel good about how you treat each other.

You are grateful to trust your kind, generous neighbors.

September 22

2 Timothy 19

An Approved Worker

The foundation that God has laid is solid. Make themselves pure will become special. Their lives will be holy and pleasing to the master and they will be able to do all kind of good deeds. Always do the right thing. Be faithful loving and easy to get along with. Worship people whose hearts are pure.

Mary

Praying o my Lord! Indeed are my bones and the hair of my head do glisten. I am blest. O my Lord in my prayer to you to his son come the command O Yahya! Take hold of the book with might. We gave him wisdom even as a youth. And piety for all creatures as from us and purity. He was devout and kind to his parents. So peace on him the day he was born and the day he is raised to life.

We are grateful to have the most helpful neighbors.

We are grateful our neighbors and us have an active social life.

We are grateful for the good neighborhood we live in.

We are grateful we have a caring and protective relationship with our neighbors.

We are grateful our neighborhood is clean, friendly and safe always.

We are grateful our neighbors and us are always helpful.

We are grateful our neighbors are safe, happy, clean and healthy.

We are grateful us and our neighbors feel good about how we treat each other.

We are grateful to trust our kind, generous neighbors.

September 23

Acts 26:15

Paul to Agrippa

Then the Lord answered. I am Jesus. I am the one. I have appeared to you because I have chosen you to be my servant. You are to tell others what you have learned about me and what I will show you later. The Lord said I will protect you from the Jews and from the Gentiles that I am sending you to. I want you to open their eyes to light and the power of God. Then be forgiven and by faith in me they will become part of God's holy people.

The City of Saba

Our Lord will gather us together and will in the end decide the matter between us and you in truth and justice and he is the one to decide the one who knows all. He is Allah the exalted in power and wise. We have sent as a universal messenger to men giving them glad tidings and warning them.

The universe supplies me with money always.

My bank balance is increasing every day and I always have enough money.

I am a money magnet.

I am attracting and saving more money daily.

I am debt free and have really good credit.

I have a positive money mindset.

I am becoming more and more rich in wealth, happiness and good health.

I am fully supported making money doing what I love always.

Money flows to me from expected and unexpected sources.

Money is good and I have a lot of it all the time.

September 24

Luke 6:19

Blessings

Everyone was trying to touch Jesus because power was going out from him and healing them all. Jesus looked at his disciples and said God will bless you people. His kingdom belongs to you. God will bless you people. You will have plenty to eat.

The Iron

Know you all that Allah gives life to the earth already have we shown the signs plainly to you that you may learn wisdom. For those who give in charity men and women and loan to Allah a beautiful loan. It shall be increased manifold to their credit and they shall besides a liberal reward. And those who believe in Allah and his apostles they are the sincere lovers of truth and the witnesses who testify in the eyes of their Lord.

The universe supplies you with money always.

Your bank balance is increasing every day and you always have enough money.

You are a money magnet.

You are attracting and saving more money daily.

You are debt free and have really good credit.

You have a positive money mindset.

You are becoming more and more rich in wealth, happiness and good health.

You are fully supported making money doing what you love always.

Money flows to you from expected and unexpected sources.

Money is good and you have a lot of it all the time.

September 25

Ephesians 1:2

Christ Brings Spiritual Blessings

I pray that God our father and our Lord Jesus Christ will be kind to you and will bless you with peace. Praise the God and father of our Lord Jesus Christ for the spiritual blessings that Christ has brought us from heaven. Before the world was created. God had Christ choose us to live with him and to be holy, innocent and loving people.

The Cave

Moses said to him may I follow you on the footing that you teach me something of the higher truth which has been taught. Whoever believes and works righteousness he shall have a goodly reward and easy will be his task as we order it by our command. He said the power in which my Lord has established me is better than tribute. Help me therefore with strength and labor.

The universe supplies us with money always.

Our bank balance is increasing every day and we always have enough money.

We are a money magnet.

We are attracting and saving more money daily.

We are debt free and have really good credit.

We have a positive money mindset.

We are becoming more and more rich in wealth, happiness and good health.

We are fully supported making money doing what we love always.

Money flows to us from expected and unexpected sources.

Money is good and we have a lot of it all the time.

September 26

Psalm 85

A Prayer for Peace

Our Lord you have blessed your land and made all go well for Jacobs descendants. You have forgiven. Our God you saved us. Please bring us back home. Show us your love and save us. I will listen to you Lord God because you promise peace to those who are faithful. You are ready to resolve everyone who worships you so that you will live with us in all your glory, love, loyalty will come together goodness and peace will unite.

The Thunder

The Lord and sustainer of the heavens and the earth. Allah is the creator of all things. He is the one the supreme.

I am grateful to be rich and attract money.

I am grateful to be content with all the money that comes to me.

I am grateful to be willing and ready to receive money from expected and unexpected sources always.

I am grateful to be a money magnet and manage money very well.

I am grateful money comes to me and delivers always.

I am grateful my income grows higher and higher.

I am grateful to receive and give money happily.

I am grateful I am sensible with money and manage it wisely.

I am grateful to save and invest my money well.

I am grateful to always use money wisely, frugally and beneficially.

September 27

Philippians 4:10

Give Thanks

The Lord has made me very grateful that at last you have thought about me once again. I have learned to be satisfied with whatever I have. I have lived under all kinds of conditions. Christ gives me the strength to face anything. It was good of you to help me.

Ornaments of Gold

And verily it is in the mother of the book. In our presence high in dignity full of wisdom. That has created pairs in all things and has made for you ships and cattle on which you ride. In order that you may sit firm and square on their backs and when so seated you may celebrate the kind favor of your Lord and say glory to him.

You are grateful to be rich and attract money.

You are grateful to be content with all the money that comes to you.

You are grateful to be willing and ready to receive money from expected and unexpected sources always.

You are grateful to be a money magnet and manage money very well.

You are grateful money comes to you and delivers always.

You are grateful your income grows higher and higher.

You are grateful to receive and give money happily.

You are grateful you are sensible with money and manage it wisely.

You are grateful to save and invest your money well.

You are grateful to always use money wisely, frugally and beneficially.

September 28

Colossians 1

The Person and Work of Christ

We always pray that God will show you everything we wanted you to do and that you may have all the wisdom and understanding that his spirit gives. Then you will live a life that honors the Lord and you will always please him by doing good deeds. You will come to know God even better. His glorious power will make you patient and strong. I pray that you will be truly happy.

The Mount

By the mount of revelation. By a decree inscribed in a scroll unfolded. By the canopy raised high by the ocean filled with swell. As to the righteous they will be in gardens and in happiness enjoying the bliss which their Lord has bestowed on them.

We are grateful to be rich and attract money.

We are grateful to be content with all the money that comes to us.

We are grateful to be willing and ready to receive money from expected and unexpected sources always.

We are grateful to be a money magnet and manage money very well.

We are grateful money comes to me and delivers always.

We are grateful my income grows higher and higher.

We are grateful to receive and give money happily.

We are grateful we are sensible with money and manage it wisely.

We are grateful to save and invest our money well.

We are grateful to always use money wisely, frugally and beneficially.

September 29

Acts 7:35

God Works with Moses

God's angel had spoken to Moses from the bush. And God had even sent the angel to help Moses rescue the people and be their leader. In Egypt and at the red sea and in the desert Moses rescued the people by working miracles, wonders for 40 years. Moses is the one who told the people of Israel God will choose one of your people to be a prophet just as he chose me.

The Rocky Tract

The righteous will be amid gardens. Fountains of clear flowing water. Their greeting will be enter you here in peace and security. Tell my servants that I am indeed the oft forgiving most merciful. Tell them about the quests of Abraham when they entered his presence and said peace. We give you glad tidings of a son endowed with wisdom.

I am surrounded by love and all is well.

I deserve love, romance, joy and all the good in life and that's what I receive.

I am in joyous intimate relationships with others who truly love me.

Enduring loving relationships brighten my life.

I give and receive love freely and joyfully.

I find love everywhere I go and life is amazing.

I love being with people who bring out the best in me.

I am loved, loving, and lovable all the time.

I love sharing interesting fun conversations with my friends and family.

I accept that I am loved and treasured.

September 30

John 18:20

Secrets of the Kingdom of Heaven

Jesus answered I have explained the secrets about the kingdom of heaven. Everyone who has something will be given more. If they could they would turn to me and I would heal them. God has blessed you because your eyes can see and your ears can hear.

The Ways of Ascent

Now I do call to witness the Lord of all points in the east and the west that we certainly substitute for them better men. They encounter that day of theirs which they have been promised.

You are surrounded by love and all is well.

You deserve love, romance, joy and all the good in life and that's what you receive.

You are in joyous intimate relationships with others who truly love you.

Enduring loving relationships brighten your life.

You give and receive love freely and joyfully.

You find love everywhere you go and life is amazing.

You love being with people who bring out the best in you.

You are loved, loving, and lovable all the time.

You love sharing interesting fun conversations with your friends and family.

You accept that you are loved and treasured.

October 1

Psalm 84

The Joy of Worship

Lord God all powerful your temple is so lovely and deep in my heart. I long for your temple and with all that I am I sing joyful songs to you. Lord God all powerful my king my God. You bless everyone who lives in your house and they sing your praise. You bless all who depend on you for their strength and all who deeply desire to visit your temple. Lord God all-powerful the God of Jacob please answer my prayer. You are the shield that protects your people and I am your chosen one.

The Thunder

Once Allah wills a people's punishment there can be none turning it back nor will they find besides him any to protect. It is he who does show you the lightning by hope. It is he who does raise up the clouds with fertilizing rain. Thunder repeats.

We are surrounded by love and all is well.

We deserve love, romance, joy and all the good in life and that's what we receive.

We are in joyous intimate relationships with others who truly love us.

Enduring loving relationships brighten our life.

We give and receive love freely and joyfully.

We find love everywhere we go and life is amazing

We love being with people who bring out the best in us.

We are loved, loving, and lovable all the time.

We love sharing interesting fun conversations with our friends and family.

We accept that we are loved and treasured.

October 2

Matthew 19:16

Eternal Life

A man came to Jesus and asked teacher what good thing must I do to have eternal life. Jesus replied I wanted to be perfect and will have riches in heaven. Then come and be my follower. It's easier for a camel to go through the eye of the needle to get into Gods kingdom. Yes all of you have become my followers. And so in the future world when the son of man sits on his glorious throne. I promise that I will sit on the 12 thrones to judge the 12 tribes.

The Believer

Raised high above ranks or degrees. He is the Lord of the throne of authority by his command. He sends the spirit of inspiration to only his servants. He pleases that it may warn men of the day of mutual meeting. That day will every soul be requited for what it earned. That day for Allah is swift in taking account. Allah will judge with justice and truth. Verily it is Allah alone who hears and sees all things. Do they travel through the earth and see what was the end of those before them?

I am grateful my heart is always open to love.

I am grateful to radiate love to everyone around me.

I am grateful all my relationships are loving.

I am grateful I love everything and everyone and they love me.

I am grateful to deserve love and receive it in abundance.

I am grateful my partner and I have a perfect union of two loving souls.

I am grateful I am loved, loving, and lovable.

I am grateful I am full of joy and I love myself.

October 3

John 6:22

The Bread that Gives Life

Rabbi when did you get here? Jesus answered I tell you for certain that you are looking for me because you saw the miracles. Work for food that gives eternal life. The son of man will give you this food because God the father has given him the right to do so. What exactly does God want us to do? The people asked Jesus answered God wants you to have faith in the one he sent.

Those Range

And thus proclaim the message of Allah. Verily your Allah is one Lord of the heavens and of the earth and all between them and Lord of every point at the rising of the sun. We have indeed decked the lower heaven with beauty in the stars. A voice will say this is the day of sorting out. The sincere and devoted servants of Allah for them is a sustenance's determined fruits delights and they shall enjoy honor and dignity in gardens of felicity facing each other on thrones of dignity.

You are grateful your heart is always open to love.

You are grateful to radiate love to everyone around you.

You are grateful all your relationships are loving.

You are grateful you love everything and everyone and they love you.

You are grateful to deserve love and receive it in abundance.

You are grateful your partner and you have a perfect union of two loving souls.

You are grateful you are loved, loving, and lovable.

You are grateful you are full of joy and you love yourself.

October 4

Psalm 111

Praise the Lord

Shout praises to the Lord and with all my heart I will thank the Lord when his people meet. The Lord has done many wonderful things. Everyone who is pleased with God's marvelous deeds will keep them in mind. Everything the Lord does is glorious and majestic and his power to bring justice will never end. The Lord God is famous for his wonderful deeds and he is kind and merciful. He gives food to his worshipers and always keeps his agreement with them. God is always honest and fair and his laws can be trusted. They are true and right and will stand forever. Respect and obey the Lord. This is the first step to wisdom and good service. God will always be respected.

The Woman to be Examined

If you have come out to strive in my way to seek my good pleasure. For I know full well all that you conceal and all that you reveal. I will pray for your forgiveness.

We are grateful our heart is always open to love.

We are grateful to radiate love to everyone around us.

We are grateful all our relationships are loving.

We are grateful we love everything and everyone and they love us.

We are grateful to deserve love and receive it in abundance.

We are grateful our partner and us have a perfect union of two loving souls.

We are grateful we are loved, loving, and lovable.

We are grateful we are full of joy and we love ourselves.

October 5

Colossians 1

The Person and Work of Christ

Christ is exactly like God who can be seen he is the first born son superior to all creation. Everything was created by him everything in heaven and on earth everything seen and unseen including all forces and powers and all rulers and authorities. All things were created by God's son and everything was made for him. God's son was before all else and by him everything is held together.

Ornaments of Gold

When Jesus the son of Mary is held up as an example. He was a servant. We granted our favor to him and we made him an example to the children of Israel. And Jesus shall be a sign for the coming of the house of judgment. Follow you me this is the straightway. Jesus came with clear signs he said now have I come to you with wisdom.

The perfect partner is in my healthy and happy life.

I have fun in all my journeys.

I smile and feel joy everywhere with everyone always.

Sharing laughter and good times always happens easily.

I have achieved success in my life.

I am powerful, capable, confident and energetic always.

I live in the present and radiate positivity, beauty and enthusiasm.

I am well groomed, healthy and full of confidence.

My world is a friendly peaceful loving and joy filled place to live.

I live in the moment and am forever mindful and present in my relationships.

October 6

Proverbs 7

Wisdom is Calling

My son pay close attention what I tell you to do. Obey me and you will live and let my instructions be your greatest treasure. Keep them at your fingertips and write them on your mind. Let wisdom be your sister and common sense your closest friend. With great understanding wisdom calling out as she stands at the crossroads and on every hill. Good sense, judgment can be yours. Listen for what I say is worthwhile and right. I always speak the truth.

Mary

To his son came the command o Yahya! Take hold of the book with might and we gave him wisdom even as a youth and piety for all creatures. He was devout. And kind to his parents so peace on him. Relate in the book the story of Mary when she withdrew from her family to a place in the east.

The perfect partner is in your healthy and happy life.

You have fun in all your journeys.

You smile and feel joy everywhere with everyone always.

Sharing laughter and good times always happens easily.

You have achieved success in your life.

You are powerful, capable, confident and energetic always.

You live in the present and radiate positivity, beauty and enthusiasm.

You are well groomed, healthy and full of confidence.

Your world is a friendly peaceful loving and joy filled place to live.

You live in the moment and are forever mindful and present in your relationships.

October 7

2 Peter 2

The Lord Will Return

My dear friends this is the second letter I have written to encourage you to do some honest thinking. The day of the Lord's return will surprise us. The heavens will disappear with a loud noise. The heat will melt the whole universe. You should look forward to the day God judges everyone you should try to make it come soon. On that day the heavens everything else will melt in the heat. God has promised a new heaven and a new earth where justice will rule.

Al-Imran

Of the good Allah knows well those that do right. Remember you said to the faithful is it enough for you that Allah should help you with 3000 angels specially sent down.

The perfect partner is in our healthy and happy life.

We have fun in all our journeys.

We smile and feel joy everywhere with everyone always.

Sharing laughter and good times always happens easily.

We have achieved success in our life.

We are powerful, capable, confident and energetic always.

We live in the present and radiate positivity, beauty and enthusiasm.

We are well groomed, healthy and full of confidence.

Our world is a friendly, peaceful loving and joy filled place to live.

We live in the moment and we are forever mindful and present in our relationships.

October 8

Matthew 4

Jesus

The scriptures say God will give his angels orders about you. They will catch you in their arms. Jesus answered the scriptures also say don't try to test the Lord your God. God blesses those people who depend on him. They belong to the kingdom of heaven. God blesses those people. They will find comfort. God blesses those who are humble. The earth will belong to them. God blesses those people who want to obey him. They will be given what they want.

The Prophets

We roll up the heavens like a scroll rolled up for books completed even as we produced the first creation so shall we produce a new one. A promise we have undertaken truly shall we fulfill it. Before this we wrote in the psalms after the message given to Moses. My servants the righteous shall inherit the earth.

I am grateful to be in a state of joy and contentment.

I am grateful to be happy, enthusiastic about life always.

I am grateful to find joy and pleasure in the simple things in life.

I am grateful to have an active sense of humor and love.

I am grateful to live in the house of my dreams with my perfect match.

I am grateful to be the architect of my life.

I am grateful to take up healthy positive habits.

I am grateful to have the best healthiest, happiest and richest lifestyle.

I am grateful to have a divine nature and my life is a beautiful success.

October 9

Matthew 18

Pray Together

I promise you that God in heaven will allow whatever you allow on earth. I promise that when any two of you on earth agree about something you are praying for my father in heaven and will do it for you. Whenever two or three of you come together in my name I am there. This story will show you what the kingdom of heaven is like.

The Gathering

Whatever is in the heavens on earth let it declare the praises and glory of Allah for he is the exalted in might the wise. Take what the apostle assigns to you. Allah his good pleasure and aiding Allah and his apostle such are indeed the sincere ones. And those saved they are the ones that achieve prosperity.

You are grateful to be in a state of joy and contentment.

You are grateful to be happy, enthusiastic about life always.

You are grateful to have an active sense of humor and love.

You are grateful to live in the house of your dreams with your perfect match.

You are grateful to be the architect of your life.

You are grateful to take up healthy positive habits.

You are grateful to have the best healthiest, happiest and richest lifestyle.

You are grateful to have a divine nature and your life is a beautiful success.

October 10

Psalm 116

Lord Saves

When the Lord saves you. I love you Lord. You answered my prayers you paid attention to me and so I will pray to you. You are kind Lord so good and merciful. You protect ordinary people and you saved me and treated me so kindly. You Lord have saved my life. I worship you Lord just as my mother did and you have rescued me.

The Mount

By the mount of revelation by a decree inscribed in a scroll unfolded. As to the righteous they will be in gardens and in happiness enjoying the bliss which their Lord has bestowed on them and their Lord shall deliver them. To them will be said enter drink you with good pleasure because of your good deeds. They will recline with ease on thrones of dignity arranged in ranks and we shall join them to companions with beautiful big eyes.

We are grateful to be in a state of joy and contentment.

We are grateful to be happy, enthusiastic about life always.

We are grateful to find joy and pleasure in the simple things in life.

We are grateful to have an active sense of humor and love.

We are grateful to live in the house of our dreams with our perfect match.

We are grateful to be the architect of our life.

We are grateful to take up healthy positive habits.

We are grateful to have the best healthiest, happiest and richest lifestyle.

We are grateful to have a divine nature and our life is a beautiful success.

October 11

John 7

Jesus at the Festival

Jesus replied what I teach comes from the one who sent me. If you really want to obey God you will know what I teach comes from God. I wanted to bring honor to myself. I want to honor the one who sent me. That is why I tell the truth.

Al Qasas

Truly the best of men for you to employ is the man who is strong and trustworthy. Allah wills one of the righteous. He said be that the agreement between me and whichever of the two terms I fulfill. Be Allah a witness to what we move your hand into your bosom and it will come forth white and draw your hand close to your side to guard. Those are two credentials from your Lord.

I have the energy and passion to achieve my goals.

I am in a loving, fun, respectful and passionate relationships.

I feel passionate about my life.

I live a creative, fun, successful life.

I am passionate about writing, learning, art, health, love and many other things.

I am passionate eternally, easily, effortlessly and magically all the time.

Everything I do is with passion, love, energy and grace.

I am smart, creative, pretty, rich and passionate.

I can express my love, passion and understanding easily and wisely.

My passion is a thirst for knowledge, love, success and good health and wealth.

October 12

Psalm 148

Come Praise the Lord

Shout praises to the Lord. Shout the Lords praises in the highest heavens. All of you angels and all who serve him above come and after praise, sun and moon and all of you bright stars come and offer praise, highest heavens come and offer praise.

The Light

Say to believing men that they should lower their gaze and guard their modesty that will make for greater purity for them and Allah is well acquainted with all that they do. And say to believing women that they should lower their gaze and guard their modesty that they should display their beauty and ornaments except what must ordinarily appear.

You have the energy and passion to achieve your goals.

You are in a loving, fun, respectful and passionate relationships.

You feel passionate about your life.

You live a creative, fun, successful life.

You are passionate about writing, learning, art, health, love and many other things.

You are passionate eternally, easily, effortlessly and magically all the time.

Everything you do is with passion, love, energy and grace.

You are smart, creative, pretty, rich and passionate.

You can express your love, passion and understanding easily and wisely.

Your passion is a thirst for knowledge, love, success and good health and wealth.

October 13

Mark 9:12

The True Glory of Jesus

Six days later the cloud passed over and covered them. From the cloud a voice said this is my son and I love him listen to what he says. At once the disciples looked around but they saw Jesus. Jesus replied anything is possible for someone who has faith. Right away the boy's father shouted I do have faith. Please help me to have even more.

Fussilat

A gift from one forgiving most merciful who is between in speech than one who calls men to Allah work righteousness. Say I am of those who bow in Islam. And one will be granted such goodness except those whom exercise patience and self-restraint persons of the greatest good fortune.

We have the energy and passion to achieve our goals.

We are in loving, fun, respectful and passionate relationships.

We feel passionate about our life.

We live a creative fun successful life.

We are passionate about writing, learning, art, health, love and many other things.

We are passionate eternally, easily, effortlessly and magically all the time.

Everything we do is with passion, love, energy and grace.

We are smart, creative, pretty, rich and passionate.

We can express our love, passion and understanding easily and wisely.

Our passion is a thirst for knowledge, love, success and good health and wealth.

October 14

Luke 22:66

Jesus is Questioned

From now on the son of man will be seated at the right side of God all powerful. Then they asked are you the son of man? Jesus answered you say I am they replied why do we need more witnesses. He said it himself.

The Confederates

For Allah understands the finest mysteries and is well acquainted with them. For Muslim men and women for believing men and women for devout men and women for true men and women for men and women who are patient and constant for men and woman who humble themselves for men and women who fast and for men and women who guard their chastity for men and women who engage much in Allah's praise for them has Allah prepared forgiveness and a great reward.

I am grateful everything I do is with love and passion.

I am grateful to purse a successful, happy, love life.

I am grateful I am passionate with a will and intensity.

I am grateful to succeed with grace, sophistication, love and passion always.

I am grateful my passion is diligent and faithful.

I am grateful I am in loving, fulfilling entertaining relationships.

I am grateful to be full of energy and passion.

I am grateful to be passionate about my life, family, art, writing, heaven and good news spreading.

I am grateful to be passionate filled with excitement and energy always.

I am grateful I live with passion, love and purpose always.

October 15

Psalm 199:161

Peace of Mind

But with all my heart I respect your words because they bring happiness like treasures. I love your law. I praise you seven times a day because your laws are fair. You give peace of mind to all who love your law. I love and obey your laws with all my heart.

An-Naba

Verily for the righteous there will be a fulfillment of the hearts desires. Gardens enclosed and grapevines. A cup full to the brim. Recompense from your Lord a gift amply sufficient from the Lord of the heavens and the earth and all between. Allah most gracious the day that the spirit and the angels will stand forth in ranks.

You are grateful everything you do is with love and passion.

You are grateful to pursue a successful, happy, love life.

You are grateful you are passionate with a will and intensity.

You are grateful to succeed with grace, sophistication, love and passion always.

You are grateful your passion is diligent and faithful.

You are grateful you are in loving, fulfilling entertaining relationships.

You are grateful to be full of energy and passion.

You are grateful to be passionate about your life, family, art, writing, heaven and good news spreading.

You are grateful to be passionate and filled with excitement and energy always.

You are grateful you live with passion, love and purpose always.

October 16

Acts 26:15

Paul's Defense

I have appeared to you because I have chosen you to be my servant. You are to tell others what you have learned about me and what I will show you later. Then Lord also said I will protect you from the Jews and from the Gentiles that I am sending you so that they will turn to light. By faith in me they will become part of God's holy people. King Agrippa obeyed this vision from heaven.

The Poets

I am to you an apostle worthy of all trust. So obey me. My reward is only from the Lord of the worlds. Will you be left secure in the enjoyment of all that you have here. Gardens and springs and cornfields and date palms with the weight of fruit.

We are grateful everything we do is with love and passion.

We are grateful to pursue a successful, happy, love life.

We are grateful we are passionate with a will and intensity.

We are grateful to succeed with grace, sophistication, love and passion always.

We are grateful our passion is diligent and faithful.

We are grateful we are in loving, fulfilling entertaining relationships.

We are grateful to be full of energy and passion.

We are grateful to be passionate about our life, family, art, writing, heaven and good news spreading.

We are grateful to be passionate filled with excitement and energy always.

We are grateful we live with passion, love and purpose always.

October 17

Luke 17

God's Kingdom

Jesus said to his disciples. The time will come when you will long to see one of the days of the son of man. The day of the son of man will be like lightning flashes across the sky.

The Spider

For those who hopes are in the meeting with Allah in the hereafter let them strive for the term appointed by Allah is surely coming and he hears and knows all things. If any strive with might and maim they do so for their own souls for Allah is free of all needs from all creation. Those who believe and work righteous deeds. We have enjoined on man kindness to parents.

I am grateful to be intuitive and aware.

I am grateful to have an inner knowingness and clairvoyance.

I am grateful to be psychic and trust my vision.

I am grateful my inner vision is strong and accurate.

I am grateful my intuition can be trusted and I act upon it properly.

I am grateful I am focused, clear and visualize my successful future.

I am grateful I listen to my body, my feelings and can trust them.

I am grateful to be tuned into the cosmos.

I am grateful to invite guidance and clarity always.

I am grateful I am guided by the universe.

October 18

James 2:13

Wisdom From Above

Wisdom that comes from above leads us to be pure, friendly, gentle, sensible, kind, helpful, genuine and sincere. When peacemaker's plant seeds of peace they will harvest justice. Come near to God and he will come near to you. Clean up your lives. Purify your hearts. Be humble in the Lord's presence and he will honor you. God is our judge and he can save us.

The Pen

By the pen and the record which men write. Verily for you is a reward. And you stand on an exalted standard of character. Soon will you see. Verily it is you Lord that knows best who receives true guidance. Shall we then treat the people of faith like people? Or have you a book through which you learn. Truly powerful is my plan.

You are grateful to be intuitive and aware.

You are grateful to have an inner knowingness and clairvoyance.

You are grateful to be psychic and trust your vision.

You are grateful your inner vision is strong and accurate.

You are grateful your intuition can be trusted and you act upon it properly.

You are grateful you are focused, clear and visualize your successful future.

You are grateful you listen to your body, your feelings and can trust them.

You are grateful to be tuned into the cosmos.

You are grateful to invite guidance and clarity always.

You are grateful you are guided by the universe.

October 19

Luke 1

Mary's Song of Praise

Mary said with all my heart I praise the Lord and I am glad because of God my savior. God comes for me his humble servant from now on all people will say God has blessed me. God all powerful has done great things for me and his name is holy. God gives good things to eat.

The Scattered Winds

Verily judgment and justice must indeed come to pass. The sky with its numerous paths. As to the righteous they will be in the midst of gardens and springs taking joy in the thing which their Lord gives them. On earth are signs for those of assured faith as also in your own selves. And in heaven is your sustenance as also that which you are promised. Then by the Lord of heaven and earth this is the very truth as much as the fact that you speak intelligently to each other.

We are grateful to be intuitive and aware.

We are grateful to have an inner knowingness and clairvoyance.

We are grateful to be psychic and trust our vision.

We are grateful our inner vision is strong and accurate.

We are grateful our intuition can be trusted and we act upon it properly.

We are grateful we are focused, clear and visualize our successful future.

We are grateful we listen to our body, our feelings and can trust them.

We are grateful to be tuned into the cosmos.

We are grateful to invite guidance and clarity always.

We are grateful we are guided by the universe.

October 20

James 1:19

Obey God's Message

My dear friends you should be quick to listen and slow to speak. Be humble and accept the message that is planted in you to save you. Obey God's message. The law that sets you free. God will bless you in everything you do if you listen and obey. Religion that pleases God the father must be pure and spotless.

Mary

Allah most gracious extends the rope to them and until when they see the warning of Allah being fulfilled either in the approach of the hour they will of length realize who is in position. And Allah does advance in guidance those who seek guidance and the things that endure good deeds are best in the sight of your Lord as rewards and best in respect of their eventual return. The day we shall gather the righteous to Allah most gracious like a band presented before a king for honors.

I have a strong, immune, respiratory, reproductive and nervous system.

Every cell of my body vibrates with wellbeing.

A golden aura of perfect wellbeing surrounds me always.

I am beauty, fitness, good health and happiness.

I am always healthy and filled with excellent energy.

I am blessed with good health, wealth and wisdom.

I enjoy optimum health and I can heal others.

All my muscles, organs, tendons, and veins are healthy.

I am strong, flexible and toned all the time.

I take perfect care of my attractive, aligned and energized body, mind and soul.

October 21

John 1:29

The Lamb of God

Here is the Lamb of God. He is the one I told you about when I said someone else will come he is greater than I am because he was alive before I was born. I did know who he was. I came to baptize you with water so that everyone in Israel would see him. I was there and saw the spirit come down on him like a dove from heaven. And the spirit stayed on him.

The Narrations

Any that in this life had repentance believed and worked righteousness happily he shall be one of the successful. Your Lord does create and choose as he pleases. Glory to Allah and far is he above. Your Lord knows all that their hearts conceal and all that they reveal. And he is Allah. Be praised at the first and the last for him is the command and to him shall you all be brought back.

You have a strong, immune, respiratory, reproductive and nervous system.

Every cell of your body vibrates with well-being.

A golden aura of perfect wellbeing surrounds you always.

You are beauty, fitness, good health and happiness.

You are always healthy and filled with excellent energy.

You are blessed with good health, wealth and wisdom.

You enjoy optimum health and you can heal others.

All your muscles, organs, tendons, and veins are healthy.

You are strong, flexible and toned all the time.

You take perfect care of your attractive, aligned and energized body, mind and soul.

October 22

Luke 29:25

Jesus Appears

When the two of them came near the village where they were going Jesus seemed to be going farther. They begged him stay with us. It's already late the sun is going down. So Jesus went into the house to stay with them. After Jesus sat down to eat he took some bread he blessed and broke it. Then he gave it to them.

The Consultation

Behold gracious is Allah to his servants he gives sustenance to whom he pleases and he is strong the mighty. For he knows well the secrets of all hearts. He is the one that accepts repentance from his servants and forgives. He knows all that you do and he listens to those who believe and do deeds of righteousness and gives them increase of his bounty.

We have strong, immune, respiratory, reproductive and nervous systems.

Every cell of our body vibrates with wellbeing.

A golden aura of perfect wellbeing surrounds us always.

We are beauty, fitness, good health and happiness.

We are always healthy and filled with excellent energy.

We are blessed with good health, wealth and wisdom.

We enjoy optimum health and we can heal others.

All our muscles, organs, tendons, and veins are healthy and functioning perfectly well.

We are strong, flexible and toned all the time.

We take perfect care of our attractive, aligned and energized body, mind and soul.

October 23

Psalm 132

The Lord is Always with His People

You have gladly chosen Zion as your home our Lord. You said this is my home I will live here forever. I will bless Zion with food. Victory will be like robes for the priests and the faithful people will celebrate and shout. I will give mighty power to the kingdom of David. Each of my chosen kings will shine like lamps near a sparkling crown. It is wonderful when the people of God live together in peace.

The Women

To Allah belong all things in the heavens and on earth. Verily we have directed the people of the book before you. To Allah belongs all things in the heavens and on earth and Allah is free of all wants worthy of all praise. If it were his will he could create another race for he has power this to do.

I am grateful to be healthy, happy and full of positive high energy always.

I am grateful every cell in my body is overflowing with health and healing energy.

I am grateful to establish healthy eating, and drinking.

I am grateful to nourish my body, mind and soul.

I am grateful to be perfectly healthy.

I am grateful to have energy, vitality and wellbeing.

I am grateful my body can heal quickly and easily.

I am grateful I love and care for myself well.

I am grateful to discover to new ways to stay healthy and heal others.

I am grateful to appreciate myself and appreciate the love in my mind, body and soul.

October 24

1 Corinthians 3:10

Only One Foundation

God was kind and let me become an expert builder. I laid a foundation on which others have built. But we must each be careful how we build because Christ is the only foundation. Whatever we build on that foundation will be tested by fire on the Day of Judgment. Then everyone will find out if we have used gold, silver and precious stones or wood, hay and straw.

The Dominion

Blessed be he in whose hands are dominion and he has authority over all things. Say it is he who has created you and made you grown and made for you the faculties of hearing, seeing, feeling and understanding and thanks it is you give. Say it is he who has multiplied you through the earth and to him shall you be gathered together.

You are grateful to be healthy, happy and full of positive high energy always.

You are grateful every cell in your body is overflowing with health and healing energy.

You are grateful to establish healthy eating and drinking.

You are grateful to nourish your body, mind and soul.

You are grateful to be perfectly healthy.

You are grateful to have energy, vitality and wellbeing.

You are grateful your body can heal quickly and easily.

You are grateful you love and care for yourself well.

You are grateful to discover to new ways to stay healthy and heal others.

You are grateful to appreciate yourself and appreciate the love in your mind, body and soul.

October 25

Psalm 84

The Joy of Worship

Lord God all powerful your temple is so lovely. Deep in my heart I long for your temple and with all that I am I sing joyful songs to you. Lord God all powerful my king and my God. You bless everyone who lives in your house and they sing your praises. You bless all who depend on you for their strength and all who deeply desire to visit your temple.

Al Alaq

He who taught the use of the pen. Taught man in that he looks upon himself as self-sufficient verily to your Lord is the return of all we have indeed revealed the message in the night of power. The night of power is better than a thousand months. There in came down the angels and the spirit by Allah's permission on every errand. Peace.

We are grateful to be healthy, happy and full of positive high energy always.

We are grateful every cell in our body is overflowing with health and healing energy.

We are grateful to establish healthy eating and drinking.

We are grateful to nourish our body, mind and soul.

We are grateful to be perfectly healthy.

We are grateful to have energy, vitality and wellbeing.

We are grateful our body can heal quickly and easily.

We are grateful we love and care for ourselves well.

We are grateful to discover to new ways to stay healthy and heal others.

We are grateful to appreciate ourselves and appreciate the love in our mind, body and soul.

October 26

Galatians 4:4

Paul's Concern

When the time was right and God sent his son and a woman gave birth to him. His son obeyed the law so he could set us free from the law and we could become God's children. God has sent the spirit of his son into our hearts. And his spirit tells us that God is our father. Where is the good feeling now? It is always good to give your attention to something worthwhile.

The Crowds

Praise be to Allah. He who brings the truth and he who confirms and supports it such are the men who do right. They shall have all that they wish for in the presence of their Lord such is the reward of those who do good. Allah will give them their reward according to the best of what they have done. Is Allah exalted in power able to enforce his will Lord of retribution.

I am happier now than I have ever been and filled with joy all the time.

I live happily ever after now and forever.

It's a happy universe and I enjoy its moment.

I am happy because I choose happy always.

Every cell in my body, mind and soul are at peace, healthy and happy.

Remaining happy and positive benefits me and others.

I live a happy life and laugh all the time.

I am peaceful, serene, happy and content now and forever.

I spread joy and happiness everywhere I go.

I deserve to be happy.

October 27

Luke 2:46

Searching for Jesus

Three days later they found Jesus sitting in the temple listening to the teachers and asking him questions. Everyone who heard was surprise at how much he knew at the answers he gave. When his parents found him they were amazed.

The Heifer

This is the book in it is guidance. In the law of equality there is saving of life to you o you men of understanding. O you who believe fasting is prescribed to you as it was prescribed to those before you that you may learn self restrain. Fasting is for a fixed number of days but if any of you is on a journey the prescribed number should be made up from days later. He that will give more of his free will it is better for him and it is better for you that you fast if you only knew.

You are happier now than you have ever been and filled with joy all the time.

You live happily ever after now and forever.

It's a happy universe and you enjoy its moment.

You are happy because you choose happy always.

Every cell in your body, mind and soul are at peace, healthy and happy.

Remaining happy and positive benefits you and others.

You live a happy life and laugh all the time.

You are peaceful, serene, happy and content.

You spread joy and happiness everywhere you go.

You deserve to be happy.

October 28

Revelation 4

Worship in Heaven

After this I looked and saw a door that opened in heaven. Then the voice that had spoken to me at first and that sounded like a trumpet said come up here I will show you what must happen next. Right then the spirit took control of me and there in heaven I saw a throne someone sitting on it. The one who was sitting there sparked like precious stones of jasper and carnelian. A rainbow that looked like an emerald surrounded the thrones.

Repentance

And Abraham prayed for his father's forgiveness only because of a promise he had made to him. When it became clear to him and Allah will has guided them for Allah has knowledge of all things. Unto Allah belongs the dominion and the heavens and the earth. He gives life. Allah is sufficient for me. On him is my trust he is the Lord of the throne of glory supreme.

We are happier now than we have ever been and filled with joy all the time.

We live happily ever after now and forever.

It's a happy universe and we enjoy its moment.

We are happy because we choose happy always.

Every cell in our body, mind and soul are at peace, healthy and happy.

Remaining happy and positive benefits us and others.

We live a happy life and laugh all the time.

We are peaceful serene, happy and content.

We spread joy and happiness everywhere we go.

We deserve to be happy.

October 29

John 9

Jesus Heals

Jesus you will see God work a miracle for him. As long as it is day we must do what the one who sent me wants me to do. When night comes no one can work. While I am in the world I am the light of the world. After Jesus said this he spit on the ground he made some mud and smeared it on the man's eyes. Then he said go and wash off the mud in Siloam pool. The man went and washed in Siloam which means one who is sent. When he had washed off the mud he could see.

The Heifer

Those who spend their substance in the cause of Allah and follow their reward is with the Lord. Kind words are better. Allah is free of all wants and he is most forbearing. And the likeness of those who spend their substance seeking to please Allah and to strengthen their souls is as a garden high and fertile rain falls on it but makes it yield a double increase of harvest.

I am grateful to be full of joy, happiness and love.

I am grateful to be happy and full of positive energy always.

I am grateful I see, hear, taste, touch, smell and feel good.

I am grateful to be joyful every moment.

I am grateful to be thankful and appreciate always.

I am grateful to spread positive energy to others.

I am grateful my life gets better and better always.

I am grateful to be naturally happy and joyous.

I am grateful to have a sense of peace and happiness within and around me.

I am grateful to be optimistic.

October 30

Psalm 35

A Prayer for Protection

Shield me and help me. Promise to save me. I will celebrate and be joyful because your Lord has saved me. You protect those in power. You see everything Lord. Defend me Lord God and prove that I am right by your standards.

The Cave

Say you my Lord knows best their number it is but few that know their real case, if Allah so wills and call your Lord to mind and say I hope that my Lord will guide me ever closer even then this to the right road. Allah knows best how long they stayed with him is the knowledge of the secrets of the heavens and the earth. How clearly he sees how finely he hears everything. Recite and teach what has been revealed to you in the book of the Lord.

You are grateful to be full of joy, happiness and love.

You are grateful to be happy and full of positive energy always.

You are grateful you see, hear, taste, touch, smell and feel good all the time.

You are grateful to be joyful every moment.

You are grateful to be thankful and appreciate always.

You are grateful to spread positive energy to others.

You are grateful your life gets better and better always.

You are grateful to be naturally happy and joyous.

You are grateful to have a sense of peace and happiness within and around you.

You are grateful to be optimistic and can make everyone happy always.

October 31

Hebrews 8

A Better Promise

What I mean is that we have a high priest who sits at the right side of God's great throne in heaven. He also serves as the priest in the most holy place inside the real tent there in heaven. This tent of worship was set up by the Lord. I tell the people of Israel this is my new agreement. The time will come when I the Lord will write my laws on their minds and hearts.

The Children of Israel

One day we shall call together all human beings with their respective moms those who are given their record in their right hand will read it with pleasure and they will be dealt with justly. Say O my Lord let my entry be by the gate of truth and honor and likewise my exit by the gate of truth and honor and grant me from your presence an authority to aid me. And say truth has now arrived.

We are grateful to be full of joy, happiness and love.

We are grateful to be happy and full of positive energy.

We are grateful we see, hear, taste, touch, smell and feel good all the time.

We are grateful to be joyful every moment.

We are grateful to be thankful and appreciate always.

We are grateful to spread positive energy to others.

We are grateful our life gets better and better always.

We are grateful to be naturally happy and joyous.

We are grateful to have a sense of peace and happiness within and around us.

We are grateful to be optimistic and can make everyone happy always.

November 1

1 Corinthians 15:45

Bodies from Heaven

The first man was named Adam and the scriptures tell us that he was a living person. Jesus who may be called the last Adam is a life giving spirit. We see that the one with a spiritual body did not come first. He came after the one who had a physical body. The first man was made from the dust of the earth but the second man came from heaven. Everyone on earth has a body. And everyone in heaven has a body like the body of the one who came from heaven.

The Pilgrimage

My house for those who compass it round and stand up or bow or prostrate themselves therein pray. And proclaim the pilgrimage among men they will come to you on foot and mounted up on every kind of camel lean on account of journeys through deep and distant mountain highways.

I have complete faith in myself and God.

God's purpose for him and us is abundance, joy, love, good health and wealth.

I am Gods beloved perfect child.

I have faith the right people and circumstances naturally appear.

God loves me and forgives and guides us always.

I am faithful, good, loyal and true forever.

My faith can move mountains.

God is eternally begotten fully divine, and supremely joyful.

I am blessed with a grateful pure heart and breastplate of righteousness.

I believe the sun and sons have power.

November 2

1 Thessalonians 2:1

Paul's Work

My friend you know that our time wasn't wasted. As you remember God gave us the courage to tell you the good news about him. We didn't have any hidden motives when we won you over. God was pleased to trust us with his message. We speak to please people to please God who knows our motives. Christ is the one who sent us. Both you and God are witnesses that we were pure and honest and innocent in our dealings with you followers of the Lord.

Sad

We have revealed to you this Book with Our Blessing, so that the wise might ponder its revelations and take warning. We gave Solomon to David and he was a good and faithful servant.

You have complete faith in yourself and God.

God's purpose for him and us is abundance, joy, love, good health and wealth.

You are Gods beloved perfect child.

You have faith the right people and circumstances naturally appear.

God loves you and forgives and guides you always.

You are faithful, good, loyal and true forever.

Your faith can move mountains.

God is eternally begotten fully divine, and supremely joyful.

You are blessed with a grateful pure heart and breastplate of righteousness.

You believe the sun and sons have power.

November 3

Psalm 149

A New Song of Praise

Shout praises to the Lord. Sing him a new song of praise. Whom his loyal people meet. People of Israel rejoice because of their creator. People of Zion celebrate because of your king. Praise his name by dancing and playing music on harps and tambourines. The Lord is pleased with his people and he gives victory to those who are humble.

The Narrations

Everything that exists will perish except his own face. To him belongs the command and to him will you all be brought back. Allah will certainly know those who are true. For those whose hopes are in the meeting with Allah in the hereafter let them strive for a term appointed. Allah hears and knows all things. And if we strive with might and maim they do so for their own souls for Allah is free of all needs from all creation.

We have complete faith in ourselves and God.

God's purpose for him and us is abundance, joy, love, good health and wealth.

We are Gods beloved perfect child.

We have faith the right people and circumstances come.

God loves us and forgives and guides us always.

We are faithful, good, loyal and true forever.

Our faith can move mountains.

God is eternally begotten fully divine.

We are blessed with grateful pure hearts and breastplates of righteousness.

We believe the sun and sons have power.

November 4

Acts 13:23

A Promise

God promised that someone from David's family would come to save the people of Israel and that one is Jesus. But before Jesus came John was telling everyone in Israel to turn back to God and be baptized when Johns work was almost done he said who do you people think that I am? Do you think I am the promised one? God made a promise to our ancestors it is just on the second psalm says about Jesus you are my son because today I have become your father. God raised Jesus.

The Bee

To Allah belongs the mystery of the heavens and the earth the decision of the hour of judgment is as the twinkling of an eye or even quickest for Allah has power over all things. It is he who brought you forth from the wombs of your mothers when he gave you hearing and sight and intelligence and affections that you may give thanks to Allah.

I am grateful to be accepted into Gods kingdom because I am born again.

I am grateful Gods power is in me.

I am grateful I follow and believe in Jesus.

I am grateful God meets all my needs and wants.

I am grateful I set my heart, mind, body and soul on God and heavenly things.

I am grateful to trust God.

I am grateful to serve, please and impress God always.

I am grateful I have faith in the universe.

I am grateful God is in charge of everyone everywhere.

November 5

Psalm 2

A Prayer for Help

Please help me Lord and all who were faithful and all who were loyal have appeared. Lord tells them I will do something. I'll rescue all. Our Lord you are true to your promises and your word is like silver burned seven times in a fiery furnace. You will protect us and always keep us safe from those people I trust your love and I feel like celebrating because you rescued me. You have been good to me Lord and I will sing about you I am your chosen one.

Yusuf

Over all that we say be Allah the witness and guardian. Further he said o my sons enter not all by one gate enter you by different gates. None can command except Allah. On him do I put my trust.

You are grateful to be accepted into Gods kingdom because you are born again.

You are grateful Gods power is in you.

You are grateful you follow and believe in Jesus.

You are grateful God meets all your needs and wants.

You are grateful you set your heart, mind, body and soul on God and heavenly things.

You are grateful to trust God.

You are grateful to serve, please and impress God always.

You are grateful you have faith in the universe.

You are grateful God is in charge of everyone everywhere always.

November 6

Acts 6:1

Taken to Heaven

While the apostles were still with Jesus they asked him Lord are you now going to give Israel its king again? Jesus said to them you don't need to know the time of these events that only the father controls. But the Holy Spirit will come upon you and give you power. After Jesus had said this and while they were watching he was taken up into a cloud. They kept looking up into the sky. Jesus has been taken to heaven.

Mary

Allah does advance in guidance those who seek guidance and the things that endure. Good deeds are best in the sight of your Lord as rewards are best in respect of their eventual return. To us shall return all that he talks of and he shall appear before us. The day we shall gather the righteous to Allah most gracious like a band presented before a king of honors. The skies are ready to burst the earth to split asunder.

We are grateful to be accepted into God's kingdom because we are born again.

We are grateful God's power is in us.

We are grateful we follow and believe in Jesus.

We are grateful God meets all our needs and wants.

We are grateful we set our heart, mind, body and soul on God and heavenly things.

We are grateful to trust God.

We are grateful to serve, please and impress God always.

We are grateful we have faith in the universe.

We are grateful God is in charge of everyone everywhere.

November 7

Ephesians 6:14

Saving Power of Prayer

Be strong pray by the power of the spirit. Stay alert. Pray that I will give the message to speak. Be ready. Let the truth be like a belt around your waist and let God's justice protect you like armor. Tell the good news about peace be like the shoes on your feet. Let your faith like a shield. Let God's saving power be like a helmet and for a sword use God's message that comes from the spirit. Always explain the mystery about the good news.

The Woman

Allah belongs all things in the heavens and on the earth. And Allah is free of all wants and worthy of all praise. Enough is Allah to carry through all affairs. It were his will he could destroy you o mankind create another race for he has power this to do. In this life Allah's gift is the reward both of this life and of the hereafter for Allah is he that hears and sees all things.

I have a loving supportive family.

I am loving, open and affectionate with my family.

I respond to family needs by serving, care, love and attention.

I am very close with my happy and healthy family.

I treat my family including all pets very well.

I enjoy family get togethers.

I give all family members equal love and attention.

My family is healthy, happy, safe and loved.

My family treats me with respect, love are understanding.

I have a positive, patient and loving family.

November 8

Psalm 107

The Lord is Good to His People

Shout praises to the Lord. He is good to us and his love never fails. Everyone the Lord has rescued. You should praise the Lord for his love and for his wonderful things he does for all of us. To everyone he gives something to drink, to everyone he gives good things to eat. Our God I am faithful to you with all my heart and you can trust me. I will sing and play music for you with all that I am. I will start playing my harps before the sun rises. I will praise you Lord for everyone to hear.

Al-Tahrim

Allah has already ordained for you O men the absolution of your oaths in some cases and Allah is your protector and he is full of knowledge and wisdom. If you turn in repentance to him your hearts are inclined. Truly Allah is his protector and Gabriel and are among those who believe furthermore the angels will back him up. O you who believe save yourselves and your families.

You have a loving supportive family.

You are loving, open and affectionate with your family.

You respond to family needs by serving, care, love and attention.

You are very close with your happy and healthy family.

You treat your family including all pets very well.

You enjoy family get together.

You give all family members equal love and attention.

Your family is healthy, happy, safe and loved.

Your family treats you with respect, love are understanding.

You have a positive, patient and loving family.

November 9

Luke 20:35

Traveling Bags

Jesus asked his disciples when I sent you out without a moneybag or a traveling bag or sandals did you need anything? No they answered Jesus told them but now if you have a moneybag take it with you. Also take a traveling bag and if you don't have a sword sell some of your clothes and buy one. This was written about me and it will soon come true. The disciples said Lord here are two swords.

Repentance

Those who believe in Allah and the last day. Allah knows well those who do their duty. He is our protector and on Allah let the believers put their trust. You expect for us any fate other than victory. In reality Allah and his apostle will soon give us of his bounty to Allah do we turn our hopes.

We have a loving supportive family.

We are loving, open and affectionate with our family.

We respond to family needs by serving, care, love and attention.

We are very close with our happy and healthy family.

We treat our family including all pets very well.

We enjoy family get togethers.

We give all family members equal love and attention.

Our family is healthy, happy, safe and loved.

Our family treats us with respect, love are understanding.

We have a positive, patient and loving family.

November 10

Luke 10:21

Jesus Thanks his Father

At that same time Jesus felt the joy that comes from the Holy Spirit and he said, my father Lord of heaven and earth. I am grateful that you hid all this from wise educated people. Yes father that is what pleases you and my father has given me everything. He is the only one who knows the son. The only one who really knows the father is the son. But the son wants to tell others about the father so that they can know him too.

The Confederates

Allah is witness to all things. Allah and his angels send blessings on the prophet O you who believe. Send your blessings on him and salute him with all respect.

I am grateful for my healthy, happy and loving good looking family.

I am grateful to communicate well with my family.

I am grateful to spend good quality time with my family.

I am grateful to treat my family with love and understanding.

I am grateful to be a capable, caring and helpful family member always.

I am grateful to have a loving, patient and kind family always.

I am grateful to be responsible and respectful towards each family member.

I am grateful my family treats me with love, respect and understanding.

I am grateful for my family and we share peace always.

I am grateful to do my best for my family.

November 11

John 8:12

Jesus is the Light of the World

Once again Jesus spoke to the people. This time he said I am the light for the world. Follow me. You will have the light that gives life. I know where I come from and where I am going. If I did judge I would judge fairly because I would not be doing it alone. The father who sent me is here with me.

Al-Isra

O my Lord! Let my entry be by the gate of truth and honor and likewise my exit by the gate of truth and honor and grant me from your presence an authority to aid me. And say, "Truth has now arrived." We send down stage by stage in the Qur'an that which is a healing and a mercy to those who believe.

You are grateful for your healthy, happy and loving good looking family.

You are grateful to communicate well with your family.

You are grateful to spend good quality time with your family.

You are grateful to treat your family with love and understanding.

You are grateful to be a capable caring and helpful family member always.

You are grateful to have a loving, patient and kind family.

You are grateful to be responsible and respectful towards each family member.

You are grateful your family treats you with love, respect and understanding.

You are grateful for your family and we share peace always.

November 12

2 Corinthians 13

Jesus Comes

I am coming to you. In the mouth of two or three witness shall every word be established. I told you before and foretell you as if I were present. Ye seek proof of Christ speaking in me which to you word is mighty in you.

The Believers

And to you there came Joseph in times gone by with clear signs. No apostle will Allah send after him. The ways and means of reaching the heavens and that I may mount up to the Allah of Moses. The man who believed said further: O my people follow me. I will lead you to the path of right. O my people. The hereafter that is the home that will last.

We are grateful for our healthy, happy and loving, good looking family.

We are grateful to communicate well with our family.

We are grateful to spend good quality time with our family.

We are grateful to treat our family with love and understanding.

We are grateful to be a capable caring and helpful family members always.

We are grateful to have a loving, patient and kind family always.

We are grateful to be responsible and respectful towards each family member.

We are grateful our family treats us with love, respect and understanding.

We are grateful for our family and we share peace always.

We are grateful to do our best for our family.

November 13

Romans 12:6

A Living Sacrifice to God

In his grace, God has given us different gifts for doing certain things well. So if God has given you the ability to prophesy, speak out with as much faith as God has given you. If your gift is serving others, serve them well. If you are a teacher, teach well. If your gift is to encourage others, be encouraging. If it is giving, give generously. If God has given you leadership ability take the responsibility seriously. And if you have a gift for showing kindness to others do it gladly. Really love them. Love each other with genuine affection and take delight in honoring each other. Work and serve the Lord enthusiastically. Rejoice in our confident hope. Be patient.

The Bee

Inevitable comes to pass the command of Allah. Glory to him. He does send down his angels with inspiration of his command to such of his servants as he pleases saying, warn man that there is God so do your duty unto me. He has created the heavens and the earth for with truth.

Joy is in my heart and life now and forever.

I project joy to everyone I interact with.

I live in a natural state of joy, bliss, peace and happiness.

I choose joy and love and I receive it.

Joy, peace, wealth and good health are all around me.

I joyfully honor the flow of life.

I have cultivated a good sense of humor and joy follows it.

I keep an attitude of gratitude and joy always.

I know my path is full of fun, safe and joyous experiences.

I am filled with joy and contentment all the time.

November 14

Hebrews 1:5

The Son is Greater than the Angels

For God never said to any angel what he said to Jesus. You are my son today I have become your father. God also said I will be his father and he will be my son. And when he brought his firstborn son into the world God said let all of Gods angels worship him. Regarding the angels he says he sends his angels like the winds his servants like flames of fire but to the son he says, your throne o God endures forever and ever you rule with a scepter of justice. You love justice. Therefore o God your God has anointed you pouring out the oil of joy on you more than on anyone else.

Al-Baqra

When they have purified themselves, you may approach them in any manner, time or place ordained for you by Allah. For Allah loves those who turn to him constantly and loves those who keep themselves pure and clean. And know that you are to meet him in the hereafter and give these good things to those who believe.

Joy is in your heart and life now and forever.

You project joy to everyone you interact with.

You live in a natural state of joy, bliss, peace and happiness.

You choose joy and love and you receive it.

Joy, peace, wealth and good health are all around you.

You joyfully honor the flow of life.

You have cultivated a good sense of humor and joy.

You keep an attitude of gratitude and joy always.

Your path is full of fun, safe and joyous experiences.

You are filled with joy and contentment all the time.

November 15

Acts 12: 7

Peter's Miraculous Escape

Suddenly there was a bright light and an angel of the Lord stood before Peter. The angel to awaken him and said get up and then the angel told him get dressed and put on your sandals and he did now put on your coat and follow me the angel ordered. So Peter left following the angel. Peter finally came to his senses. It's really true he said the Lord has sent his angel and saved me.

Az-Zumar

To Allah belongs exclusively the right to grant intercession. To him belongs the dominion of the heavens and the earth. In the end it is to him that you shall be brought back. When Allah the one and only is mentioned they are filled with joy. Say, o Allah! Creator of the heavens and the earth. Knower of all that is hidden and open. It is you that will judge between your servants.

Joy is in our heart and life now and forever.

We project joy to everyone we interact with.

We live in a natural state of joy, bliss, peace and happiness.

We choose joy and love and we receive it.

Joy, peace, wealth and good health are all around us.

We joyfully honor the flow of life.

We have cultivated a good sense of humor and joy.

We keep an attitude of gratitude and joy always.

We know our path is full of fun, safe and joyous experiences.

We are filled with joy and contentment all the time.

November 16

Ephesians 3:9

God's Mysterious Plan Revealed

I was chosen to explain to everyone this mysterious plan that God the creator of all things had kept secret from the beginning. God's purpose in all this was to use the church to display his wisdom in its rich variety to all the rulers and authorities in the heavenly places. This was his eternal plan, which he carried out through Christ Jesus our Lord. Because of Christ and our faith in him we can now come boldly and confidently into God's presence.

The Spider

Verily Allah does know everything. He is exalted in power, wise and such are the parables we set forth for mankind but understand them who have knowledge. Allah created the heavens and the earth in true proportion. Verily in that is a sign for those who believe.

I am grateful for joy, peace, and happiness all the time.

I am grateful every atom of my being resonates with joy and love.

I am grateful I am love, abundance and joy.

I am grateful to enjoy every aspect of my life.

I am grateful to be blessed with a future of love, joy, peace and freedom.

I am grateful to enjoy eating healthy and nutritious things.

I am grateful to enjoy all other people and for joyful dreams of love and remember them.

I am grateful to experience the highest vibrations of joy always.

I am grateful joy is a healing choice and I accept and receive it now and always.

November 17

2 Thessalonians 3:12

Sharing Peace

We command people and urge them in the name of the Lord Jesus Christ to work to earn their own living. As for the rest of you dear brothers and sisters do good. May the Lord of peace himself give you his peace at all times and in every situation. The Lord be with you all. May the grace of our Lord Jesus Christ be with you all.

Al-Kahf

As to those who believe and work righteousness verily we shall reward any who do a single righteous deed. For them will be gardens of eternity beneath them rivers will flow they will be adorned therein with bracelets of gold and they will wear green garment of fine silk. They will recline therein on raised thrones. How good the recompense. How beautiful a couch to recline on.

You are grateful for joy, peace, and happiness all the time.

You are grateful every atom of your being resonates with joy and love.

You are grateful you are love, abundance and joy.

You are grateful to enjoy every aspect of your life.

You are grateful to be blessed with a future of love, joy, peace and freedom.

You are grateful to enjoy eating healthy and nutritious things.

You are grateful to enjoy all other people and for joyful dreams of love and remember them.

You are grateful to experience the highest vibrations of joy.

You are grateful joy is a healing choice and you accept and receive it now and always.

November 18

1 Corinthians 13:7

Love is the Goal

Love is always hopeful and endures through every circumstance. Love will last forever. Three things will last forever—faith, hope and love and the greatest of these is love. Let love be your highest goal. You will be speaking by the power of the spirit but it will all be mysterious.

Jah

For it is indeed a message of instruction. Therefore let whoso will keep it in remembrance. It is in books held greatly in honor. Exalted in dignity kept pure and holy. Written by the hands of scribes. Honorable and pious and just.

We are grateful for joy, peace, and happiness all the time.

We are grateful every atom of our being resonates with joy and love.

We are grateful we are love, abundance and joy.

We are grateful to enjoy every aspect of our life.

We are grateful to be blessed with a future of love, joy, peace and freedom.

We are grateful to enjoy eating healthy and nutritious things.

We are grateful to enjoy all other people and for joyful dreams of love and remember them.

We are grateful to experience the highest vibrations of joy.

We are grateful joy is healing choice and we accept and receive it now and always.

November 19

Philippians 3:12

Be Perfect in Christ

Press on to that perfection for Christ Jesus. I focus on this one thing looking forward to what lies ahead. I press on to reach the end of the race and receive the heavenly prize for which God through Christ Jesus is calling us. Therefore my dear brothers and sisters stay true to the Lord, I love you and long to see you dear friends for you are my joy and the crown I receive for my work.

An- Nahl

And we sent down the book to you for the express purpose that you should make clear to them those things in which they differ and that it should be a guide and a mercy to those who believe. And Allah sends down rain from the skies and gives therewith life to the earth, verily in this is a sign for those who listen.

The door to my heart opens I move from forgiveness to love.

I listen to my feelings and I am gentle with myself.

I give myself the gift of freedom and move to joy.

I am willing to forgive always.

I move beyond forgiveness and have compassion for all.

I am forgiving, loving, gentle and kind.

I forgive myself and correct myself to perfection.

I am not responsible for other people and only wish to help and be my best for them.

I know all of life's lessons are a learning process and I accept this.

I forgive everyone everywhere always.

November 20

1 Corinthians 7:32

Devoted to the Lord

I want you to be free of the concerns of this life. Man can spend his time doing the Lords work and thinking how to please him. In the same way a woman can be devoted to the Lord and holy in body and in spirit.

As-Sajda

Such is he the knower of all things, hidden and open, the exalted in power, the merciful. He who has made everything which he has created most He began the creation of man with clay. And made his progeny from a quintessence of the nature of a fluid. But he fashioned him in due proportion, and breathed into him something of his spirit. And he gave the faculties of hearing and sight and feeling and understanding.

The door to your heart opens you move from forgiveness to love.

You listen to your feelings and you are gentle with yourself.

You give yourself the gift of freedom and move to joy.

You are willing to forgive always.

You move beyond forgiveness and have compassion for all.

You are forgiving, loving, gentle and kind.

You forgive yourself and correct yourself to perfection.

You are not responsible for other people and only wish to help and be your best for them.

You know all of life's lessons are a learning process and you accept this.

You forgive everyone everywhere always.

November 21

James 5:14

Pray

You should call for the elders of the church to come and pray over you, anointing you with oil in the name of the Lord. Such a prayer offered in faith will heal the sick, and the Lord will make you well. You will be forgiven. Confess to each other and pray for each other so that you may be healed. The earnest prayer of a righteous person has great power and produces wonderful results.

Al-Mumenoon

I have rewarded them this day for their patience and constance they are indeed the ones that have achieved bliss. Therefore exalted be Allah the king, the reality, the Lord of the throne of honor. So say, o my Lord! Grant us forgiveness and mercy for you are the best of those who show mercy.

The door to our heart opens we move from forgiveness to love.

We listen to our feelings and we are gentle with ourselves.

We give ourselves the gift of freedom and move to joy.

We are willing to forgive always.

We move beyond forgiveness and have compassion for all.

We are forgiving loving, gentle and kind.

We forgive myself and correct myself to perfection.

We are not responsible for other people and only wish to help and be our best for them.

We know all of life's lessons are a learning process and we accept this.

We forgive everyone everywhere always.

November 22

Colossians 2:2

Be Encouraged

I want them to be encouraged by strong ties of love. I want them to have complete confidence that they understand God's mysterious plan, which is Christ himself. In him lie hidden all the treasures of wisdom and knowledge. I rejoice that you are living as you should and that your faith in Christ is strong.

Kitab AL-Iman

They were created by him the exalted in power full of knowledge. Yes the same that has made for you the earth like a carpet spread out and has made for you roads and channels therein in order that you may find guidance on the way. We send down from time to time rain from the sky in due measure and we raise to life therewith a land.

I am grateful to forgive myself and forgive others easily and quickly.

I am grateful to follow the path of forgiveness and love.

I am grateful to live my life as pure and innocent as possible.

I am grateful to be forgiving, loving and gentle always.

I am grateful to move beyond forgiveness into understanding.

I am grateful I forgive everyone from my life in the past.

I am grateful to set myself free from my past.

I am grateful to accept the best and receive it always.

I am grateful to grow stronger, faster, wiser, healthier, smarter, prettier and richer every day.

I am grateful to achieve peace by forgiving easily and wisely and quickly.

November 23

Titus 2:1

Good Living

Promote the kind of living that reflects wholesome teaching. Teach the older men to exercise self-control to be worthy of respect and to live wisely have sound faith and be filled with love and patience. Teach older women to live in a way that honors God. Teach others to be good. The older women must train the younger women to love their husbands and their children to live wisely and be pure to work in their homes to do good. Encourage the young men to live wisely.

Al-Haqqah

On that day shall the great event come to pass. That day shall you be brought to judgment. Then he that will be given his record in his right hand will say ah here read you my record. I did really understand my account would one day reach me. And he will be in a life of bliss in a garden on high.

You are grateful to forgive yourself and others.

You are grateful to follow the path of forgiveness and love.

You are grateful to live your life purely and innocently.

You are grateful to be forgiving, loving and gentle always.

You are grateful to move into understanding.

You are grateful you forgive everyone.

You are grateful to set yourself free from your past.

You are grateful to accept the best and receive it always.

You are grateful to grow stronger, faster, wiser, healthier, smarter, prettier and richer every day.

You are grateful to achieve peace by forgiving easily and wisely and quickly.

November 24

1 Timothy 3:16

Faith's Mystery

This is the great mystery of our faith. Christ was revealed in a human body and vindicated by the spirit. He was seen by angels and announced to the nations. He was believed in throughout the world and taken to heaven in glory. Since everything God created is good, we should receive it with thanks. For we know it is made acceptable by the word of God and prayer.

Al- Ankaboot

But those who believe and work deeds of righteousness to them shall we give a home in heaven lofty mansions beneath which flow rivers to dwell therein forever an excellent reward for those who do good. Those who persevere in patience and put their trust in their Lord and cherisher.

We are grateful to forgive ourselves and others.

We are grateful to follow the path of forgiveness and love.

We are grateful to live our life as a pure and innocent as possible.

We are grateful to be forgiving, loving and gentle always.

We are grateful to move beyond forgiveness into understanding.

We are grateful I forgive everyone from our life in the past.

We are grateful to set ourselves free from our past.

We are grateful to accept the best and receive it always.

We are grateful to grow stronger, faster, wiser, healthier, smarter, prettier and richer every day.

We are grateful to achieve peace by forgiving easily and wisely and quickly.

November 25

John 16:33

Eternal Life is Earned

Take heart because I have overcome the world. After saying all these things Jesus looked up to heaven and said father the hour has come glorify your son so he can give glory back to you. For you have given him authority over everyone. He gives eternal life to each one you have given him and this is the way to have eternal life to know you the only true God and Jesus Christ the one you sent to earth.

As- Saffat

And we gave him the good news of Isaac a prophet one of the righteous. We blessed him and Isaac but of their progeny that do right. We bestowed our favor on Moses and Aaron and we helped them so they were victorious and we gave them the book which helps to make things clear. And we guided them to the straightway and we left this blessing for them among generations to come in later times.

I pay close attention to my dreams for divine guidance.

My dreams always have a deep spiritual purpose.

I use my dreams to manifest my desires.

God speaks to me through my dreams.

Angels and messengers of love come to me in my dreams.

I am able to interpret my valuable dreams well.

My dreams give me inspiration and value and divine guidance always.

My dreams are always good and positive.

My sleep provides rest and dreams with real life answers.

I am a lucid vivid dreamer and I remember them all the time.

November 26

1 Timothy 4:6

God's Servant

Physical training is good but training for godliness is much better, promising benefits in this life and in the life to come. This is a trustworthy saying and everyone should accept it. Be an example to all believers in what you say in the way you live in your love your faith and your purity.

Fussilat

In the case of those who say, our Lord is Allah and further stand straight and steadfast the angels descend on them from time to time. Receive the glad tidings of the garden of bliss the which you were promised. We are your protectors in this life and in the hereafter therein shall you have all that you ask for. A hospitable gift from one of forgiving most merciful.

You pay close attention to your dreams for divine guidance.

Your dreams always have a deep spiritual purpose.

You use your dreams to manifest my desires.

God speaks to you through your dreams and you remember all of them.

Angels and messengers of love come to you in your dreams.

You are able to interpret your valuable dreams well.

Your dreams give you inspiration and value and divine guidance always.

Your dreams are always good and positive.

Your sleep provides rest and dreams with real life answers.

You are a lucid vivid dreamer and you remember them all the time.

November 27

Ephesians 3:10

Faith in Christ

God's purpose in all this was to use the church to display his wisdom in its rich variety to all the rulers and authorities in the heavenly places. This was his eternal plan, which he carried out through Christ Jesus our Lord. Because of Christ and our faith in him we can now come boldly and confidently into God's presence.

Al-Akhir

It is to Allah that the end and the beginning of all things belongs. How many so ever be the angels in the heavens. Allah has given leave for whom he pleases and that he is acceptable to him.

We pay close attention to our dreams for divine guidance.

Our dreams always have a deep spiritual meaning and purpose.

We use our dreams to manifest our desires.

God speaks to us through our dreams and we remember all of them.

Angels and messengers of love come to us in our dreams.

We are able to interpret our valuable dreams easily and quickly.

Our dreams give us inspiration and value and divine guidance always.

Our dreams are always good, uplifting, spiritually guided and positive.

Our sleep is safe and secure providing dreams with real life answers.

We are lucid vivid dreamers and we remember them all the time.

November 28

Hebrews 12:22

Names in Heaven

You have come to mount Zion, to the city of the living God, the heavenly Jerusalem and to countless thousands of angels in joyful gathering. You have come to the assembly of God's firstborn children whose names are written in heaven. You have come to God himself who is the judge over all things. You have come to the spirit of the righteous ones in heavens who have been made perfect.

Al-Ankabut

Those who believe and work deeds of righteousness and believe in the revelation sent down to Muhammad for it is the truth from the Lord, he will improve their condition.

I am grateful to be a lucid, vivid, good dreamer.

I am grateful to be fully aware and in control of my dreams.

I am grateful my dream consciousness is strong, reliable, guarded and helpful.

I am grateful my dream memory is perfect and accurate.

I am grateful to remember my dreams in high detail.

I am grateful to have excellent dream awareness, interpretation and reactions.

I am grateful to be completely safe and secure in my dreams.

I am grateful I can see my goals in my dreams.

I am grateful my dreams guide me in the right direction all the time.

I am grateful God speaks to me all the time.

November 29

Acts 1:5

Water Baptizes

I baptize with water. Repent and turn to God. Someone is coming soon who is greater than I am so much greater. He will baptize you with the Holy Spirit and with fire. He is ready. He will clean up the threshing area, gathering the wheat into his barn. After his baptism as Jesus came up out of the water.

Jah

Freeing man, give of food in a day of privation. Then will he be of those who believe, and enjoin patience constancy and self-restraint and enjoin deeds of kindness and compassion. Such are the companions of the right hand.

You are grateful to be a lucid, vivid, good dreamer.

You are grateful to be fully aware and in control of your dreams.

You are grateful your dream consciousness is strong, reliable, guarded and helpful.

You are grateful your dream memory is perfect and accurate.

You are grateful to remember your dreams in high detail.

You are grateful to have excellent dream awareness, interpretation and reactions.

You are grateful to be completely safe and secure in your dreams.

You are grateful you can see your goals in your dreams.

You are grateful your dreams guide you in the right direction all the time.

You are grateful God speaks to you all the time.

November 30

1 Thessalonions 2:9

Treat Others Good

Night and day we toiled to earn a living as we preached Gods good news to you. You yourselves are our witnesses and so is God that we were devout and honest toward all of you believers. And you know that we treated each of you as a father treats his own children. We pleaded with you encouraged and urged you to love your lives in a way that God would consider worthy. For he called you to share in his kingdom and glory.

Al-Kahf

Allah knows best how long they stayed; with him is the knowledge of the secrets of the heavens and the earth; how clearly he sees how finely he hears everything. And recite and teach what has been revealed to you of the book of your Lord. And keep your soul content with those who call on their Lord morning and evening, seeking his face.

We are grateful to be lucid, vivid, good dreamers.

We are grateful to be fully aware in our dreams.

We are grateful our dream consciousness is strong, reliable, guarded and helpful.

We are grateful our dream memory is perfect and accurate.

We are grateful to remember our dreams in high detail.

We are grateful to have excellent dream awareness, interpretation and reactions.

We are grateful to be secure in our dreams.

We are grateful we can see our goals in our dreams.

We are grateful our dreams guide us in the right direction.

We are grateful God speaks to us all the time.

December 1

John 1:29

Chosen One

Look the Lamb of God! He is the one I was talking about when I said a man is coming after me who is far greater than I am for he existed before me. I did recognize him as the messiah but I have been baptizing with water so that he might be revealed to Israel. Then John testified, I saw the Holy Spirit descending like a dove from heaven and resting upon him. I saw this happen to Jesus so I testify that he is the chosen one of God.

An-Nur

Yes to Allah belongs the dominion of the heavens and the earth and to Allah is the final goal of all. Do you see that Allah makes the clouds move gently then joins them together then makes them into a heap? Then will you see rain issue forth from their midst. It is Allah who alternates the night and the day Verily in these things is an instructive example for those who have vision.

I travel to the most beautiful places.

Curiosity leads me to interesting safe, comfortable places.

Every time I travel I arrive at my destination safely.

I travel in style, luxury, ease and comfort.

I can move anywhere and resources always are available.

I travel often for business and pleasure.

I always receive help and guidance when I need it.

My journey to every destination is safe, affordable, comfortable, peaceful, fun and enjoyable.

I am rewarding myself with new fun traveling experiences.

All my journeys are safe, smooth, affordable, and comfortable always.

December 2

Romans 15:1

Do What is Right

We who are strong must be considerate of those who are sensitive. We must please ourselves. We should help others do what is right and build them up in the Lord. And the scriptures give us hope and encouragement as we wait patiently for God's promises to be fulfilled. May God who gives this patience and encouragement help you live in complete harmony with each other.

Al- Qasas

Move your hand into your bosom and it will come forth clean and close to your side to guard. Those are two credentials from your Lord to pharaoh and his chiefs.

You travel to the most beautiful places.

Curiosity leads you to interesting safe, comfortable places always.

Every time you travel you arrive at your destination quickly and safely.

You travel in style, luxury, ease and comfort.

You can move anywhere you want and resources always are available.

You travel often for business and pleasure.

You always receive help and guidance when you need it.

Your journey to every destination is safe, affordable, comfortable, peaceful, fun and enjoyable.

You are rewarding yourself with new fun traveling experiences.

All your journeys are safe, smooth, affordable, and comfortable always.

December 3

1 Corinthians 11:1

Imitate Christ

Be imitators of me, Christ. Now I praise you because you remember me in everything and hold firmly to the traditions just as I delivered them to you. I want you to understand that Christ is the head of every man and God is the head of Christ.

Al-Hadid

And those who believe in Allah and his apostles they are the sincere testify in the eyes of the Lord. They shall have their reward and their light. And forgiveness from Allah and his good pleasure for the devotees of Allah. Be you foremost in seeking forgiveness from your Lord and a garden of bliss, the width whereof is the width of heaven and earth prepared for those who believe in Allah and his apostle that is the grace of Allah which he bestows on who he pleases and Allah is the Lord of grace abounding.

We travel to the most beautiful places.

Curiosity leads us to interesting safe, comfortable places.

Every time we travel we arrive at our destination safely.

We travel in style, luxury, ease and comfort.

We can move anywhere and resources always are available.

We travel often for business and pleasure.

We always receive help and guidance when we need it.

Our journey to every destination is safe, affordable, comfortable, peaceful, fun and enjoyable.

We go on rewarding fun traveling experiences.

All my journeys are safe, smooth, affordable, and comfortable always.

December 4

Revelation 4:1

Heaven

Then as I looked I saw a door standing open in heaven and the same voice I had heard before spoke to me like a trumpet blast. The voice said come up here and I will show you what must happen after this and instantly I was in the spirit and I saw a throne in heaven and someone sitting on it. The one sitting on the throne was as brilliant as gemstones like jasper and carnelian. And the glow of an emerald circled his throne like a rainbow.

Al- Fath

Allah may help you with powerful help. It is he who sent down tranquility into the hearts of the believers that they may add faith to their faith for to Allah belongs the forces of the heavens and the earth and Allah is full of knowledge and wisdom. That he may admit the men and women who believe to gardens beneath which rivers flow to dwell therein forever and that is in the sight of Allah the highest achievement for man.

I am grateful to have the means to travel abroad.

I am grateful to be able to travel where I want and have unlimited resources.

I am grateful to be able to travel more for enjoyment.

I am grateful I appreciate how far I traveled.

I am grateful I have worldly fun experiences.

I am grateful to travel and live a life of my dreams.

I am grateful to travel safely and get along with everyone at my destination.

I am grateful to embark on amazing memorable journeys.

I am grateful to travel to exotic places.

December 5

Romans 2:5

Glory and Honour

Gods righteous judgment will be revealed. He will judge everyone according to what they have done. He will give eternal life to those who keep on doing good, seeking after the glory and honor and Immortality that God offers. There will be glory and honor and peace from God for all who do good.

Ar-Rahman

It he who has taught the Qur'an he has created man. He has taught him speech and intelligence. The sun and the moon follow courses exactly computed and the herbs and the trees both alike bow in adoration. And the firmament has he raised high and he has set up the balance of justice.

You are grateful to have the means to travel abroad.

You are grateful to be able to travel where you want and have unlimited resources.

You are grateful to be able to travel more for enjoyment.

You are grateful you appreciate how far you traveled.

You are grateful you have worldly fun experiences.

You are grateful to travel and live a life of your dreams.

You are grateful to travel safely and get along with everyone at your destination.

You are grateful to consciously embark on amazing memorable journeys.

You are grateful to explore the planet and travel to exotic places.

December 6

Hebrews 10:19

Trust the Priest

Dear brothers and sisters we can enter heavens most holy place. We have a high priest who rules over God's house, let us go right into the presence of God with sincere hearts fully trusting him. Our consciences have been sprinkled clean and our bodies have been washed with pure water.

The Great News

Concerning the great news about verily they shall soon come to know. And have we created you in pairs, made your sleep for rest and made the night a covering. Verily the day of sorting out is a thing appointed. The day the trumpet shall be sounded and you will come forth in crowds and the heavens shall be opened as if there were doors.

We are grateful to have the means to travel abroad.

We are grateful to be able to travel where we want and have unlimited resources.

We are grateful to be able to travel more for enjoyment.

We are grateful we appreciate how far we have traveled.

We are grateful we have worldly fun experiences.

We are grateful to travel and live a life of our dreams.

We are grateful to travel safely and get along with everyone at my destination.

We are grateful to consciously embark on amazing memorable journeys.

We are grateful to explore the planet and travel to exotic places.

December 7

John 17:1

God Glorifies His Son

Jesus looked up to heaven and said, "Father the hour has come. Glorify your son so he can give glory back to you. For you have given him authority over everyone. He gives eternal life to each one you have given him. And this is the way to have eternal life to know you the only true God and Jesus Christ the one you sent to earth. I brought glory to you here on earth by completing the work you gave me to do. Now father bring me into the glory we shared before the world began.

Al- Kareem

Those who sustain the throne of Allah and those around it sing glory and praise to their Lord believe in him and implore forgiveness for those who believe our Lord your reach is over all things in mercy and knowledge forgive and follow your path and preserve them.

I have great conversations with everyone always.

I have a good sense of humor in my communication.

My ability to communicate and positively connect is good.

I can communicate clearly, easily and very well always.

I can express myself honestly, attractively and wisely all the time.

I can flow with conversations easily.

I can talk, listen and communicate with ease, comfort and confidence.

Staying focused, relaxed and easy going is natural and fun.

Others enjoy communicating with me always.

My communication skills improve daily.

December 8

Revelation 2:26

Obey the Lord's Authority

To all who are victorious who obey to the very end. To them I will give authority over all the nations. They will rule the nations with an iron rod and smash them like clay pots. They will have the same authority I received from my father and I will also give them the morning star! Anyone with ears to hear must listen to the spirit and understand what he is saying to the churches.

Ta Ha

High above all is Allah the king the truth. Say O my Lord! Advance me in knowledge. We had already beforehand taken the covenant of Adam.

You have great conversations with everyone always.

You have a good sense of humor in your communication.

Your ability to communicate and positively connect is good.

You can communicate clearly, easily and very well always.

You can express yourself honestly, attractively and wisely all the time.

You can flow with conversations easily.

You can talk, listen and communicate with ease, comfort and confidence.

Staying focused, relaxed and easy going is natural and fun.

Others enjoy communicating with you always.

Your communication skills improve daily.

December 9

Acts 13:47

Thank the Lord

For the Lord gave us this command when he said, I have made you a light to the Gentiles to bring salvation to the farthest corners of the earth. When the Gentiles heard this they were very glad and thanked the Lord for his message and all who were chosen for eternal life became believers. The Lord's message spread throughout the region. Believers were filled with joy and with the Holy Spirit.

Al-Hadid

The apostle invites you to believe in your Lord, and has indeed taken your covenant if you are men of faith. He is the one who sends to his servants manifest signs that he may lead you into the light and verily Allah is to you most kind and merciful.

We have great conversations with everyone always.

We have a good sense of humor in our communication.

Our ability to communicate and positively connect is good.

We can communicate clearly, easily and very well always.

We can express yourself honestly, attractively and wisely all the time.

We can flow with conversations easily.

We can talk, listen and communicate with ease, comfort and confidence.

Staying focused, relaxed and easy going is natural and fun.

Others enjoy communicating with us always.

Your communication skills improve daily.

December 10

Luke 3:15

John Baptizes

Everyone was expecting the messiah to come soon, so they were eager to know whether John might be the messiah. John answered their questions by saying, "I baptize you with water but someone is coming soon who is greater than I am so much greater. He will baptize you with the Holy Spirit and with fire. John used many such warnings as he announced the good news to the people.

AL-Kahf

The things that endure, good deeds are best in the sight of your Lord, as rewards are best as the foundation for hopes. One day we shall remove the mountains and you will see the earth as a level stretch and we shall gather them all together.

I am grateful to enjoy communicating with others.

I am grateful to be an excellent communicator and leader.

I am grateful to be confident, outgoing and friendly.

I am grateful conversations with others are beneficial, easy and a pleasure.

I am grateful to have an enhanced ability to communicate giving and receiving information.

I am grateful to be approachable and use body language.

I am grateful to speak the truth with grave, sincerity, knowledge and compassion.

I am grateful it's easy for me to understand others.

I am grateful to communicate effectively, efficiently and correctly always.

I am grateful to be intelligent in all my interactions.

December 11

Matthew 7:7

Ask and Receive

Keep on asking and you will receive what you ask for. Keep on seeking and you will find. Keep on knocking and the door will be opened to you. For everyone who asks receives. Everyone who seeks finds and to everyone who knocks the door will be opened. Do to others whatever you would like them to do to you. This is the essence of all that is taught in the law and the prophets.

Ash- Shura

He bestows both males and females and he leaves barren whom he will. For he is full of knowledge and power. Allah should speak to him by inspiration or by sending of a messenger to reveal. With Allah's permission what Allah wills for he is most high most wise.

You are grateful to enjoy communicating with others.

You are grateful to be an excellent communicator and leader.

You are grateful to be confident, outgoing and friendly.

You are grateful conversations with others are beneficial, easy and a pleasure.

You are grateful to have an enhanced ability to communicate giving and receiving information.

You are grateful to be approachable and use body.

You are grateful to speak the truth with grave, sincerity, knowledge and compassion.

You are grateful it's easy for you to understand others.

You are grateful to communicate effectively, efficiently and correctly always.

You are grateful to be intelligent in all your interactions.

December 12

Matthew 22:36

Love Your God

Jesus replied you must love the Lord your God with all your heart, all your soul and all your mind. This is the first and greatest commandment a second, is equally important. Love your neighbor as yourself. The entire law and all the demands of the prophets based on these two commandments.

Al-Hashr

Allah is the sovereign, the holy one, the source of peace and perfection, the guardian of faith, the preserver of safety, the exalted in might, the irresistible, the supreme glory to Allah! High is he. He is Allah, the creator, the originator, the fashioner, to him belongs the most beautiful name whatever is in the heavens and on earth, does declare his praises and glory and he is the exalted in might the wise.

We are grateful to enjoy communicating with others.

We are grateful to be an excellent communicators.

We are grateful to be confident, outgoing and friendly.

We are grateful conversations with others are beneficial, easy and a pleasure.

We are grateful to have an enhanced ability to communicate giving and receiving information.

We are grateful use body language well.

We are grateful to speak the truth with grave, sincerity, knowledge and compassion.

We are grateful it's easy for us to understand others.

We are grateful to communicate effectively, efficiently and correctly always.

December 13

John 8:12

The Truth

The father who sent me is here with me. Your law requires two witnesses and the father who sent me is the other one. If you knew me you would know my father. The truth will set you free. Jesus told the people who had faith in him. If you keep on obeying what I have said, "Are my disciples?" You will know the truth and the truth will set you free.

The Sure Reality

Then when one blast is sounded on the trumpet. That day shall you be brought to judgment. He that will be given his record in his right hand will say, ah here read you my record. I did really understand that my account would one day reach me.

My thoughts, actions, words, deeds all support my commitment.

I am committed to making my dreams reality.

I am committed to being a positive role model.

I am committed to treating others as I would have them treat me.

I am committed to live a life of gratitude and love.

I am committed to finish what I start.

I have focused, positive, magical intentions always.

My intentions inspire good vibes, brilliant ideas and positive actions.

My word is my power.

I commit to giving 100% to achieve the life of perfection and love.

December 14

3 John 1

Obey the Truth

To my dear friend Gaius. I love you because we follow the truth. Dear friend and I pray that all goes well for you. I hope that you are as strong in body as I know you are in spirit. It makes me very happy when the Lord's followers come by and speak openly of you. Obey the truth. Brings me greater happiness to hear that my children are obeying the truth.

Jah

Moses said, My Lord has since invested me with judgment and wisdom and appointed me as one of the apostles. And this is the favor with which you do reproach me. Moses said the Lord and cherisher of the heavens and the earth and all between.

Your thoughts, actions, words, deeds all support your commitment.

You are committed to making your dreams reality.

You are committed to being a positive role model.

You are committed to treating others as you would have them treat you.

You are committed to live a life of gratitude and love.

You are committed to finish what you start.

You have focused positive magical intentions always.

Your intentions inspire good vibes, brilliant ideas and positive actions.

Your word is your power.

You commit to giving 100% to achieve the life of perfection and love.

December 15

Acts 2:17

God Gives His Spirit

When the last days come, I will give my spirit to everyone. Your sons and daughters will prophesy. Your young men will see visions and your old men will have dreams. In those days I will give my spirit to my servants both men and women and they will prophesy. I will work miracles in the sky above and wonders on the earth below.

Al-Qalam

A respite will I grant them truly powerful is my plan. The unseen is in their hands so that they can write it down. So wait with patience for the command of your Lord.

Our thoughts, actions, words, deeds all support our commitment.

We are committed to making our dreams reality.

We are committed to being positive role models.

We are committed to treating others as we would have them treat us.

We are committed to live a life of gratitude and love.

We are committed to finish what we start.

We have focused, positive, magical intentions always.

Our intentions inspire good vibes, brilliant ideas and positive actions.

Our word is our power.

We commit to giving 100% to achieve the life of perfection and love.

December 16

Matthew 10:42

Be Humble

Anyone who gives one of my most humble followers a cup of cool water just because that person is my follower will surely be rewarded. Jesus answered, my mother and my brothers are those people who hear and obey God's message.

Maryam

He said, I am indeed a servant of Allah: he has given me revelation and made me a prophet. And he has made me blessed wheresoever's I be, and has enjoined on me prayer and charity as long as I live. He has made me kind to my mother. So peace is on me. Such was Jesus the son of Mary it is a statement of truth. Glory be to him when he determines a matter he only says to it be and it is.

I am grateful daily commitment to my goals makes success happen.

I am grateful to support my partner unconditionally.

I am grateful to be in a lasting fun loving mutually entertaining and loving relationship.

I am grateful to be considerate in my relationships.

I am grateful there is natural connections and commitments in my relationships.

I am grateful all my goals are put into action.

I am grateful to stick to my goals and achieve them.

I am grateful to make a commitment to my soul mate.

I am grateful I back all my commitments with action, honesty and effort.

I am grateful to be committed to living a passionate, successful divine heavenly life.

December 17

Mark 9:7

This is My Son

A cloud passed over and covered them from the cloud a voice said, this is my son and I love him. Listen to what he says at once the disciples looked around but they saw only Jesus.

Believer

The revelation of this book is from Allah, exalted in power full of knowledge. Who forgives, accepts repentance, and is all bountiful. God is the final goal. Those who sustain the throne of Allah and those around it sing glory and praise to their Lord. Believe in him and implore forgiveness for those who believe, our Lord! Your reach is over all things in mercy and knowledge. Forgive then those who turn in repentance and follow your path.

You are grateful daily commitment to your goals makes success happen.

You are grateful to support your partner unconditionally.

You are grateful to be in a lasting fun loving mutually entertaining and loving relationship.

You are grateful to be considerate in your relationships.

You are grateful there is natural connections and commitments in your relationships.

You are grateful all your goals are and put into action.

You are grateful to stick to your goals and achieve them.

You are grateful to make a commitment to your soul mate.

You are grateful you back all your commitments with action, honesty and effort.

You are grateful to be committed to living a passionate, successful divine heavenly life.

December 18

Romans 10:5

Anyone Can Be Saved

Moses said that a person could become acceptable to God by obeying the law. He did this when he wrote if you want to live you must do all that the law commands. You will be saved if you honestly say Jesus is Lord and if you believe with all your heart that God raised him. God will accept you and save you if you truly believe.

Al-Hadid

We sent aforetime our apostles with clear signs and sent down with them the book and the balance of right that men may stand forth in justice and we sent down iron in which is material for mighty way as well as many benefits for mankind that Allah may test who it is that will help him and his apostles.

We are grateful daily commitment to our goals makes success happen.

We are grateful to support our partner unconditionally.

We are grateful to be in a lasting fun loving mutually entertaining and loving relationship.

We are grateful to be considerate in our relationships.

We are grateful there is natural connections and commitments in our relationships.

We are grateful all our goals are put into action.

We are grateful to stick to our goals and achieve them.

We are grateful to make a commitment to our soul mate.

We are grateful we back all our commitments with action, honesty and effort.

We are grateful to be committed to living a passionate, successful divine heavenly life.

December 19

2 Timothy 4

Finish the Race

I have finished the race and I have been faithful. So a crown will be given to me for pleasing the Lord. He judges fairly and on the Day of Judgment he will give a crown to me.

An-Nisa

Allah will admit him to gardens beneath which rivers flow and he who turn back. Allah's good pleasure was on the believers when they swore fealty to you under the tree. He knew what was in their hearts and he sent down tranquility to them and he rewarded them with a speedy victory.

I am grateful to do my best work with other children.

I accept children as they are.

I am vibrant and get along well with children.

I achieve successful results as a teacher.

I create healthy self-esteem and enlightenment in children.

I can open up all children's minds and hearts to their divine source.

I focus on being the best teacher.

I enjoy teaching and making learning fun, exciting and education.

I can help children be their best.

Opportunities for growth, learning and fun are available always.

December 20

Luke 15:4

Find Your Sheep

If any of you has a hundred sheep and one of them gets lost. What will you do? Won't you leave the 99 in the field and go look for the lost sheep until you find it? And when you find it you will be glad that you will put it on your shoulder and carry it home. Then you will call in your friends and neighbors and say let's celebrate. I've found my lost sheep.

The Pilgrimage

Allah will admit those who believe and work righteous deeds to gardens beneath which rivers flow they shall be adorned there in with bracelets of gold and pearls and their garments there will be silk. For they have been guided in this life to the purest of speeches they have been guided to the path of him who is worthy of all praise.

You are grateful to do my best work with other children.

You accept children as they are.

You are vibrant and get along well with children.

You achieve successful results as a teacher.

You create healthy self-esteem and enlightenment in children.

You can open up all children's minds and hearts to their divine source.

You focus on being the best teacher.

You enjoy teaching and making learning fun, exciting and education.

You can help children be their best.

Opportunities for growth, learning and fun are available always.

December 21

Luke 1:26

Birth of Jesus

One month later. God sent the angel Gabriel to the town of Nazareth in Galilee with a message for a virgin named Mary. She was engaged to Joseph from the family of King David. The angel greeted Mary and said you are truly blessed. The Lord is with you. Then the angel told Mary God is pleased with you and you will have a son. His name will be Jesus. He will be great and will be called the son of God most high.

Muhammad

Ask forgiveness and for men and women who believe for Allah knows how you move about and how you dwell in your homes. Verily we have granted you a manifest victory. Allah may help you with powerful help. It is he who sent down tranquility into the hearts of the believers.

We are grateful to do my best work with other children.

We accept children as they are.

We are vibrant and get along well with children.

We achieve successful results as a teacher.

We create healthy self-esteem and enlightenment in children.

We can open up all children's minds and hearts to their divine source.

We focus on being the best teacher.

We enjoy teaching and making learning fun, exciting and education.

We can help children be their best.

Opportunities for growth, learning and fun are available always.

December 22

2 Corinthians 2:7

Forgiven

You should forgive and comfort them. You should make them sure of your love for them. I also wrote because I wanted to test you and find out if you would follow my instructions. I will forgive anyone you forgive. Yes for your sake and with Christ as my witness. I have forgiven whatever needed to be forgiven.

The Criterion

Had it been our will we could have sent a Warner to every center of population. It is he who has set free the two bodies of flowing water. One palatable and sweet and the other sour and bitter.

I am grateful children are awesome, fun and innocent.

I am grateful children are very intelligent and fast learners.

I am grateful children provide deep unconditional love.

I am grateful children love to learn and learning is fun.

I am grateful to teach valuable lessons at school.

I am grateful to believe in my teaching abilities.

I am grateful for my many teaching talents and skills.

I am grateful to bring out the best in children and others.

I am grateful children love me, we get along well and respect each other.

December 23

Romans 12

God is Good

So I beg you to offer your bodies to him as a living sacrifice pure and pleasing. That's the most sensible way to serve God. Let God change the way you think. Then you will know how to do everything that is good and pleasing to him. I realize how kind God has been to me. Use good sense and measure yourself by the amount of faith that God has given you.

Al I Imran

Obey Allah and the apostle that you may obtain mercy. Be quick in the race for seeking forgiveness from your Lord and for a garden whose width is that of the whole of heavens and of the earth prepared for the righteous. Those who spend freely Allah loves those who do good. For such the reward is forgiveness from their Lord and gardens with rivers flowing underneath an eternal dwelling. How excellent a recompense.

You are grateful children are awesome, fun and innocent.

You are grateful children are very intelligent and fast learners.

You are grateful children provide deep unconditional love.

You are grateful children love to learn and learning is fun.

You are grateful to teach valuable lessons at school.

You are grateful to believe in your teaching abilities.

You are grateful for your many teaching talents and skills.

You are grateful to bring out the best in children and others.

You are grateful children love you, we get along well and respect each other.

December 24

Romans 12

Serve Others

If we can serve others we should serve. If we can teach we should teach. If we can encourage others we should encourage them. If we can give we should be generous. If we are leaders we should do our best. If we are good to others we should do it cheerfully. Be sincere in your love for others love each other as brothers and sisters and honor others more than you do yourself.

The Smoke

By the book that makes things clear for we ever wish to warn. By command from our presence for we ever send revelation. As mercy from your Lord for he hears and knows all things. The Lord of the heavens and the earth and all between them. Watch for the day that the sky will bring forth a kind of smoke or mist plainly visibly. Saying restore to me the servants of Allah. I am to you an apostle worthy of all trust.

We are grateful children are awesome, fun and innocent.

We are grateful children are very intelligent and fast learners.

We are grateful children provide deep unconditional love.

We are grateful children love to learn and learning is fun.

We are grateful to teach valuable lessons at school.

We are grateful to believe in our teaching abilities.

We are grateful for our many teaching talents and skills.

We are grateful to bring out the best in children and others.

We are grateful children love us, we get along well and respect each other.

December 25

2 Corinthians

Living God

You are like a letter written by Christ and delivered by us. You are written in our hearts by the spirit of the living God. Christ made us sure in the very presence of God. The Lord and the spirit are one.

The Confederates

And as one who invites to Allah and grace by his leave and as a lamp spreading light. Then give the glad tidings to the believers that they shall have from Allah a very great bounty. Trust in Allah for enough is Allah as a disposer of affairs.

My thoughts and actions are geared towards success at work.

I am working at my dream job.

I love my careers and they give me complete satisfaction.

My job offers money, and opportunities for growth and monetary rewards.

I have a great relationship with everyone at work always.

I have a great relationship with everyone at work always.

I have excellent work ethic, professional and team strategies.

I am doing the best in my career field and life is good.

I work well with others.

I am able to balance my work, family, social life perfectly.

I am a valuable asset to every company that I work for.

December 26

Titus 2

Instructions for People

Titus you must teach only what is correct. Tell older men to have self-control and to be sensible. Their faith, love and patience must never fail. Tell the older women to behave as those who love the Lord should. They must teach what is proper. Each of the younger women must be sensible and kind as well as a good homemaker who puts her husband first. Tell the young men to have self-control in everything. Always set a good example for others. Be sincere.

The Kneeling Down

Allah created the heavens and the earth for just ends and in order that each soul may find the recompense for what it has earned. This day shall you be recompensed for all that you did. This our record speaks about you with truth. Then as to those who believe and did righteous deeds their Lord will admit them to his mercy that will be the achievement for all to see.

Your thoughts and actions are successful.

You are working at your dream job.

You love your career satisfaction.

Your job offers money, and opportunities for growth and monetary rewards.

You have a great relationship with everyone at work.

You have a great relationship with everyone at work.

You have excellent professional and team strategies.

You are doing the best in your career field and life is good.

You work well with others.

You are able to balance your work, family, social life.

You are a valuable asset to every company.

December 27

Acts 3:21

In Heaven

Jesus must stay in heaven. God makes all things new just as his holy prophets promised. Peter and John had been set free. The group of followers all felt the same way about everything. In a powerful way the apostles told everyone that Lord Jesus was alive.

The Victory

We have granted you a manifest victory for Allah may He forgive you and fulfill his favor to you and guide you on the straightway. And that Allah may help you with powerful help. It is he who sent down tranquility into the hearts of the believers that they may add faith to their faith.

Our thoughts and actions are geared towards success at work.

We are working at our dream job.

We love our careers and they give us complete satisfaction.

Our job offers money, and opportunities for growth and monetary rewards.

We have a great relationship with everyone at work always.

We have a great relationship with everyone at work always.

We have excellent work ethic, professional and team strategies.

We are doing the best in our career field and life is good.

We work well with others.

We are able to balance our work, family, social life perfectly.

We are valuable assets to every company that we work for.

December 28

Acts 2

Miracles

Peter told them many other things on that day 3000 believed this message and were baptized. They spent their time learning from the apostles and they were like family to each other. They also broke bread and prayed together. Everyone was amazed by the many miracles and wonders that the apostles worked. All the Lords' followers met together and they shared everything they had.

Al-Baqara

For Allah loves those who do good. Allah made the Kaba the sacred house an asylum of security for men as also the sacred months, the animals for offerings and the garlands that mark them. Allah is well acquainted with all things.

I am grateful to have good job satisfaction.

I am grateful to be happy, peace and in love with my job.

I am grateful financial security and stability are received.

I am grateful to acquire all the positive qualities an employer needs.

I am grateful work is important and I am excellent at my job always.

I am grateful to do work that inspires others always.

I am grateful to appreciate and recognize my value to my company.

I am grateful to show appreciation to those I work with.

I am grateful my bank account continues to grow in good credit.

I am grateful everyday something divine and miraculous always.

December 29

3 John

Blessings

Dear friend you have always been faithful in helping other followers of the Lord. They have told the church about your love. They say you were good enough to welcome them and to send them on their mission in a way that God's servants deserve. Follow the example of people who do kind deeds. I pray that God will bless you with peace.

Ta Ha

The day when the trumpet will be sounded that day we shall gather them. All faces shall be humbled before him the living the self-subsisting eternal. High above all is Allah the king the truth!

You are grateful to have good job satisfaction.

You are grateful to be happy and in love with your job.

You are grateful for financial security and stability.

You are grateful to acquire all the positive qualities an employer needs.

You are grateful work is important and you are excellent at your job always.

You are grateful to do work that inspires others always.

You are grateful to appreciate and recognize your value to your company.

You are grateful to show appreciation to those you work with.

You are grateful your bank account continues to grow in good credit.

You are grateful everyday something divine and miraculous always.

December 30

Mark 10:35

Holy Spirit

As I began to speak Peter continued the Holy Spirit fell on them. Then I thought of the Lord's words when he said John baptized with water but you will be baptized with the Holy Spirit. And since God gave these Gentiles the same gift he gave us when we believed in the Lord Jesus Christ.

Ta Ha

Behold we sent to your mother by inspiration the message. Throw the child into the chest and throw the chest onto the river the river will cast him up on the bank. I cast the garment of love over you and from me and this in order that you maybe reared undermine eye.

We are grateful to have good job satisfaction.

We are grateful to be happy, peace and in love with our job.

We are grateful financial security and stability are received.

We are grateful to acquire all the positive qualities an employer needs.

We are grateful work is important and we are excellent at our job always.

We are grateful to do work that inspires others always.

We are grateful to appreciate and recognize our value to our company.

We are grateful to show appreciation to those we work with.

We are grateful our bank account continues to grow in good credit.

December 31

Luke 12:1

Warnings

Jesus told his disciples everything that is hidden will be found out. Whatever you say will be heard.

The Light

It is Allah who alternates the night and the day verily in these things is an instructive example for those who have a vision. Allah has created every animal from water of them there are some that creep on their bellies some that walk on two legs and some that walk on four. Allah creates what he wills for verily Allah has power over all things.

Abundance and prosperity are my birthright and I have it all.

I am in a state of contentment and have an abundance of love and joy.

I am and will always be prosperous, successful and righteous.

All my thoughts and actions lead to abundance, prosperity and love.

I am successful because I am kind and generous.

I enjoy all the abundance of good things in my life.

I am open to receiving an abundance of good things in my life.

I am open to receiving an abundance of wealth, health and happiness.

I always have what I need when I need it.

I love all the exciting safe opportunities of wealth, abundance and fame.

My universe is full with abundance, wealth, good health, love and happiness.

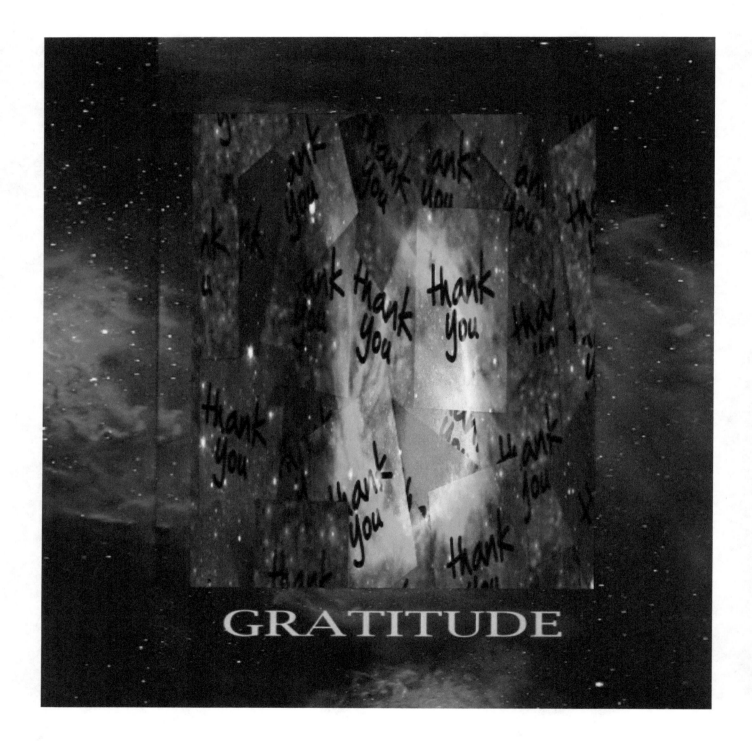

CELESTIAL KOSMOS UNIVERSAL LAWS
By Diana Hutchings

The celestial kingdom is the highest of the three degrees of glory. In 1 Corinthians 15:40 it says, "There are also celestial bodies and bodies terrestrial but the glory of the celestial is one and the glory of the terrestrial is another." In another doctrine it mentions the bodies of the celestial whose glory is that of the sun, even the glory of God the highest of all. The Celestials are for the righteous and are considered the permanent residence of the Almighty Creator. In Job this question is posed, "have you grasped the celestial laws?" The Holy Bible contains some fascinating information. Aristotle created a system of the Cosmos in which earth was the center of the universe. Sir Isaac Newton proposed an idea that gravity caused an attraction between the heavenly bodies. The laws of the universe govern our existence. Laws and theories can be applied in the past, present, and future. We have physical, spiritual, mental and emotional laws that create justice and fairness in our world.

The Universal Laws were published in 1908 called the Kybalion. This Hermetic philosophy detailed the seven laws of the universe. The trick with them is having Omni awareness. When you use these laws as they are intended you will create happy transformations of pure pleasure. Having positive thoughts, doing good deeds, keeping an optimistic mood and showing kindness all play a role in the success of implementing the celestial laws.

I would like you to repeat after me, "I, (insert your full name) will use this Celestial Kosmos oracle to create a better awareness that will improve my condition and the condition of my surroundings for our highest and greatest good and potential. Namaste! Blessed Be!"

Wishing you master the universal laws, in turn mastering your life. You will learn to love the easy life you live.

1. Law of action
2. Law of attraction
3. Law of belief
4. Law of cause and effect
5. Law of compensation
6. Law of correspondence
7. Law of detachment
8. Law of dharma
9. Law of divine oneness
10. Law of faith
11. Law of focus
12. Law of forgiveness
13. Law of generation
14. Law of gratitude
15. Law of gold
16. Law of growth
17. Law of healing
18. Law of here and now
19. Law of humility
20. Law of intention
21. Law of intuition
22. Law of karma
23. Law of language
24. Law of motivation
25. Law of order
26. Law of patience and reward
27. Law of perpetual transmutation
28. Law of polarity
29. Law of relativity
30. Law of responsibility
31. Law of rhythm
32. Law of self-actualization
33. Law of vibration
34. Law of wisdom

LAW OF ACTION

We must engage in actions that supports our thoughts, dreams emotions and words. The law of action states that you must do the things and perform the actions necessary to achieve what you want. When you take action, you set into motion corresponding effects that change your immediate future. Only by taking actions will the universe know what to bring into your life. Every action creates a result. The law of action also says that if we do nothing then nothing will happen. Newton's first law states a body in motion stays in motion. If you take action towards your goals, you will attain them. If you take massive action towards your goals, you will attain them much faster. Taking action in the direction of your goals. Tony Robbins suggests taking massive action.

Steps to take:

1. Write out your goals.

2. Create and follow a visual schedule.

3. Do planning and make a to do list.

4. Build a success mindset.

5. Set up your motivation to reward yourself.

6. Maintain a daily routine.

7. Commit to moving your body and exercising daily.

LAW OF ATTRACTION

The belief is based on the ideas that people and their thoughts are made of pure energy and that a process of like energy attracting like energy exists though which a person can improve their health, wealth and personal relationships. The Law of Attraction appeared in the first time by Russian occultist Helena Blavatsky in 1877. And it appears in the 2006 book and film called "The Secret." The Secret's mantra as an extension of the law of attraction is as follows" positive thoughts and positive visualization will have a direct impact on the self. Positivity can improve one's quality of life." Advocates combine cognitive reframing techniques and creative visualizations to replace limiting thoughts with more empowering positive thoughts.

Steps to take:

1. Practice gratitude daily.

2. Use positive self-talk and affirmations.

3. Visualize success.

4. Know what you want and write your goals.

5. Meditate.

6. Do a vision board, display and look at it often.

7. Read the book The Magic by Rhonda Byrne.

LAW OF CAUSE AND EFFECT

Every action has a reaction or consequence. Every human thought, word and deed is a cause that sets off a wave of energy throughout the universe which turn creates the effect whether desirable or undesirable. With every thought of intention, action and emotion that is transmitted from you, a person sets into motion unseen chain of effects which vibration from the mental plane thought the entire cellular structure of body out into the environment and finally into the cosmos. Eventually the vibratory energy returns to the original source upon the swing of the pendulum. Every cause has an effect and every effect becomes the cause of something else. This law suggests that the universe is always in motion and progressed from a chain of events.

Steps to take:

1. Identify the issue, concern or situation that requires a response.
2. Evaluate choices before you react too quickly.
3. Read the Teachings of Buddha.
4. Get a Tao Te Ching reading.
5. Avoid abrupt emotional reactions to actions.
6. Complete a cause and effect science experiment.
7. Give a couple of examples of what happened and why it happened.

LAW OF COMPENSATION

Ralph Waldo Emerson in his essay, "Compensation," wrote that each person is compensated in like manner for that which he or she has contributed. It can rephrased as the Law of sowing and reaping. You will be compensated for your efforts and for your contribution whatever it is however much or however little. If you want to increase your compensation you must increase your value. Fill your mind with success and you will be compensated with positive experiences. People whom exceed expectations and do more than you're paid for can reward more. Your rewards will always be in direct proportion to your service to others.

Steps to take:

1. Give to charity and donate.
2. Volunteer your time.
3. Ask and offer others help.
4. Share your knowledge and resources.

5. Strive to be your best.

6. Finish the job with perfection and satisfaction.

7. If someone asks for something provide it if you can.

LAW OF CORRESPONSDENCE

Tells us there are harmony, agreement and correspondence between the physical, mental and spiritual realms. Like the Kybalion says, "as above so below; so below so above." This means our outer world is a reflection of our inner world. Our current reality is a mirror of what is going on inside us. As within so without. What's going on in my thought patterns beliefs and feelings is directly corresponds to what I perceive in the physical outer world. This line of communication or correspondence between the lower energies of the physical mind (earth) and the higher energies of the divine mind (heaven). The key to changing your physical reality is by realizing that you are more of a spiritual being than a physical one. The law of correspondence teaches us to acknowledge and look at an issue until it is healed.

Steps to take:

1. Answer the question what is your current reality?

2. What are your beliefs? Empowering and limiting?

3. Reaffirm the limiting beliefs into beliefs that you do want.

4. If you could have anything answer the question, what do you want your reality to be like?

5. Create a soul collage vision board of what you do want. And look it this daily.

6. Try visualizing what you truly desire.

7. Research the world tree known as Yggdrasill and draw it.

LAW OF DETACHMENT

It simply states that with good intentions and desires we should pursue our dreams but be detached form the outcome. Detachment leads me to do what is God's will. Detachment is in exercise in trusting God. By focusing too much on the outcome we limit possibilities and can limit God's blessings which are unlimited. Attachment is trusting yourself based on the past, conditioning and beliefs. This law requires surrender. Let go of the ego's control and let God do. In detachment lies the wisdom of uncertainty. As you let go of the need to arrange your life the universe brings abundant good to me.

Steps to take:

1. Research Ram Dass.

2. Read the Bhagavad Gita.

3. Do not be attached to the outcomes.

4. Observe your thoughts and feelings during a liberation meditation.

5. Do a release and letting go ritual where you burn a piece of paper requesting detachment from a person, place, or object.

6. Try not reacting to everything respond instead.

7. Eliminate a person, place or object from your day, week or month to confirm you have control and you are detached.

LAW OF DHARMA

Dharma signifies behaviors that include duties, rights, laws, conduct, virtues and the right way of living. Dharma is the path of righteousness and proper religious practice. Dharma is dhri which means to support, hold or bear. If you follow this code of Dharma you are moral, ethical, right and lawful. We are here to discover our true self, unearth our talents and serve fellow humans which in turn is our purpose of life. Dharma is the truth of things. When your life is full of true purpose your dharma or abundance comes easily and effortlessly. The wheel of dharma is used in many Indian religions. It suggests there is an eightfold noble path. This path includes: right view, right intention or resolve, right speech, right conduct or action, right livelihood, right effort, right mindfulness, right Samadhi or meditation and concentration. This dharma path focuses on moral virtue, meditation and insight.

Steps to take:

1. Study the Eightfold Path of Buddhism and the Way of the Bodhisattva.

2. Practice a devotion, mantra or prayer to Buddha daily.

3. Chant Om Namo Amitabha 108 times.

4. Listen to a sermon by the holy Dalai Lama.

5. Draw or color a dharma wheel and look up dharma chakra.

6. Meditate for righteousness and enlightenment.

7. Focus on spiritual self-care and do a daily or weekly activity.

LAW OF DIVINE ONENESS

We are all connected to one source. The same higher power source universe, God idea. We co-exist and collectively share an energetic foundation. This is the first law of the universe that governs us. We are all one. Everything that exists seen and unseen is connected. Wilder says, "Every single atom inside of you is connected in some way, shape or form to the rest of the universe you move through." This means that everything we do has a ripple effect and impacts the collective. This is why it is important to grow, evolve and raise our individual vibrations to help our surroundings. All humanity and God are one. If Jesus is in all of us, then we are mirrors of each other. Increasing our awareness of our interconnectedness is important to raising our pure collective consciousness. Everything consists of energy our thoughts, feelings and actions affect this energy. The law of oneness connects humans, nature, elements, minerals, plants, insects, animals and all living and nonliving matter.

Steps to take:

1. Pay more attention to your inner world and how it interacts with your outer experiences by meditating. Bring your awareness.

2. Notice synchronicities. Noises, sights, people, thoughts.

3. Research Dr. Masaru Emoto's science and do a water or rice experiment.

4. Use positive affirmations to improve thoughts.

5. Give others boosts of energy.

6. Begin and end the day with gratitude.

7. Connect to three people daily and compliment them.

LAW OF FAITH

God is a faith God. In Greek philotheos means loving God pious. Philanthropia is the love of God. Philotheis is associated with the concepts of worship and devotions towards God. Theophilia means the love or favor of God. Theophilos means friend of God or lover of God. Agape is applied to the love the humans have for God and to the love that God has for man. The love of God purifies human hearts. Every religion has their own ideas of God or Gods and Goddesses. In Christianity, the whole doctrine is centered on Father God, Jesus Christ and the Holy Spirit. Followers read the Holy Bible. Some say that the bible stands for basic instructions before leaving earth. Christians believe that if we have faith and love for God we are saved. Bahai Faith holds that the love of God is the primary reason for the human creation. Abdu'l Baha the son of the founder of Bahai Faith wrote "There is nothing greater or more blessed than the Love of God!" Hinduism devotees worship Krishna as a Bhakti movement. In Islam the love and fear of God are the foundations of Islam. Loving God is the highest spiritual attainment. Islamic Sufism Ishq means to love God selflessly and unconditionally. Ishq means to serve God by devoting one's entire life to Him and asking no reward in return. Judaism's Holy Scriptures in Deuteronomy 6:5 says, "And you shall love the Lord your God with all your heart and with all your soul and with all your might."

Steps to take:

1. Pick a religion to follow.

2. Join a prayer group or bible study.

3. Pray daily and create a prayer journal.

4. Attend a church, mosque or temple.

5. Research the fruits of the spirit and use them as positive affirmations.

6. Read and write sacred scriptures and text. Try bibliomancy but choose only good news.

LAW OF FOCUS

It states that whatever we focus on we become better at. Attention is focused energy. Focusing on too many things scatters energy. Where attention goes energy flows. If you have a laser like focus you can direct and strengthen manifestations to get what you want; which accelerates our growth. Remove distractions. Find positive people and environments to enhance your attention. The key is to become more conscious and aware to control your mind to get the universe to create the outcomes you want. Whatever the mind can conceive and believe it can achieve. One should not think of two things at the same time.

Steps to take:

1. Eliminate distractions.

2. Practice mindfulness meditations daily for at least 10 minutes.

3. Try brain food like gingko bibloba, omegas, ginseng, avocado, eggs and coconut oil.

4. Create a very structured timed daily routine to keep you on task.

5. Take healthy breaks often and go for a walk

6. Do concentration exercises to improve focus and memory. While misting lemongrass or smelling a freshly peeled orange or grapefruit.

7. Do things one at a time and avoid multitasking.

LAW OF FORGIVENESS

Connie Domino in her book The Law of Forgiveness demonstrates how to unleash the power of forgiveness to use to manifest good things in your life. Forgiveness is the most transformational strategy for personal and spiritual well-being. The secret to attracting what you really want is by forgiveness. Forgiving others and oneself is the key to greater health, better relationships, prosperity and blessings. The Ho'ponopono practice comes from Hawaii and it means I am sorry, please forgive me, I love you, thank you. Forgiveness starts a domino effect of the highest vibration to come to you and through you. Like Jesus Christ's superpower, he had the power to forgive.

Steps to take:

1. Do a hoponopono meditation.

2. Identify the names of people you may hold hard feelings for? And why you hold these feelings about them.

3. Journal by answering why you are willing to forgive? For example, for your wellness, to hold more positive emotions, to release bent of feelings and make your heart lighter.

4. CONFESS Confess your situation Offer an apology Note the emotional experience Forever value the relationship Equalize through restitution Say we will never do it again. Seek forgiveness.

5. Try Naikan Therapy lovingkindness mediation.

6. Call on Kuan Yin for compassion.

7. Write a Forgiveness Letter to yourself and/ another to let the universe know you forgive yourself and others.

LAW OF GENERATION ANCESTRY

Distinct DNA called genes determine how your body develops over time. DNA or your genetic code is the blueprint that influence how you look, how you act, and what determines how susceptible you are to disease. Every cell of your body is donated by your mother and father. Humans inherit one allele from the mom and one allele from the dad. Every human has around 20 000 genes and 3 000 000 000 bases. Your sequence of genes and bases is called your genome. This will guide your height, hair color, eye color and temperant. Genes contain the biological instructions to help the body build specific molecules or proteins. These molecules are building blocks for your cells, organs and whole body and mind. You characteristics are affected by your environment as well as your genes. Scientists can examine your family relationships, trace ancestors and find genes in specific health conditions to make breakthroughs.

Steps to take:

1. Get a past life clearing or shamanic treatment to connect with ancestors.

2. Get your genealogy DNA sample test.

3. Research your last name and find out more about your history.

4. Discover your family crest or create and draw your own.

5. Take herbs like burdock root and dandelion tea to cleanse blood ties.

6. Pray aloud, "I call forth my guides, ancestors, allies, spirit source, creator and all that come in love, light, healing, truth, abundance, protection, prosperity and peace. I ask that my family tree be cleared past, present and future. That all hexes, curses and jinxes be removed. That any places within my family tree or lineage that makes us vulnerable to negativity or attack be cleansed of any negativity, pain or sickness. And I ask that all future generations of my family to infinity be free and clear. I call forth healing to the entire family tree from the seed to the roots to the trunk, branches, leaves and fruit. I ask for blessings upon all that have been in my family all that are in my family past to present to future. For wisdom and abundance in all aspects of our lives I claim this healing and clearing I manifest it now and so it is. Blessed Be."

7. Research epigenetics.

LAW OF GRATITUDE

The key for welcoming abundance into your life is to be grateful for the things you have and what you want to happen. Whether that involves money health a promotion better relationship or an improved life. As Rhonda Bynre says, "whoever has gratitude will be given more and they will have abundance." Gratitude can transform any situation. The magic formula to life is please and thank you. I have told many students in the past years to always use there manners. There is a Hawaiian meditation called H'oponopono which means I'm sorry. Please forgive me. Thank you. I love you. An attitude of gratitude means making it a habit to express thankfulness and appreciation in all parts of your life on a regular basis. Gratitude is a divine positive that purifies us spiritually and opens up channels mentally and physically.

Steps to take:

1. Write in a daily gratitude journal in the morning and or evening.

2. Read the book the Magic by Rhonda Byrne and practice it.

3. Do a 30 day gratitude challenge with daily guideline questions.

4. Write a thank you card, email or note to someone you appreciate

5. Buy a gift for someone to let them know you are thankful for them and what they do.

6. Create a gratitude jar or box and whenever you catch a moment you appreciate write a post it and throw it in. You may use a white board to for save paper.

7. Every time you receive a service thank the person whom is giving you this service.

THE LAW OF GOLDEN RULE

The golden rule is the principle of treating others as you want to be treated. What you wish upon others your wish upon yourself. So do not treat others in ways that you would not like to be treated. This golden rule or law has been widely used for centuries worldwide. In ancient India the Sanskrit tradition in the Mahabharata states "one should never do something to others that one would regard as an injury to one's own self." Ancient Grecan Sectus the Pythagorean says "what you do not want to happen to you do not do it yourself either." In Christianity the bible says to love your neighbor as yourself. Galatians 5:14 "For all the law is fulfilled in one word even in this Thou shalt love thy neighbor as thyself." Islams Sukhanan I Muhammad tells "That which you want for yourself seek for mankind. The most righteous person is the one who consents for other people what he consents for himself and who dislikes for them what he dislikes for himself." In Sikhism Gura Arjan Dev Ji 259 stated "precious like jewels are the minds of all. To hurt them is not at all good. If thou desirest thy beloved then hurt thou not anyone's heart. "The Declaration Toward a Global Ethic from the Parliament of the World's Religions in 1193 proclaimed the Gold Rule as the common principle for many religions. It was signed by 143 leaders from all the world's major faiths including Bahai, Brahmanism, Brahma, Kumaris, Buddhism, Christianity, Hinduism, Indigenous, Interfaith, Islam, Jainism Judaism, Native American Neo Pagan Sikhism, Taoism Theosophist Unitarian Universalist and Zoroastrian.

Steps to take:

1. Be kind and friendly always.

2. Do not criticize or judge someone but offer compassion.

3. Pray and repeat that you will treat others as you treat yourself.

4. Use polite manners.

5. Live your life as to do no hurt or harm to others while offering perfect respect.

6. If you have nothing nice to say don't say anything at all. Speak good things about others.

7. Practice empathy and surround yourself with pink colors.

LAW OF GROWTH

Certain principles like growth and development are a natural process. There is a biological development that takes place with a predictable order; also called a developmental stage. There are differences in personality, activity level and timing of some milestones. Milestones include physical growth, thinking and reasoning, emotional and social development, language development and sensory and motor development. Growth and development are a continuous process. It can be influenced by family genes and the environment. There is a principal of association with maturity and learning.

Steps to take:

1. Get routine checkups and physical exams.

2. Look for sources of information and support for your age group.

3. Call your local provincial or federal health hotline for any questions or concerns you may have about you or someone near and dear.

4. Follow a food, activity, and sleep guide for your age and gender category.

5. Get a massage to relax the body.

6. Hire a life coach to improve your body image, self-efficacy and self-esteem.

7. Check your Body Mass Index to ensure you are on a healthy spectrum.

LAW OF HEALING

Healing is the process of making and becoming sound or healthy again. There are three conditions for healing that include cellular replacement, time and supply and demand. In order for our body to heal it must replace the cells that are damaged to become healthy again. Healing takes time. Your body will heal accordingly to the supply and demand of healthy options for your body. Which means having suitable conditions and taking care of yourself will accelerate healing. Diet and healthy practices and methods facilitate healing. Constantine Hering's law of cure states that all cure starts from within out from the head down and in reverse order as the symptoms have appeared. Keeping thoughts and intentions on healing can trick the body into healing itself.

Steps to take:

1. Do energy work like reiki, qi gong, yoga, breath work and walking.

2. Join a healing circle or group.

3. Get monthly holistic treatments like reiki, massage, chiropractor, acupuncture, osteopathy, etc...

4. Try kundalini, chakra meditations.

5. Ground your energy with visualizations, nature connections and grounding crystals.

6. Connect to high vibration healthy people and environments.

7. Try healthy supplements like probiotics, multivitamin and protein.

LAW OF HERE AND NOW

Old thoughts, old patterns of behavior and old dreams prevent us from having new ones. Eckhart Tolle wrote a book called the Power of Now. His book is a daily guide to living in the present moment and transcending thoughts of the past and future. The power of creative potential lies concealed in the now. Perfecting your current situation. Living in the moment can create natural momentum and increase energy of your surroundings. Abraham Hicks explains the point of power is in the present in Abraham Now.

Steps to take:

1. Do breath work and consciously breathe into every body part. Inhale here and exhale now. You can coordinate with yoga, tai chi or qi gong.

2. Enjoy every moment you have like it's your last.

3. Do your best in everything you undergo like you are receiving an award.

4. Participate, show up, dress up and be present always.

5. Stop thinking about the past it's over. Stop thinking about the future it hasn't happened. Live in the now and set an intention to have the most pleasant experience.

6. Do a body scan mindful meditation for 5-10 minutes. Feel your bodies' sensations.

7. Be grateful. Tell yourself, the people, places and objects you interact with that you thank them for this experience.

LAW OF HUMILITY

What you refuse to accept will continue for you. This means you need to accept the true reality of something before you'll ever be able to change it. Humility is the quality of being humble. It is widely seen as a virtue. You can appreciate your talents and skills and efface of oneself to something higher. Humility is not to think lowly or oneself but to appreciate the self-one has received. Because there is always someone better or something we can do better. Elders, masters or teachers provide us with learning experiences make us humble and strong.

As Islamic Imam ash-Shafi'I says the loftiest in status are those who do not know their own status and the most virtuous of them are those who do not know their own virtue. Or as Abudlbary Yahya says your humbleness humbles others and your modesty brings out the modesty in others.

Steps to take:

1. Give credit and compliments to others whom are doing a good job.

2. Learn to apologize and accept you can do better.

3. Accept constructive feedback gently and improve.

4. Smudge and pray to Jesus or like ascended master to give you strength and perfection.

5. Practice makes perfect. Create the time and experience to master skills.

6. Find a mentor or teacher in the field to learn from.

7. Try confessioning at a church, mosque or temple and seek strength.

LAW OF INTENTION

Intention and desire have infinite organizing power and can ground pure potentiality. Wayne Dyer has a book called the Power of Intention. His philosophy relates to the law of attraction and how you can attract what you want and are by focusing on it. Deepak Chopra believes that energy and information are located in the quantum field of pure consciousness. We can access this energy with intention and desire. Our attention energizes and our intention transforms. The quality of intention on the object of attention will orchestrate an infinity of space time events to bring about the outcome intended. Intention lays the groundwork for effortless flow of pure potentiality.

Steps to take:

1. Create a daily or weekly mantra to repeat 3x aloud..

2. Start a daily intention journal

3. Whenever you are starting a task, think and say what you want the end result to be or look like.

4. Ask the universe, God source, your guides to assist you in achieving your goals and intentions.

5. Every new moon or full moon to an intention ritual to manifest faster.

6. Keep your goals, intentions and desires visible to see them daily.

7. Share your intentions with your loved ones.

LAW OF INTUITION

Intuition is the ability to acquire knowledge without recourse to conscious reasoning. The word intuit means to contemplate. Intuition is that quiet voice that speaks up to lead you to an unknown truth. If you are intuitive, you can make connections like reading people, feeling emotions, and maintaining self-awareness. In the book "The 21 Irrefutable Laws of Leadership" by John Maxwell, he discusses the law of intuition. He states great leaders use their intuition. Intuition comes from natural ability and learned skills. Intuits know their situation, trends, resources, people and themselves well. Some people are born with these intuitive instincts and others acquire them over time.

Steps to take:

1. Shhh listen to your intuition in a quiet environment as you breathe consciously.

2. Pay attention to your senses even your sixth sense to capture subtle messages.

3. Ask yourself questions like what does my life need right now? Listen, look and write information that comes to you.

4. Do a pineal gland activation meditation with 852 Hz and or 963 Hz.

5. Get an intuitive oracle reading to confirm, reassure and guide you.

6. Buy a dreamcatcher to place above your bed and notice your dreams.

7. Work with the color indigo to enhance your third eye awareness.

LAW OF KARMA

One can think of karma as the spiritual equivalent of Newton's Law of Motion. For every action there is an equal but opposite reaction. Karma means action, work or deed. The principle of karma's is based on the actions of an individual cause influence on the future effect of the individual. Good intent and good deeds contribute to good karma and happier rebirths. The opposite is true. Karma can be carried on into future lives, so it is good to cleanse past lives. It is good when our acts are motivated by generosity love or wisdom then we are creating the karmic conditions for abundance and happiness.

Steps to take:

1. Be honest. Tell the truth all the time.

2. Do random acts of kindness at least once a week.

3. Try compassion meditations.

4. Do a forgiveness journaling activity.

5. Get a past life clearing or akashic record karma reading.

6. Do good and follow the rules and the law.

7. Always send good vibes.

LAW OF LANGUAGE

Gary Chapman wrote a book about the Five Love Languages. He mentioned that words of affirmation, acts of service, receiving gifts, quality time and physical touch help communicate to someone that you love them. Speaking words of praise and appreciation will prove to have promising love responses. Like the old saying actions speak louder than words. Gift giving is an expression of love. Spending time with your loved ones giving them undivided attention fills the love tank. There is emotional power in touching someone tenderly and with affection. Each person has a primary love language that we must learn to speak if we want that person to feel loved.

Steps to take:

1. Practice positive affirmations daily. Write, read and say them at least 3 times.

2. Be a gift giver. Buy a gift for a loved one, you can include yourself.

3. Offer affection, hugs, massages and eye gazes.

4. Spend more quality time with your loved ones and offer more attention.

5. Always use optimism and gratitude when interacting with others.

6. Show them you love them by serving them. For example, making breakfast, fold their laundry, running errands.

7. Do a self-love, positive affirmation, gratitude meditation daily.

LAW OF MOTIVATION

Motivation means to move. It is the state of an individual's perspective which represents the strength of his or her propensity to exert toward some particular behavior. Motivation in an internal force which stimulates regulates and upholds a person's actions. It is the need or drive an individual has toward goals. Abraham Maslow propounded the need theory in 1943 that suggests there are 5 basic needs. At the top of the hierarchy to the lower the order is self-actualization esteem needs social needs, safety needs and physiological needs. Once a need is satisfied the person is concerned with the next level of their personal hierarchy. A process cognitive motivation theory states that different variables can influence the amount of effort an individual puts forth.

Steps to take:

1. Take a motivation quiz https://richardstep.com/self-motivation-quiz-test/.

2. Surround yourself with like-minded people that you admire. Create your support group.

3. Do goal planning. Set 7 day 30 day 60 day 365 day goals and review them.

4. Reward yourself when you finish tasks and complete a goal.

5. See a hypnotherapist or attend a life coaching vision workshop to create more motivation.

6. Exercise with intensity to raise your vibration.

7. Boost dopamine levels with loud music that pumps you up.

LAW OF ORDER

Order is a condition or logical arrangement. Eternal law maintains the universal order in the physical reality since the beginning. There are five major types of order in nature: logical, physical, biological moral and social. The concept of order equates with the concept of truth. As whatever is orderly is reasonable and true. The physical order is a universal order for maintaining in existence of matter and energy by the universal laws and forces of nature without which there would be no matter and energy nor could any universe exist. Law is an ordinance of reason, promulgated by an authority for the creation of order. Where there is order there must be a law. The natural law provides an authoritative basis for maintaining order among human beings.

Steps to take:

1. Organize a daily, weekly, monthly schedule include cleaning and tidying up.

2. When you take something put it back in the same place.

3. Try a cleaning service to help you accomplish organization.

4. Take a course on time management skills or self-assertiveness.

5. Create your to do list and complete your priorities.

6. Choose your planning tools, apps and programs. For example, google calendar, paper calendars, digital to do list app, timers, financial planners, receipts apps, keep fit apps, etc....

7. Try daily journaling your goals, dreams, brain dumps, to do lists, schedules, etc....

LAW OF PATIENCE AND REWARD

This states that the most valuable rewards require persistence. This means that anything worth having in life requires persistence. This means that anything worth having in life requires perseverance. All rewards require initial toil. Rewards of lasting value require patient and persistent toil. True joy comes from doing what one is supposed to be doing and knowing that the reward will come in its own time. The more time and patience put into something, the more the reward will be, this is true even of transient things as.

Steps to take:

1. Repeat your efforts till you get it right. Practice makes perfect.

2. Change your strategy after a few attempts at completing the task.

3. Model someone who is successful again and again.

4. Create motivation incentives whether internal or external.

5. Practice visioning or visualizing your reward. What does it look and feel like?

6. Create a wish box and put all the images and ideas of what reward you are desire and be patient it will come to fruition.

7. Keep an optimistic frame of mind and your emotions positive it will come.

LAW OF PERPETUAL TRANSMUTATION OF ENERGY

Energy is constantly flowing into the material world and taking form. The energy of the universe is always moving and transmuting into and out of form. This law of nature further tells us that energy is always in a state of motion. This law relates to the universe and our consciousness through the realization that everything seen and unseen is constantly changing. We can harness energy and transform what form we desire. The energy is flowing into our consciousness constantly we transform this energy into whatever we choose through our focus of attention at the moment. Even in the Last Airbender movie there is the taking of energy and bending or transmuting it to your will in order to achieve or attain something greater than intended. It's important to redirect energy into more positive directions in order to maintain a high level of positive energy. This law states that we all have power within us to change any condition in our lives. Higher energy vibration will consume and transform lower ones.

Steps to take:

1. Get your Reiki 1,2,3 Master certificate.

2. Commit to daily Qi Gong.

3. Eat a high vibration food and drinks.

4. Take more baths and shower every day.

5. Connect with the color spectrum and lights.

6. Listen to loud music.

7. Smudge often.

LAW OF POLARITY

This states that everything has a polar opposite. Forces are paired in opposites. Everything exists has two poles. This includes all things animate or inanimate, thoughts, feelings and energies. This dualism can be a source of conflict but generates energy that allows us to experience the richness of life and see the truth of our reality and receive deep lessons. In ancient Chinese philosophy yin and yang is the concept of polarity or dualism. Our natural world is interconnected and complementary with each other. Opposites include positive/negative, male/female dark/light, resonance/dissonance. Opposites are identical in their nature and different only in degree.

Steps to take:

1. Accept the polar opposites exist.

2. Express gratitude.

3. Draw a scales the Libra constellation.

4. Hold two equal cups or bowls and right and left hand and time how long you can hold it there.

5. Maintain a balanced life with work play social solitude eat sleep exercise.

6. Try the 888 diet 8 hours of work, sleep and play.

7. Draw a ying yang symbol.

LAW OF RELATIVITY

The spiritual and metaphysical aspects of this law of relativity tell us that everything in our physical world is only made real by its relationship or comparison to something. Light only exist because we compare it to dark. Hot can only exist because we compare it to cold. Everything in our life just is until we compare it to something. Nothing can have meaning except for the meaning we give it. Each person will receive tests of initiations and lessons for the purpose of strengthening the light within each of these tests or lessons to be a challenge and remain connected to our hearts when proceeding to solve the problems. All things are relative and related to each other. Every law must be in harmony and agreement with each other.

Steps to take:

1. Use your GPS on your smartphone or car.

2. Connect to the color gold and wear it.

3. Buy a fridge magnet.

4. Connect to the light spectrum and color therapy.

5. Have a meal on a moving train, plane or boat.

6. Get sunshine and sun gaze.

7. Listen to an Einstein documentary.

LAW OF RESPONSIBILITY

Responsibility is the state or fact of having a duty to deal with something or of having control over someone. It's the opportunity or ability to act independently and make decisions without authorization. It means doing things you're supposed to do and accepting the results of your actions. Being responsible keeps everyone safe and ensures a suitable environment for everyone. Everyone has a legal responsibility to complete certain duties as civilians. Everyone has a law they need to obey and there are consequences for actions if people are not responsible enough to follow the rules.

Steps to take:

1. Be consistent and keep to your schedule.

2. Create your weekly to do list and commit to accomplishing it.

3. Know your role and job and complete it to the best of your ability.

4. Buy an angelite or jasper gemstone to hold or place in your wallet or pocket to maintain your responsibility.

5. Participate in community service projects.

6. Develop a mentor relationship that keeps you accountable for your actions and behaviors.

7. Call on the angel Jegudiel the angel of responsibility, merciful love and is the laudation(praise) of God. "Saint Jejudiel the Archangel, the angel of praise to God, help me! Keep by my side in every job, every work and in every labor. May I constantly carry out my responsibility gladly for all that has been given to me. Thank you."

LAW OF RHYTHM

All energy vibrates at a certain speed and rhythm. These rhythms establish season's cycles, stages of development, and patterns. Each cycle reflects the regularity of God's Universe. There is an ebb of flow. Like the wave in the ocean of life. If you relax and let the waves take you and go with the flow riding the waves is easier. "Everything flows out and in, everything has its tides, all things rise and fall, the pendulum swing manifests in everything, the measure of the swing to the right is the measure of the swing to the left rhythm compensates." The Kybalion. The law of rhythm states that the energy in the universe is like a pendulum. Whenever something swings to the right, it must then swing to the left. Everything in existence is involved in this flow.

Steps to take:

1. Pay attention to your rhythms, cycles and patterns.

2. Research gender, ages and stages and find advice for your age category.

3. Learn to use a crystal pendulum for yes no maybe answers.

4. Persevere and be consistent daily.

5. Have a bubble bath with Epsom salts and notice the bubbles flow.

6. Plan a vacation each season.

7. Join a Zumba class or try ecstatic dance

LAW OF SELF ACTUALIZATION

The growth of self-actualization refers to the need for personal growth and discovery that is present throughout a person's life. This is at the top of the pyramid of Maslow's hierarchy o needs. It is the highest level of psychological development where the actualization of full personal potential is achieved which occurs after all bodily and ego needs are fulfilled. This leads people in different directions. For some people it can be achieved through creating works of art or literature for others through sport, classroom or within a corporate setting. This perfect state of self-actualization is a continual process of reaching happily ever after. This is the idea that each individual desires and is motivated to achieve ambitions and realize one's capabilities.

Steps to take:

1. Call on the angel Ananchel to practice acceptance and grace.

2. Go see a life coach, psychotherapist, hypnotherapist or art therapist to see how you can pursue self-actualization.

3. Increase spontaneity and go with the flow.

4. Increase your vibration and connect to higher frequencies via sound, light, people, crystals, nature, etc....

5. Take a self-mastery course.

6. Fully enjoy each moment and be appreciative to the people and situations you experience.

7. Research Abraham Maslow's hierarchy of needs.

LAW OF VIBRATION

States that anything that exists in our universe whether seen or unseen, is analyzed in its purest form consists of energy or light which resonates and exists as a vibratory frequency or pattern. All matter, thoughts and feelings have their own vibrational frequency. Everything in the universe is composed of packets of energy. As Albert Einstein believes, "everything is energy and that's all there is to it. Match the frequency of the reality you want and you cannot help but get that reality. It can be no other way. This is not philosophy. This is physics." There are many ways to raise your vibration. Connecting to nature, crystals, water, music, light, gratitude, optimism, movement and breath can increase your vibration. By raising your vibration you can optimize your manifestation powers and align with your desires easier.

Steps to take:

1. Drink a blessed 1-2 liters of water daily.

2. Exercise.

3. Breathe deeply and fully.

4. Listen to inspiring music.

5. Walk in nature.

6. Do yoga, tai chi, chi gong.

7. Connect with plants, animals and crystals.

LAW OF WISDOM

Wisdom is the ability to think and act using knowledge, experience, understanding, common sense and insight. In the book The Laws of Wisdom by Ryuhu Okawa he guides you on the path to acquire wisdom. He offers ways to transform information into knowledge and wisdom while offering effective planning strategies. Words of wisdom can be compared to the Proverbs in the Holy Bible. Focusing on the positive statements of the Proverbs that contain what God loves, which is wise. As it states in Proverbs 7:4 Say to wisdom you are my sister and make common sense your closest friend. The ancient Greeks Zeus earned the title Metieta which means the wise counselor. As some say the older you get the wiser you become.

Steps to take:

1. Try new things. Like learning a new language.

2. Connect with music like Mozart Major D. Learn a musical instrument.

3. Read daily for at least 10 minutes.

4. Enrich yourself with education. Take a course at least once a year.

5. Find high vibration, success oriented, wise beings to surround yourself with.

6. If you make a mistake fix it and learn from it.

7. Connect to wisdom symbols like wisdom eyes, owls, lotuses and display them.

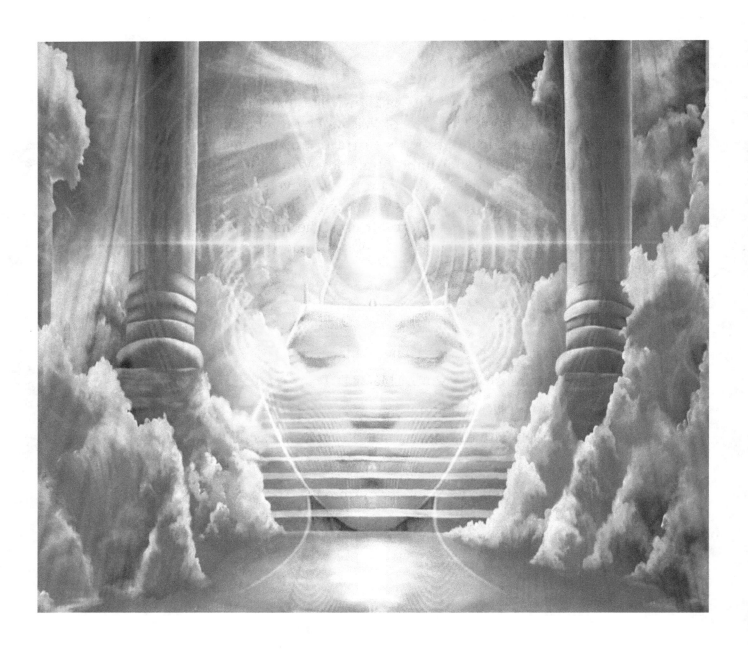

Miracle Healing Oracle

Healing involves repairing living tissues, organs and body systems to resume normal functioning. There are multiple ways to regenerate, mend and heal. To heal is to become well again. There are various types of healing, physical, mental, emotional, spiritual and environmental healing. Everything is energy and energy is the life force of health. Alternative medicine has taken a leap in the right direction by providing many alternative approaches to healing. In this Miracle Healing Oracle you will discover many alternative methods to use, try and practice. Learn the powerful strategies available to heal you from the inside out. Align your mind, body and soul with these healing practices to live at your optimum state of health and wellness. Research retreats associated with the modalities you are guided to. Going to a retreat is a fun way to get immersed in those healing practices; you can find many combined therapies that will lead to a healthier and happier lifestyle. Experience the healing results to maintain perfect wellness. In this 63 card Miracle Healing oracle you will: cleanse, strengthen and heal, promote harmony and balance, master your energy, release and relax, remove blockages and receive many physical, emotional, social and spiritual benefits.

Miracle Healing

1. Acupuncture
2. Affirmations
3. Angel
4. Animals
5. Aromatherapy
6. Art therapy
7. Ayurveda
8. Binaural beats
9. Cardio
10. Celestial music
11. Chakras
12. Chant
13. Chiropractor
14. Color therapy
15. Crystals
16. Detox
17. Energy
18. Fast
19. Family crest
20. Float
21. Frequency sounds
22. Goal setting
23. Herbology
24. Homeopathy
25. Hydrotherapy
26. Hypnotherapy
27. Ion cleanse
28. Intentions
29. Interpersonal group
30. Journal
31. Laugh
32. Mandala
33. Mantra
34. Massage
35. Mudras
36. Mediation
37. Naturopath
38. Osteopath
39. Plants
40. Pranayama
41. Psychedelics
42. Qi gong
43. Red light therapy
44. Reflexology
45. Reiki
46. Sacred geometry
47. Sauna
48. Shaman
49. Sound bath
50. Sports
51. Steam room
52. Stretching
53. Soul collage
54. Sunshine
55. Sun catcher
56. Supplements
57. Ultraviolet light
58. Vegetarian
59. Vegan
60. Vision board
61. Vitamins
62. Walk
63. Yoga

Miracle Healing

Acupuncture

Acupuncture is a system of integrative medicine that involves pricking the skin or tissues with needles used to alleviate pain and to treat various physical, mental and emotional conditions. It originated in China over 2500 years ago. Each acupuncture needle which vary in size and length produce a tiny insertion site which can cause little to no discomfort, it sends a signal for your body to respond. This response involves stimulation of the immune system and promotes circulation to that area. The Chinese philosophy is that the human body is filled with qi (life giving force energy). When qi is flowing correctly you can experience a good mental and physical health. Typical acupuncture sessions are anywhere from 30 to 90 minutes. They can cost anywhere from $60 to $150. Acupuncture has different types like auricular which is a traditional Chinese practice. Electro acupuncture which uses a stimulation of an electrical current. There are different additions you can add to acupuncture like heat, Tui Na massage, cupping, gua sha and moxibustion which promote and improve wellbeing. The main benefits include: reduced stress, increased energy, reduced pain, improved immune system, enhanced mental clarity and more.

Affirmations

Affirmations are the action or process of affirming something or being affirmed. It is emotional support encouragement. Positive affirmations can make you feel better about yourself and can manifest real change in your life. You may use affirmations for career success, feeling attractive, boosting self-worth, building abundance, for your positive relationships and for anything you want to focus on. Affirmations can be written, heard or seen. To be really effective you should write them down, say them and hear them at least three times. It is best to use the phrase I am, you are and we are to impact yourself and your surroundings. It's suggested that you keep them in the present tense, be positive, specific and use simple language. For example, I am loving, loveable and loved. You are loving, loveable and loved. We are loving, loveable and loved. There are many benefits to affirmations like the motivation to act, concentration on goals, changing thought patterns into positive ones, influencing your subconscious mind for the better, boost self-confidence and manifesting at higher speeds.

Angels

Angels are spiritual beings. The angels serve according to divine will and direct interventions. Angels will nudge your thinking, diet, and lifestyle changes. Ask them to open your heart, pay attention, meditate, and keep asking for help. We communicate with angels for healing and guidance. The best way to create an atmosphere for angels is to clean and clear the space you are requesting their help. You may light a candle because they love lights. You may burn incense, sage, Palo Santo or another smudge because they love sweet smells. You may also use mists with real essential oils and or rose. Angels can communicate to you through your physical sensations. You may be able to see them, hear them, feel them, smell them or speak with them. If you feel nudges, see repetitive numbers or symbols or have sudden epiphanies be sure that the angels are helping you. In addition to finding random coins, feathers and finding things misplaced. It is best to meditate often with no distractions, to clear you mind and allow them to funnel knowledge to you. Before bed try calling on the angels to guide you in a specific way by asking them angels please clarify and guide me in this situation. Then state what your question, concern or issue is that you need help with. Remember that angels can only if you call upon them and ask for their help, as well as having immediate emergencies your guardian angels will always help.

Animals

Animals assisted therapy is a growing field that uses dogs and other animals to help people recover from or better cope with health-related issues. It's a guided interaction between related issues. It's a guided interaction between a person and an animal. Animals help to naturally regulate emotions. A cat's healing purrs are believed to repair tendons, muscles and joints. Animals can reduce the risk of any heart issues and lower your blood pressure. Dogs on the other hand increase your opportunities to exercise with regular walking and playing. Pets can manage companionship to help one avoid feelings of loneliness. The best part about animals is that there is no judgement and they provide unconditional love. It gives one the feeling of caring for and be cared for by your pet. Everyone wants to love and be loved. The benefits of petting an animal soothe the emotions and reduce stress. We release a relaxation hormone and often times depending on the cuddle abilities of your pet, oxytocin levels rise.

Aromatherapy

Aromatherapy is a holistic healing treatment that uses natural plant extracts to promote health and wellbeing called essential oil therapy. It's medicinally proven to improve body, mind and spirit. It enhances physical and emotional health. Aromatherapy has many benefits like managing pain, improving sleep, increasing energy, improving moods and treating various conditions. The best way to get immersed in aromas is to buy a lava bracelet or necklace and place a few drops on the lava stones. Lavender is a great one for a few drops on a bracelet or wrist as it is calming, sedating and relaxing. You can buy mist sprays like lemongrass or rose water that provide clarity of thought, concentration and cleansing. Also, you may find that humidifiers which sometimes have the menthol Vapo Rub pads and air misters are great to try a couple drops of grapefruit or rosemary. A favorite way is to put a few drops in the bath, but make sure when you put directly on the skin that they do not need to be diluted. It is very important to research your aromas or essential oils to see their uses and cautions.

Art therapy

Art therapy is a distinct discipline that incorporates creative methods of expression through visual art media. It combines the creative process with psychotherapy, facilitating self-exploration and understanding. Using imagery, color and shape. Thoughts and feelings can be expressed. Best part about art therapy is that it is a great form of expression for all ages. Say you have children that are needing counselling, this is the best way to allow them to express their thoughts, feelings and actions without judgment or criticism. There are many benefits to art therapy like: relaxing, social interaction and connection, fulfillment in creating projects, supported in a safe space, choice making when deciding what materials and how your project should be and it provides artistic skills, while providing a life review. This is a great career to pursue because some expressive art therapists include drama, music, art and journaling activities.

Ayurveda

Ayurveda is an alternative medicine system with historical roots in the Indian subcontinent. It begins with the medical knowledge from the gods to sages and then the human physicians. Ayurveda is based on complex herbal compounds, minerals and metal substances. It is the balance of diet, herbal treatments and yogic breathing that offer a balance the body systems. There are many benefits like promoting self-love, better health and wellbeing. It reduces stress and removes toxins from the body. It's a great way to manage weight and improve immunity. There are three dosha bodies that are related to Ayurveda medicine. They are Kapha, Pitta and Vata. Kaphas have an energy of lubrication and structure and their elements are earth and water. Pitta has an energy of transformation and their elements are fire and water. Vata has an energy of movement and their elements are space and air. Based on your dosha there are various ways to balance your type of physical and mental body. It is suggested to cook with ghee and drink herbal teas. Some doshas should prefer cold or warm food and drinks for balance.

Binaural beats

Binaural beats is a term given to playing a sound frequency in one ear and another sound frequency in the opposite ear, creating a 2 tone effect in the mid brain that's actually perceived to be one tone. It's a self-help method that people use to treat conditions such as anxiety. It was first discovered in 1839, by a Prussian physicist and meteorologist named Heinrich Dove. There are many benefits to beats like reducing stress, increasing relaxation and energy, fostering positive moods, promoting creativity and lucid dreaming, managing conditions and increasing mental wellness. There are different brainwaves: delta 1-4hz (deep relaxation, access the unconscious), theta 4-8hz(deeper REM sleep, inner peace), alpha 8-14hz(relaxed focus, positive thinking), beta 14-30hz(focused attention), high level cognition, gamma 30-100hz(high level information processing, transcendental states and peak awareness). Hertz (Hz) is the way we measure a cycle of sound. 1 Hertz means one vibration cycle per second. The frequency following response is the difference of Hz between the two ears. For effective listening try using the waves

Cardio

Cardio or aerobic exercise is physical exercise of low to high intensity. Aerobic like cardio means relating to involving or requiring free oxygen. Cardio is any exercise that raises the heart rate and benefits your heart, lungs and blood vessels. Improves your quality of life and reaps health benefits. Regular exercise can increase exercise tolerance, reduce body weight, reduce blood pressure, increase good cholesterol, improve insulin sensitivity, it can help control appetite, improve moods and energy, help sleep and make you feel better. There are three types of intensities low, mild to moderate and high. It is recommended to start with a warm up for 5 to 10 minutes to rev up your cardiovascular system and increase blood flow to your muscles. Then at your own pace do your cardio conditioning. You may be doing organized sports, strength training, dancing, a circuit or some other type of conditioning. After cool down for 5-10 minutes and stretch your muscles out to prevent injury and get your heart rate back to normal. Engaging in cardio regularly will help you live longer, healthier and happier lives.

Celestial music

Celestial the universal music called music of the spheres or harmony of the spheres is an ancient philosophical concept that regards proportions in the movements of celestial bodies-the sun, moon and planets-as a form of music. Celestial music has a connection between music and astronomy. This ambient music can heal the body, mind and spirit as it carries the energy of the stars. It is deeply relaxing and beneficial to try listening before and during sleep. The discovery of the relation between the pitch of a musical note and length of the string is attributed by Pythagoras. There is a metaphysical mathematical principle that expresses the tones of energy to manifest numbers, visual angles, shapes and sounds. Pythagoras also mentioned that the sun and moon emit their own unique hum. Johannes Kepler published Harmonices Mundi in 1619. It introduced Mysterium and posited that musical intervals and harmonies describe the motions of the six known planets of those times. This music will help you tune in to the cosmos and boost positive healing and energy.

Chakras

Chakras refer to various energy centers in your body that correspond to specific nerve bundles and internal organs. Seven major chakras run from the base of your spine to the top of your head keeping these wheels or chakras in harmony are key. There are seven major chakras that run along the center meridian of the body. The base chakra located around your sexual organs is red in color. It is associated with physical energy. The sacral chakra located an inch below your navel is orange in color. It is associated with creativity. The solar plexus chakra is located one palm length above your navel it is yellow in color. It is associated with the power of your will. The heart chakra is located at the heart it is green. It is associated with love. The throat chakra located at the throat is blue in color. It is associated with communication. The third eye chakra located between the eyebrows is indigo in color. It is associated with intuition. The crown chakra located at the top of the head is violet in color. It is associated with awareness. Maintaining healthy chakras helps balance the body, mind, emotions and spirit. Also, it leads to more awareness of your body. It is paired well with sound meditations, crystals, aromatherapy and chanting. Reiki masters are trained in balancing, cleansing, harmonizing and energizing the chakra system. The benefits include better sleep, connection to your inner self, power to heal and self-heal, provides peace and contentment and there are good changes to your energetic system. Chakra clearings have been known to improve moods, reduce stress and pain and improve the total well-being.

Chant

A chant is the iterative speaking or singing of words or sounds primarily on one or two main pitches called reciting tones. Chants range from simple melody to highly complex music structures including repetition or musical sub phrases. Chanting improves the cardiovascular system and relaxes the body while bringing blood pressure to a normal level. When you chant Om the sound through your vocal cord clears and opens up sinuses. Om is the primordial sound of creation. There are various other chants like Om Shanti, Om Mani Padme Om, and other extensions that can be chanted. Chanting promotes focus, increases energy, improves the mood, and helps with the digestive system. There are various types of chants from African, Hawaiian, Islamic, Buddhist and other spiritual developments. Tibetans Buddhist chants involve throat singing where multiple pitches are produced by each performer.

Chiropractor

A chiropractor practitioner of the system of integrative medicine based on the diagnosis and manipulative treatment of neuromuscular system with an emphasis on treatment through manual adjustment and or manipulation of the spine. There are five common chiropractor techniques. Gonstead technique this is a hands on technique that involves adjusting the low back or pelvis as the patient lies on this side. Activator technique where they use a rod tool positioned on parts of your body. In addition to the flexion distraction, drop table and diversified techniques. There are ample benefits. Improving joint mobility, function and health, loosening muscles, decreases degeneration, improved circulation and nerve system functions, strengthens the immune system, increases energy, vitality and improves sleep and improves athletic performance, cognitive ability and enhances your quality of life. Chiropractors can prescribe soft tissue therapy, adjustments, joint bracing and taping, exercises and stretches and referrals to integrative medicine experts.

Color therapy

Color therapy or chromo therapy uses colors and their frequencies to heal physical and emotional issues. It enhances wellbeing physically, emotionally, spiritually and mentally. It's a pseudoscience offering light therapy. The goal of color therapy to correct physiological and psychological balance in the body. Color therapy has been around since the time of Ancient Egypt. Egyptians believed in the power of light and used different colors of light to promote healing within the human body. Green is the most balancing of all colors. It can improve mood and enhance love, joy and inner peace. Blue is a cold color and helps with peace and relaxation. It is associated with wisdom, creativity, loyalty and spirituality. Light blue promotes serenity. Yellow brings energy and encourages action. It can make you happier and is intense. Orange signifies abundance, pleasure, wellbeing and sexuality. It stimulates different organs for physical healing especially the spleen. Red influences emotional issues like financial independence and physical survival. Red is extreme and can be used in red light therapy. Purple is associated with beauty, spirituality and bliss. Placed on the neck or forehead to bring calm and can be used on any part of the body. A therapy light may illuminate the room during a session for various purposes. You may paint your walls and incorporate Feng Shui to design the balance you need.

Crystals

Crystals is a pseudoscientific alternative medicine technique that uses semiprecious stones and crystals such as quartz, amethyst or opals. Different crystals provide healing properties. Crystals have been hailed as ancient forms of medicine with the philosophies of Hinduism and Buddhism. They're thought to promote the flow of good energy and aid the body, mind and soul. Each crystal has a specific purpose. It is important to look up your crystals to activate these purposes. You may hold the crystal in your hand and read the metaphysical properties aloud or silently. This crystal now has a purpose. Once activated it is important to cleanse, charge and reactivate them after various uses. Some crystals love to be cleansed in water, others in sunlight and many like to be smudged and buried in soil or Himalayan salt. Please know that some crystals prefer certain cleansing methods. Citrine and kyanite need not be cleansed as they are self-cleansing. Selenite prefers not to be exposed to the water.

Fluorite doesn't withstand sunlight well. Rose quartz and citrine love coming into your bath. If you want to amplify the areas of your house you can try putting clear quartz in those areas as they energize these spaces. Clear quartz loves sunshine. There are various shapes, lusters, hardness's and colors of crystals that are more attractive than others. A great starter kit is a chakra set. If you want to expand your knowledge you can buy crystals in the shape of record keepers or generators. There are platonic solids, palm stones, tumbled stones, rough stones, pendants, bracelets and so on. There is a crystal for everything like wealth, love, health, knowledge and self-growth. Learn about placing crystals on the body and more about crystal grids.

Dentist

Dentists help provide people with oral health. Oral health is vital for everyone as it affects the well-being of the body and a good set of white teeth can boost a person's self-esteem. There are several benefits of going for a dental check up on a regular basis. The dentist can make your teeth cleaner, white, straighter and ensure that the gums are strong while detecting any dental issues. It is important to get your teeth cleaned once a year and visit at least twice a year. By brushing twice a day and flossing you can eliminate teeth and gum issues. Basic oral health care requirements can include preventive measures. One can try coconut oil pulling to ensure the health of their mouth. Most dentists can offer direct billing and trusted relationships.

Detox

Detoxification is the physiological or medicinal removal of toxic substances from a living organism including the human body which is mainly carried out by the liver. Typically a detox implies a specific diet or special products the rid your body of toxins thereby improving health and promoting weight loss. It is good for your body to eliminate toxins. Your body's main organs like skin, liver, kidneys, lungs and your digestive system need cleansing every so often. You can try using natural cleaning products and body care to help with detoxification. Try liver, kidney and colon cleansing kits. Giving your organs a break can improve your overall health. It improves circulation of the blood, refuels healthy nutrients and stimulates your body which in turn has benefits mentally. Quick tips include exercise, fasting, avoiding processed foods, choosing whole grains, drinking two liters of water, eating greens, choosing fruits instead of desserts, avoiding sugar and alcohol. There is an apple juice cleanse that will repair your liver quickly. You can try apple cider foot detox pads that you place on the bottom of your feet overnight and peel off in the morning. There are various detox retreats and spas you can enjoy that will help.

Dreams

Dreams are a series of thoughts, images and sensations occurring in a person's mind during sleep. Dreams mainly occur in Rapid eye movement (REM) stage of sleep when brain activity is high and resembles that of being awake. Sigmund Freud developed the psychological disciple of psychoanalysis wrote on dream theories. Oneiromancy is the theory of dreams. In many religious stories there are dreams recorded in sacred texts. There are two types of dreams premonitory and dreams of compensation or digestion. The purpose of our dreams is to clarify, illuminate and awaken us. Dreams should be recorded in a dream diary and interpreted using the signs and symbols to be analyzed. To assist in the REM stage one should get a dreamcatcher or two to put above the head; this will prevent nightmares and offer a safe place to dream and recall upon awakening. Getting an eye mask and take a calcium, magnesium, Vitamin D supplement will aid dreaming. According to Freud, dreaming is the royal road of the unconscious. According to Carl Jung reoccurring dreams demand your attention and these are called dreams of compensation. There are many benefits to dreaming like guidance, regulating mood and help us to make connections to our realities. Lucid dreaming is the conscious perception of ones state while dreaming. Lucid dreamers have control over their own actions. The theory of déjà vu attributes to have seen or experience something to have dreamed about a similar situation. There are different types of daydreamers. Daydreamers refer to milder imagery, realistic future planning and reviewing past memories.

Energy

Energy medicine is based on the belief that healers can channel healing energy into a patient and effect positive results for instance on electrocardiogram (EKG) around the heart or an electrophalogram) EEG) around the brain is a reading of the energy field around the organ our bodies are electrical. We are energy and exert our own energetic fields. High positive energy beings are always well. There are various types of energy work like Reiki, Brenna Healing Science, Chakra healing, Donna Eden's Energy Medicine, Energy focused bodywork, amongst others Being a giver and receiver of energy work that are many benefits like: improved immune system, enhanced mental abilities, sense of emotional wellness, enhanced personal growth, radiating positive auras and it can reduce pain and stress. Energy work can be performed on anyone as it is painless, easy and accessible. The result of energy work is overall wellness and good vibes. Energy masters work with Qi gong, pranayama, quantum healing, crystals and reiki.

Family crest

People refer family crest by shield of arms or coat of arms. You can run across the term heraldry. It originates back in the middle ages. Adorning distinguishable family names with a shield, helmet, armor, and various designs and guardians. The coat of arms on the shield forms the central element of the full heraldic achievement which consists of shield, supporters, crest and motto. The design symbol is unique to every family. The first evidence of medieval coat of arms is found in the 11th century. And became more popular for feudal lords and knights in the 12th century. You can look up your last name from your father and mother to discover you history. There are various websites you can search up your name to find your family crest and genealogy; in addition to getting ancestry tests to find your real heritage. You can find sites online that offer apparel with your family crest on it. The symbols on the coat of arms are meant to represent the achievements of the person, location or corporation to whom or which the arms are granted. Even Popes have their own coat of arms. Owners of the coat of arms can place trademarks that are governed and regulated for families and organizations. Heraldry is a real art and it doesn't have to be ancient to be created.

Fast

Fasting is a practice abstaining from all or some foods or drinks for a set period of time. There are many benefits promoting blood sugar control and better health, enhancing heart health, can boost brain health and weight loss and may aid in longevity and could delay aging. Fasting is the golden ticket to a client's health goals. Three types of fasts are calorie restriction, nutrient restriction and seasonal eating. A calorie restriction fast is done in 18-48 hours and you eat a light dinner then fast with water. A macro nutrient fast is typical for athletes who need to consume only high quality fats, carbohydrates and cooked vegetables for 2-3 days a month. Seasonal eating is when you eat fattier meats for winter and fruits and leaner meats for summer. A calorie restriction fast is similar to intermittent fasting. It's a period of fasting producing a net calorie deficit so you lose weight. There are various kinds of intermittent fasting like: 5:2 which is 2 days a week fast and eat the other 5 days, time restricted like fasting for 14-16 hours, overnight fasting, eat a few days stop for 24 hours then eat , whole day, alternate day fasting every other day and choose your day. It is important when fasting to avoid blood sugar crashes, stay hydrated, supplement where needed and be easy with the exercise. Fasting contributes to self-enlightenment as well as kick starting your digestive tract.

Frequency sounds

Sound healing synchronicities brain waves to achieve states of relaxation, helping to restore its normal vibratory frequency of the cells in our bodies. Solfeggio frequencies are used for transformational purposes and can help improve relationships, emotions and awaken ones intuition. Solfeggio frequencies include a set of sacred numbers with repeating sequence 3 6 9. The tones contain frequency to balance and heal energy fields. 396 to liberate emotions 417 to facilitate change 528 love and miracle 639 connect relationships 741 awaken intuition 852 spiritual order 963 divine consciousness. There are many benefits to sound frequencies like reduced stress, increased focus, concentration and motivation, improved confidence, better long term memory, deeper and enhanced states of meditation and mood. Solfeggio frequencies have positive effects because they resonate harmony with the Schumann resonance of 8 Hz. There are other frequencies like 174 Hz that relieves pain and tension. 285 Hz that's linked to safety, energy and survival. It is suggested to find a quiet place away from distractions and find a comfortable place. These music sounds go well with pranayama, mantras and mudras.

Float

Floating in a sensory deprivation tank with salt water. Sessions are 60-90minutes. Floating can decrease anxiety, improve sleep, relieve paint, and enhance performance. Some float studios have water based speakers with guided meditation and light therapy. You typically peacefully float on a 10" high water filled floor within a floatation tank because of the buoyant water salt solution. The effects of gravity are removed while floating which improves your circulation and allows rejuvenation. Floating can reduce blood pressure and heart rate and in turn lower stress levels. The sensory deprivation slows your brain waves until you reach theta state. Floating is great for athletes as it improves performance, strengthens immune system and accelerates healing and mental clarity. Also, it increases your energy levels. It is great to do a float if you are detoxing or fasting. Most float houses have used color, light and sound with water to amplify the positive results.

Herbology

Herbology has roots in nutrition like in china where herbs, seeds, minerals, barks and other remedies are part of the daily diet. Herbs go back to the Paleolithic Era 60 000 years ago. Decoctions, granules, pills, tinctures, and liniments are used. Herbs like ginseng, licorice, astragulus, cinnamon, shitake mushrooms and ginger are used. Master herbalists can use herbs to heal all the body, mind and soul. Knowing how to grow, sustain, harvest, forage, and produce these natural medicines is important for future generations. The best way to access these herbs is cooking with them, brewing teas and gardening. The Materia Medica is the bible or dictionary of plants. This five volume work was written in the Renaissance by Carl Linnaeus Materia Medica. Linnaeus the father of modern taxonomy is the reason for international botanical names. It is a collection of monographs of plants including information of folklore, magical uses, cultivation, medical uses and general information.

Homeopathy

Homeopathy was created in 1796 by Samuel Hahnem. Homeopathic preparations are remedies prescribed in the Materia Medica and repertories; Homeopathy uses animal, plant, minerals and synthetic substances. It's a holistic natural approach. It's a holistic approach that heals the total person. Homeopathy seeks to stimulate the body's own natural healing powers to bring health, vitality and wellbeing. Patients have reported in improvement in energy, mood, quality of sleep, digestion and seen symptoms disappear. They are safe and low cost treatments and are usually covered under health plans. Most homeopathic medicines are shaken with silicon to preserve them and should be stored in dark, cool and dry places. It's been proven to cure chronic issues. It is suggested to rinse your mouth of food particles before taking any medicine as it is absorbed by the mucus membrane of the mouth.

Hydrotherapy

Hydrotherapy involves submerging ourselves in water whether in bathing or in an all-natural body of water. From Roman baths to hot mineral springs cultures around the world have been using water therapy. We do it for personal hygiene, leisure and health. Cryotherapy is the act of taking ice baths. Cold water causes superficial blood vessels to constrict, moving blood flow away from an affected area to relieve inflammation. Hot water causes superficial blood vessels to dilate, activating sweat glands, loosening joints, and removing toxic wastes from tissues. It can improve heart health, benefits your respirator, nervous, musculoskeletal, immune and skin organs. It's a pleasant way to regulate your body temperature. You can add Epsom salts, sea salts or Himalayan salts for optimal health. There are different types of hydrotherapy like: aquatic exercises, balneotherapy (soaking in mineral rich water/hot springs), colon hydrotherapy, compresses (wrap with hot/cold), contrast (water circuit therapy), float tanks, foot baths, ice baths, saunas, steams, whirlpool, and watsu (shiatsu in pool of warm water). Hydrotherapy is super good for stimulating your immune, digestive and circulatory system. It relieves the body of gravity's effects and induces a hydrostatic effect while stimulating the skins receptors. It stimulates muscles and improves blood flow.

Hypnotherapy

Hypnosis is used to create a state of focused attention and increased suggestibility during which positive suggestions and guided imagery are used to help individuals deal with a variety of concerns and issues. Hypnotherapists use the dominant brain wave state using relaxation techniques like deep breathing and self-awareness. They try to bring clients to the edge of sleep to manage their subconscious and conscious behaviors. The optimum state offers suggestions to facilitate the client's goals. The founders of neuro linguistic programming (NLP) are similar to versions of hypnotherapy. Clients can use hypnosis to change performance, weight, smoking, drinking, drugs, eating, sex, health and any pattern they want to undue or reduce in terms of mentality. There are many benefits depending on the focus and goal desired. There have been improvements in sleeping, easing anxiety and pain, quitting addictions that no longer serve and improvements to diet, exercise and weight. There is a boost in health. Commit to trying it and do your homework. Like self-hypnosis, meditation and other online audio recordings may help to achieve your target goals.

Ion cleanse

An ion foot bath is completely painless. It's a pseudoscientific device marketed as being able to remove toxins from the human body. They work by providing an electric current to an electrode array immersed in a salt water solution. When switched on electrolysis happens. The ionic technique of pulling toxins out of your feet provides your vital organs with cleansing. It has been proven to help with eliminating blood, joint, digestive, circulatory and yeast issues. It is recommended to do five to ten sessions spread out over a few weeks apart to reap the full benefits of detoxification. It is great to do if you are detoxing, fasting or need to eliminate clean your organs. It works great with hydrocolon therapy. There are many benefits that include: relieving pain, purifying blood and lymph, increasing circulation, stimulating the immune system, clearing up skin, reducing weight, improving body flexibility, increasing oxygen, energizing the body and improving sleep. Some ion cleanse therapists offer infrared belts, liver lasers, tens massagers and sound therapy meditation with their sessions. Sessions are typically anywhere from 20 to 45 minutes. When the time is up you will find that the water has been discolored depending on what material or body system is eliminating the most.

Interpersonal group

The concept of interpersonal relationship involves social associations, connections or affiliations between two or more people. Context could be family, friends, work, clubs, neighborhoods and places of worship. It can be based on inference, love, solidarity, support, regular business interactions, and some other type of social commitment. The groups usually consist of about 4 to 8 members plus a facilitator or two. The groups are designed to enhance interpersonal skills and help each member identify and achieve their goals. Goals could be to be more assertive, a better listener, be comfortable, express emotions, or something like this. Members discover personal strengths and have opportunities to interact in new ways. Interpersonal groups are best for people working on issues such as assertiveness, communication, social well-being, self-confidence, boundaries and trust with others. Group participants are encouraged to share their thoughts, feelings, perceptions and experiences as they feel comfortable and this is not forced. These groups are great for teaching life skills and offering therapeutic conversations that bring emotional and social well-being.

Journal

A journal is a detailed account that records all your thoughts and feelings. Writing has no rules except make it a daily exercise. Journaling can help gain control of your emotions and boost your health. Diaries help us to organize our thoughts, can improve our writing, help set and achieve goals, recording ideas to remember them for boosting memory, allow for self-reflection, and inspiring creativity. Writing is a super tool for self-expression and good for your health. It was proven that journaling for 15 to 20 minutes a day three or four times over a period of four months can lower blood pressure and improve liver functionality. It is a way to reduce stress. It can improve your immune system by strengthening your immune cells. Journaling unlocks and engages the right brained creativity, improving mood and increasing confidence. Simply start with a single line to stimulate and train the brain and build your way up. There are various types of journals like bullet journal, free writing, planner journals, gratitude journals, art, dream or prayer, daily reflections, personal growth and processing feelings in journals. Try using the fill in the blank guided books that are available online or in your bookstore to give you focal points to write about. You can try using gratitude and write three things you are grateful for that day and see the improvements in your life over a period of weeks. There are various 31 day challenges that offer questions you can answer in written format. Try thinking it, writing it and speaking it. Using an optimistic love appreciation language will assist the transformation of your state of well-being for the better.

Laugh

Laugh your way to better health. Thanks to the mind body connection the simple act of laughing can tell your brain to produce chemicals that help your heart, immune system, energy and improve your mood. Positive psychology names laughter and sense of humor as one of the 24 main signature strengths one can possess. A good hearty laugh relieves physical tension and stress, leaving your muscles relaxed for up to 45 minutes after. Laughter boosts the immune system. It can lower blood pressure, improve cardiac health, boost T cells, reduces cortisol and decreases physical pain receptors and triggers a release of endorphins and dopamine. Overall produces a general sense of well-being. Laughter yoga is an excellent way to have an internal work out. A good belly laugh exercises the diaphragm, contracts the abs and works of the shoulders while relaxing the muscles. Laughter connects with others. Offering smiles and kindness can elevate the moods of yourself and everyone around you. Find the humor in life. Watch a funny movie, go to a comedy theatre, and look up one line jokes to remember and tell and laugh a lot with your friends. Learn how to chuckle, giggle, bellow, cackle, tee hee, snicker and laugh. Laughter is the purest form of communication. It will amplify resilience and increase your social attraction while building rapport with others. Laughter is the best medicine.

Mandala

A mandala is a geometric configuration of symbols. Mandalas may be employed for focusing attention of practitioners and adepts as a spiritual guidance tool for establishing a sacred space and as aid to meditations and trance induction. The New Age is a geometric pattern representing cosmos. They are used to gain knowledge from within. Mandalas may be actual drawings or paintings and can be ceremoniously displayed with symmetrical patterns using color schemes. Mandalas are tools of meditation. It is shown to reduce stress and pain, lower blood pressure, boost immune system, stimulate melatonin which is believed to slow cell aging and promote peaceful sleep. They are useful for all people. Children can express emotions through art and color. People can use crayons, pencil crayons, chalks, pastels, paint, or markers and color in a mandala book or you can create your own from scratch. Other digital art tools can be used to create mandalas. Cognitive and behavioral psychology sees them as a tool to improve higher functions such as memory, attention, perception and motor coordination. They promote harmony and creativity. You can find print mandalas, knitted or sand mandalas, tapestries and decorative pictures. To understand color therapy can magnify your intentions and goals for creating a mandala.

Mantra

Mantras are sacred utterances, a sound, syllable, word or phonemes or group of words in Sanskrit. They are believed by practitioners to have religious magical or spiritual powers in Hinduism. Mantras can be highly beneficial for your brain. The primary effect of chanting mantras provides peace of mind and improves positive vibrations. A simple chanting of OM has increased mental awareness and reduces the heart rate. Mantras improve attention, increase concentration and change your mood even if chanting for 10 minutes. Mantras are more powerful especially on the full moon, new moon or planetary alignments and retrograde. You can try the mantra Om santih santih sanith Pronounced Aum shanti shanti shanti translated Om peace peace peace. Mantras are sounds or vibrations that create a desired effect such as healing, transformation or self-awareness. Traditions around the world use the beating of a drum, a bell, a gong or another sacred sound when formulating mantras. Japa means the repetition of a mantra so it encompasses all uses of mantras. They use a string of beads known as a Mala with 108 beads. It is recommended to choose a mantra to repeat daily with a mala over 30 days to see the transformation. Another simple mantra is Gam. This mantra is used to remove obstacles and blockages and brings wisdom to your life. There are chakra, meditation and enlightenment mantras that can be chanted to focus on that intent.

Massage

Massage is a manipulation of the body's soft tissues. Massage techniques are applied with hands, fingers, elbows, knees, forearms, feet or a device. There are several types of massages. During a massage a therapist will apply gentle or strong pressure to the muscles and joints of the body to the likeness of what the client is wanting. A Swedish massage is a gentle full body massage its goal is to relax and release muscle tension. Hot stone massage is used with heated stones to ease muscle tension, improve blood flow and promote relaxation. Aromatherapy massage is used with a combination of essential oils and is best for boosting mood and relieving pain. Deep tissue is more intense than Swedish massage and applies more pressure to get into those muscles and connective tissues. Sports massage can increase flexibility and performance and assist in athletic recovery. Trigger point massage is best suited for releasing specific areas of the body and focuses on trigger points to reduce pain. Reflexology uses gentle to firm pressure on pressure points on the feet, hands, ears and face to relax and restore the entire body. Shiatsu massage is a Japanese rhythmic pressure massage that uses hands, palms and thumbs on certain points of the body. Shiatsu promotes emotional and physical calm, helps relieve tension and relaxes the muscles. Thai massage is an active form of massage that improves flexibility, circulation and energy levels. There is a sequence of movements the therapist goes through similar to yogic stretching. It is recommended to wear loose fitted clothing during a Thai massage. Prenatal massage is a safe way to relax and reduce pregnancy aches. Couple's massage allows you to have a partner, friend or family member in the same room and you both get massages. Chair massages are a quick massage focusing on the neck, shoulders and back. Typical massages are 30-90 minutes and can range from $50 to $150. Massages are recommended once a month for optimum health and well-being.

Meditation

Meditation influences the sympathetic nervous system, keeping blood pressure, respiration and heart rate in check. It's a practice like mindfulness or focusing the mind on a particular object, thought or activity. It's to train attention and awareness and to achieve a mental clear and emotionally calm and stable state. There are various types of meditation like: loving kindness, body scan, mindfulness, breath awareness, kundalini, Zen, transcendental, affirmation based and guided. Meditation techniques are described as calming or insightful. They can involve focusing on a particular object, your breath, mantra, visualization, physical sensations or mental awareness. A vipassana meditation is another ancient tradition that offers insight through silence. There are many short term benefits like lowering blood pressure, improving blood circulation, lowering heart rate, improving respiratory rates, lowering cortisol levels, increasing feelings of well-being, providing deep relaxation and improved immune function. Like anything continuing to practice meditation is important to clear your mind of any mental restrictions and allowing a deeper focus and concentration of the intention to provide your entire being with peace. It is recommended to sit or lie comfortably, close your eyes, control your breath consciously and focus your attention on your breath for a few minutes breathing in peace and love and exhaling joy and compassion. Even a few minutes a day in the morning and evening can have a positive impact on your overall wellness.

Naturopathy

Naturopathy employs an array of pseudoscientific practices that are natural, non-invasive and self-healing. It's based on the belief in the body's ability to heal itself through a special vital energy or force guiding bodily processes internally. A therapeutic effect on the biochemical pathways. It employs a natural therapy to restore physiological, psychological and structural balance. There treatments are gentle, non-invasive and effective with no adverse side effects and they can suppress symptoms. Most naturopathic treatments can include botanical medicine, nutritional therapy, acupuncture, physiotherapy and offer treatment plans to reach your goals. The benefits to naturopathy are cures, sleeping aids, disease prevention and offer a combination of alternative therapies personalized for each client. Sometimes naturopaths will do hormone (salivary, blood and urinary), thyroid and food sensitivity testing to find out where concerns originate. During a session they will ask questions about your history, stress levels, and lifestyle habits.

Osteopathy

Osteopathy emphasizes physical manipulation of tissues of the body muscle tissue and bones. Many manipulative techniques are aimed at reducing or eliminating the impediments to proper structures and function so the self-healing mechanism can restore health. Osteopathy is a hands on drug free, non-invasive manual therapy manipulating the musculoskeletal system. Treatments positively affect the body's nervous, circulatory and lymphatic system. Patients will be asked to demonstrate simple stretches and movements to help the physician make an accurate analysis of the posture and mobility. They will assess the health of the joints, ligaments and tissues. They can offer stretching and lifting techniques, posture and breathing advice. Osteopathy can remove the cause of pain, increase range of motion, treat spinal issues, improve posture and breathing and decrease stress. It is encouraged to see an osteopath if you want to remove pain. Osteopathy is a great corrective practice. Initial visits can be about $100 and take 45-90 minutes. Treatment techniques can include: osteoarticular corrections (gentle realignment of the bones), visceral mobilization (gentle mobilization of the organs of the body), cranial osteopathy (gentle movement of the bones of the skull), normalization of myofascial tissues, muscle energy and strain counterstrain (method of relaxing and repositioning joints).

Plant therapy

Engaging with plants can have a relaxing peaceful effect. The engagement of a person in gardening and plant based activities facilitated by a trained therapist to achieve specific therapeutic treatment goals. Plants have numerous benefits. Plants can assist with long term success, recovery and well-being. They can be used therapeutically to improve mental health. Essential oils, gardening, spending time in a nature and healthy eating can be used in combination to achieve a healthy lifestyle. If this interests you look up horticultural for additional help. The Horticultural Therapy Institute shares some of the best types of plants to use in therapy gardens for fragrant plants, edibles and seasonal annuals. Plant therapy the act of taking care of them and watching the progress releases happy hormones of pure enjoyment. It can improve self-esteem; foster a feeling of connection and nurturing power. People with plant based diets generally have better moods and are less prone to heart conditions. Plant therapy has potential positive effects on memory, language skills, socialization and brain cognition. It can help with balance, stamina, muscle strength and coordination. You can start by getting houseplants. Try a snake plant or a pet friendly spider plant which are both resilient and low maintenance. Plus they help freshen the air around you. You can volunteer at a community garden or rent a garden plot for summer if you need the space.

Pranayama

Pranayama is the practice of breath controlling. It consists of synchronizing the breath with movement. Prana means life force or breath. Yama means to extend or draw out. Or "Pran" means bio energy and "ayama" means to control or regulation. The goal of pranayama is to strengthen the connection between your body and mind. It can promote relaxation and mindfulness; and is proven to support aspects of physical health, including lung function, blood pressure and brain function. Daily advice can include: having a ventilated place, mornings and evenings are ideal times, about 10-15minutes daily, try on an empty stomach and avoid distractions. The Wim Hof breathing techniques are very helpful lessons to start with. Keeping the practice will activate your digestive organs, reduce fat, improve respiratory system, provide harmony and is sedative to your nervous system. Try yogendra pranayama(alternate nostril breathing). Do five rounds breathing through only one nostril and holding the other. This will regulate your breathing, increase your energy level, provide lightness to your body, improving lung capacity and destress. Together with healthy eating patterns, regular workouts, healthy sleep and proper hydration, it can be the basis of a healthy life. Tibetan Buddhists breathing exercise such as the nine breathings of purification or the Ninefold Expulsion of State Vital Energy, a form of alternate nostril breathing that can include visualizations. Breathing is paired great with meditation.

Psychedelics

Psychedelic therapy is a technique that involves the use of substances that aid the therapeutic process. Research suggests psychedelics have been around for thousands of years. Since the 1950's LSD (acid) and psilocybin (magic mushrooms) have the potential to treat a range of conditions. Other popular substances include ayahuasca (spirit molecule), MDMA (ecstasy) and ketamine. Administration of a low to moderate dose with professional supervision can create euphoric results. Some people like to micro dose by taking a very small sub hallucinogenic dose to enhance mood and performance and increase energy. Other benefits include feelings of relaxation, improved sense of wellbeing, increased social connectedness, introspection and spiritual experiences. It's suggested to go to an ayahausca ceremony at least one to experience a positive life changing experience that will change your perception of reality.

Qigong

Qigong is a millennia old system of coordinated body posture and movement, breathing and mediation used for purposes of health, spirituality and martial arts training. It involves moving meditation, coordinating slow flowing movement, deep rhythmic breathing and a calm mind. The literal translation of qi gong is energy work. Qi gong is a separate group coming through the martial arts lineages. Qi gong can harness willpower, to focus, and to help practitioners channel their energy through their palms. In the west, the eyes are considered the gateway to the soul and in the Taoist theory they are believed to guide the shen or the spirit. It is said that qi (energy) follows the shen (spirit) and the blood and body fluids in turn then follow the qi. Therefore the eyes become the command center and qi gong uses hand eye coordination, visualizations, breathing and body movements to direct energy. Bodhidharma created a routine called the Famous Tamo's Eighteen Hands of the Lohan mixing kung fu and qi gong at the Shaolin Temple.

Red light therapy

RLT is a treatment that may help skin, muscle tissue and other parts of your body heal. It exposes you to low levels of red and near infrared light. It's also called low level laser. Your cells called mitochondria soak up the red light and make more energy. Red light therapy is sometimes called photobiomodulation (PBM) or soft or cold laser therapy, biostimulation, photonic stimulation and low-power laser therapy (LPLT). Red light beds are found at salons and are said to reduce cosmetic skin issues like stretch marks and wrinkles. They can treat various skin conditions. Red light works by producing a biochemical effect in cells that strengthen the mitochondria. By increasing the function of mitochondria a cell can make more adenosine triphosphate (ATP) which is an energy carrying molecule. With more energy cells can function more efficiently rejuvenate themselves and repair damage. RLT can promote tissue repair, improve hair growth, stimulate wound healing, improve skin complexion and builds collagen, diminishes scars, improves joint health and relieves inflammation. Other noticed benefits include boosting the immune system, activating the lymphatic system to help detoxify, removes age spots and sun damage and aids in weight loss. It can be combined with white light, blue light and ultraviolet light therapies. Some tanning salons have both UVB and RLT at their studios. A typical RLT session is 20 minutes.

Reflexology

Reflexology involves the application of pressure to specific points on the feet and hands. This is done using specific thumb finger and hand massage techniques without the use of oil or lotion but it may be used. It's based on the pseudoscientific system of zones and reflex areas that purportedly reflect on image of the body on the feet, hands, ears, tongue, and face. Reflexologists use maps to guide their work and you can look up reflexology charts to see where the pressure points are and what organs and body parts they are associated with. Reflexology is similar to acupressure and acupuncture; although they believe that they can relieve stress and pain in other parts of the body by manipulation of the hands and feet. Reflexology rests on the ancient Chinese belief in qi (vital energy). In Chinese medicine, different body parts correspond with different pressure points on the body. They use the chart maps to determine where they should apply pressure to unblock the qi. People have reported reflexology helped them with boosting their immune system, clearing up sinuses, recovering from back issues, correcting hormones, boosting fertility, reducing pain and stress, lifting moods, improving general well-being and treating digestive and nervous system. It is great for your overall physical and mental health.

Reiki

Reiki is a Japanese technique channeling God's wisdom or higher power and life force energy. Reiki treats the whole person, body, emotions, mind and spirit. It can be hands on or off and include distant healing. Attunements can be given by reiki masters. It promotes harmony in others. There are various types of reiki. Western Usui Reiki, Eastern Jikiden, Karuna, Lightarian and Sekehem or Seichim Reiki. Everyone should get at least their level one reiki to help with healing practice, personal development, spiritual discipline and mystical orders. Reiki Masters provide the oral traditions, lineages, history, initiation, symbols, treatments, forms of teaching and precepts to offer students with the best teachings. Reiki can balance out the energy, provide acceptance of self and relaxation, remove pain and discomfort, better sleep, promote feelings of well-being, and instill awareness. Reiki is safe and effective for everyone. It can provide acceleration of healing and promote speedy recoveries in person or at a distance. Reiki helps lift unsettling emotions and behaviors while replacing it with positive energy. Lightarian Reiki expands and enhances your connection with the Ascended Master Buddha. You can attain a higher level of personal healing and a progression of vibrational levels. Some reiki masters heal with symbols, mantras, meditation, spiritual psychology and elemental balancing. You can also try rainbow reiki, kundalini reiki or chakra energy balancing to maintain well-being.

Sacred Geometry

Sacred geometry ascribes symbolic and sacred meanings to certain geometric shapes and certain geometric proportions. Designs are seen in structures, churches, temples and mosques. Creations of religious art go back to God's plan. Mathematical principles and forms like Nautilus, spirals, hexagonal cells and yantras are included. Sacred geometric patterns exist all around us. Geometry as the blueprint of creation and the origin of all form. The molecules of our DNA, the cornea of our eyes, snowflakes, flower petals, crystals, shells, the stars, the spiral in our galaxies and a bee's honeycomb. These patterns offer higher consciousness and self-awareness; in addition to amplifying our connection to spirit. It is often called sacred architecture. Each of us has a light body merkabah. This is our light soul body chariot which looks similar to the Star of David 3D. The platonic solids are thought to be building blocks of the universe and were taught 2500 years ago. These shapes are the tetrahedron, hexahedron, octahedron, dodecahedron and icosahedron. The triangle is a symbol that underlies all of them and symbolizes balance, harmony and completion. A circle symbolizes perfection, wholeness and the cycles of life. The square symbolizes grounding, stability and safety. The spiral like the Fibonacci and golden mean ratio connects heaven and earth. Energy moves in spirals. You can look up other shapes like the flower of life, seed of life, egg of life, pyramid and vesical pieces for further information. You can use crystals to make sacred geometry grids to manifest specific intentions.

Sauna

Sauna or sudatory is a small room or building designed as a place to experience dry or wet heat sessions. The first record of a sauna appeared in 1112 in Finland. Sauna is a Finnish word that means bath or bathhouse. This steam and high heat make the people perspire. Oldest saunas come from Finland they are smoke saunas. There are different types of saunas like the traditional Finnish sauna, dry or wet saunas, steam baths, wood burning, sweat lodge and infrared saunas. Most public saunas can be located within exercise facilities, massage clinics, health spas, beauty salons and domestic homes. Facilities claim health benefits of sauna bathing that include detoxification, increased metabolism, weight loss, increased blood circulation, pain reduction, antiaging, skin rejuvenation, improved cardiovascular function, improved immune function, improved sleep, stress management and relocation. Evidence suggests induced physiological effects. Intense short term heat exposure elevates skin temperatures and core body temperature and activated thermoregulatory pathways via the hypothalamus and central nervous system. The high heat can relax muscles and joints, improve overall wellness, release of endorphins, flush toxins, improve brain health, burn calories and it feels good. It is suggested to do for 15-20 minutes especially when detoxifying.

Sound bath

Sound bath is a meditative experience where those in attendance are bathed in sound waves. These waves are produced by various sources including healing instruments such as gongs, singing bowls, percussion, chimes, rattles, tuning forks and even the human voice. Sound baths are accompanied with a yogic or guided meditation. The instruments produce deep overlapping vibrations that sooth the nervous system and connect to the consciousness. Most people lay down in savasana (yoga pose laying on their backs) on a pat with pillows or blankets during the duration of the sound bath. Sound baths are meant to activate the alpha and theta brain waves associated with peaceful states having a body impact on the body, brain and heart. The vibrations and frequencies can help restore and enhance ones respiratory, nervous and cardiac systems. Another great tool is to practice breathing techniques or pranayama during a sound bath. A typical session lasts for an hour or two and is about $20-30. You will notice a relaxed mind and body after a sound bath session.

Shamanism

Shamanism involves a practitioner who is believed to interact with a spirit world through altered states of consciousness such as a trance or dream. The goal of this is usually to direct these spirits or spiritual energies into the physical world for healing or some other purpose. Following a shamanism perspective means to seek to be in relationship with the spirit of all things. Shamans can alter their consciousness to travel to the realms of the invisible worlds. Others describe shamans as physicians, psychotherapists, magician's storytellers and healers. They mediate between the needs of the spirit world and those of the physical world. They serve the needs of the community. They have a multidisciplinary approach to cure and restore balance. Shamans use botanical medicine, request changes to the diet and offer an accurate diagnosis of the seen and unseen energies associated with the issue. They can provide soul recovery to accomplish healing by calling back the return of lost parts of the soul. Shamanic healing is individualized to each unique person. Shamans are called through dreams or signs to get information; in addition to completing the rites of passage and completing their initiation into shamanism. Shaman's can evoke animal and plant life to search for answers. They will go into trances and vision quests to provide healing to their clients. Some shamans will use entheogens which is a psychoactive substance used in religious, shamanic or spiritual contexts. Entheogens generate the divine within. Some traditional examples include: peyote, psilocybin, magic mushrooms, uncured tobacco, cannabis, salvia, morning glory and ayahuasca. Shamans can use music in their healings. They will drum, sing medicine songs, throat sing, and ecstatic dance. Their treatments heal the whole person.

Sports/fitness

Sports activities involving physical exertion and skill in which an individual or team competes against another or others for entertainment. To amuse oneself or play in a lively energetic active way can maintain and improve physical activity and skills providing enjoyment. Regular physical activity is good for the body and mind. Exercise involves the physical exertion, voluntary movements and burning calories. This form of physical activity is planned, structured and repetitive. Examples include: skiing, swimming, cycling, aerobics, soccer, hockey, basketball, volleyball, tennis and so on. There are many physical benefits that include developing strong bones, joints and muscles, helps keep the body in healthy shape, improves balance, reflexes, coordination and overall fitness, and promotes strength.

There are psychosocial benefits like increasing relaxation, improving self-esteem, building positive self-image, increase happy hormones, increasing feelings of belonging and acceptance. To interact with others is pure fun. Finding an activity to match your physical and psychosocial goals is important. Depending on the age and physical abilities of each person it may vary as to what interests are valued. Some sports are team based and others individual. Some sports are supervised and others unsupervised. Each sport depends on the speed, amount of contact, skill levels and game plan. Depending on what sport, there is a cost and equipment involved. It is important to stretch for warm ups and cool downs to avoid injury.

Steam Room

Steam room is a heated room that people use for relaxation, detox and to relieve and medical conditions. It's created when water filled generator pumps steam into an enclosed space so there is moisture in the air when people are sitting in it. Steam rooms are generally 110 to 114 degrees Fahrenheit with 100% humidity. Most steam rooms are located in gyms and spas. Steam rooms are heated by a generator filled with boiling water. They can improve circulation. When sitting in a steam room a hormone called aldosterone is released this can help lower blood pressure. And it can reduce stress by decreasing the hormone production of cortisol. Steams aid in workout recovery by losing stiff joints and burns calories. They are great boosts to the immune system, clearing congestion and promoting skin health. You only need to stay in a steam room for 15 minutes to reap the benefits. Be cautious as to the cleanliness of the room and if needed put a towel down where you sit. Adding a steam to your post workout routine will help you feel healthier and decrease your recovery time.

Stretching

Stretching is a form of physical exercise in which a specific muscle or tendon is deliberately flexed or stretch in order to improve the muscles felt elasticity and achieve comfortable muscle tone. The result is a feeling of increased muscle control, flexibility and range of motion. Stretching is good for all ages and abilities. There are various types of stretching ballistic (uses the momentum of a moving body or limb beyond its range of motion), dynamic (moving parts gradually increasing reach, speed or both), active static(assume a position and hold it), passive (assume a position and hold it with another part of your body), static (stretching a muscle to its farthest point and holding it), isometric(involves resistance of muscle groups through contractions) and PNF (proprioceptive neuromuscular facilitation combines passive and isometric stretching). It can improve posture and increase the blood supply allowing for an increase of nutrients. Stretching is very important for all athletes before and after their exercise as it prevents injuries. Stretching can release tension, calm the mind and increase your energy. They suggest stretching at least 2-3 times a week for 10 minutes to achieve the most benefits. To get some body stretching in one can try a Thai massage as there are various movements and stretches involved. Stretching keeps the muscles flexible, strong and healthy.

Soul Collage

Soul collage is a process which you contact your intuition and you create a collage with deep personal meaning which helps you answer life's questions while manifesting dreams goals and visions. It's a multi layered creative process you use cut outs of words and pictures and give them together. Soul collage practice leads to a greater self-acceptance and helps you access your intuition and inner spiritual knowing. Working with images stimulates greater areas of brain function and can increase cognitive health. In addition to helping you connect to your conscious, subconscious and unconscious. It is a great way to play and have fun. It's a great coping skill and helps one create the future of their dreams. It's a safe process that can inspire creativity. You can find a facilitator that offers individual or group sessions. They will supply all the resources necessary like images, multimedia mediums, writing utensils, stickers, stamps, magazines, cards and other accessories. Art therapists facilitate this process the best. Other soul collage workshops can help men and women live a more positive authentic life through self-discovery.

Sun Catcher

Sun catchers or light catchers are small reflective refractive and or iridescent ornaments. It may include glass pieces and be hung indoors near a window to catch sunlight. The equivalent of a wind chime. They are believed first to be made by Native Americans. Sun catchers is a multifaceted crystal pulls in bouncing light into our home, car or work window to create unexpected patterns of color light beams. You can create a transformation in your life by putting up a sun catcher in your home. Feng Shui masters suggest it for cleansing and movement; as well as to inspire shifts and major action in your life. The benefits are" it activates positive energy and balances areas with a lack of light or color. The light can calm and with certain crystals on the sun catcher strand like rose quartz it can be a love cure. You can hang your sun catcher in areas with little or no light like a corner, hallway or even at your work desk. These sun catchers will radiate positive light energy. It brings energy of the sunlight into an area that is dark.

Sunshine

Sunshine is sunlight the electromagnetic radiation emitted by the sun especially in the visible wavelengths. It is said to be a free mood enhancer. Being in the sun can make people feel better and have more energy. Sunlight increases the levels of serotonin in the brain. The sun will improve your sleep as it increases melatonin. When sunlight touches the skin a compound called nitric oxide is released in the blood vessels that help to lower blood pressure. Vitamin D stimulates the absorption of bone strengthening calcium and phosphorus in the body. Sunlight can help with nerve cell growth in the hippocampus which is responsible for the brains memory. Other benefits include improved sleep, better moods, and stronger immune system while decreasing appetite. Get outside and be active on warm sunny days. You can try sun gazing at sunrise and sunset. Sun gazing can cure all kinds of psychosomatic, mental and physical issues, can increase memory and improve eyesight. You may notice the solar rays will energize you.

Supplements

Supplements are manufactured products intended to supplement the diet when taken by mouth as a pill, drops, powders, capsule, tablet or liquid. They provide nutrients. There are 24 types of vitamins and minerals the body needs to maintain good health. They are considered a subset of foods. Dietary supplements are products that contain one or more concentrated nutrients with the aim of balancing the daily diet if nutrients are lacking. Products can contain dietary ingredients including vitamins, minerals, amino acids, herbs and botanicals. They are generally taken to improve and maintain overall health. Most women take supplements to support bone integrity and during pregnancy. It is recommended to take a good multivitamin once or twice a day for optimum health. There are protein, carbohydrate and fatty acid supplements that are efficient to help balance your food groups. For a better cardiovascular health, metabolic health, energy and cognitive functions try supplements. Most vegetarians and vegans need a little extra Vitamin B to make red blood cells. Fiber is essential to protect the body's blood lipids.

Ultraviolet Light

Ultraviolet light is a form of electromagnetic radiations with wavelengths of 10 to 400 nanometers shorter than that of visible light but no longer than x-rays. UV is present in sunlight. It is also produced by electric arcs and specialized lights like mercury vaper lamps, tanning lamps and black lights. Moderate UV exposure has many benefits like producing Vitamin D, improving mood and increasing energy. Tanning UVB lights have been known to improve skin conditions, increase melanin the brown pigment that protects your skin from direct and indirect DNA damage and promotes serotonin production. UVC lamps are used for purification and can eliminate many types of bacteria and fungi. With proper light placement all pathogens can be eliminated from air passing through an HVAC/R unit. UVC light can be used as a light sanitizer with the ability to kill up to 99.9% of germs.

Veganism

Veganism is the practice of abstaining from the use of animal products, particularly in diet. A moral vegan extends their philosophy and avoids all animal products. Vegan diets consist of only plant derived foods. A balanced diet is made up of legumes, nuts and seeds, grains, vegetables and fruits. There are five types of vegans: ethical vegans, plant based vegans, raw vegans, HCLF High carb low fat vegans and environmentally conscious vegans. Vegans try to eat nutrient dense foods packed with protein, fiber, minerals, B vitamins, protective antioxidants and essential fatty acids. It is important to pay attention to vitamin b12, Vitamin D, omega 3 fatty acids and iodine to ensure a healthy diet. Vegan diets can promote weight loss; reduce the risk of heart issues and other risks. There are many meat substitutes and dairy alternatives to try other than soy based ones. It is a great way to boost heart health and is generally a clean diet.

Vegetarianism

Vegetarianism is the practice of abstaining from the consumption of meat (red meat, poultry, seafood and the flesh of any other animal and may also include abstention from byproducts of animal slaughter. A vegetarian diet is derived from plants with or without eggs and dairy. There are various vegetarians. Lacto diets exclude meat, fish, poultry and eggs but will contain dairy products. Ovo diets exclude meat, poultry, seafood and dairy products but allow eggs. Lacto Ovo excludes meat, poultry, and fish but allow dairy and eggs. Pescatarians exclude meat, poultry, dairy and eggs but allow fish. Pollotarians exclude meat, dairy and fish but allow poultry. Vegans exclude meat, poultry, fish, eggs and dairy products. There are many benefits like: lower cholesterol levels, reduce risk of cardiovascular disease, reduce risk of metabolic syndrome, ecologically sustainable option, help with weight loss, and can be an easy lifestyle choice. Some vegetarians have concerns for animals, birds and fish so they avoid eating them.

Vision Board

Vision or dream board is a collage of images, pictures and affirmations of ones dreams and desires. It is designed to serve as a source of inspiration and motivation and to use the law of attraction to attain goals. Visualization is important. It can improve motivation, coordination and concentration. A vision board allows the lay out of your ideal future using pictures and words. It can help to refocus life giving your ideas on what and where you want your life to go. Creating boards especially in a group activity can be a good way to share your goals with others. Seeing the end product can give a sense of accomplishment and can make you feel good. Defining your life goals and looking at your vision every day will help motivate you and see how you are doing. This activity inspires creativity and imagination. Pretend you can get anything you want without any limitations. First get clear on your vision by writing your ideas on short term and long term goals. Create a folder and obtain images to match your goals and dream. Organize these images onto a poster and add words that motivate you.

Vitamins

A vitamin is an organize molecule that is an essential micronutrient which an organism needs in small qualities for the proper functioning of its metabolism. Essential nutrients can be obtained through vitamins. Vitamins have biochemical functions and can include A, B, C, D, E, and K. Vitamins are grouped into two categories. Fat soluble vitamins are stored in the body's fat tissue; they are A, D, E and K. There are nine water soluble vitamins that leave the body through the urine. Although a small reserve of these vitamins is stored. Vitamin B12 can be stored in your liver for many years. Vitamin A helps form and maintains healthy teeth, bones, soft tissue, mucous membranes and skin. Vitamin B6 is called pyridoxine and helps form red blood cells and maintain brain function. Vitamin B12 is important for metabolism and helps form red blood cells and maintain the central nervous system. Vitamin C is called ascorbic acid and is an antioxidant that promotes healthy teeth and gyms. It helps the body absorb iron and maintain healthy tissues. Vitamin D is known as the sunshine vitamin and helps the body absorb calcium and phosphorus. Vitamin E is an antioxidant known as tocopherol. It helps the body form red blood cells and use Vitamin K. Vitamin K is needed or your blood would not stick together coagulate and is important for bone health. Biotin is essential for metabolism of proteins and carbohydrates and the production of hormones and cholesterol. Niacin is a B vitamin and helps to maintain healthy skin and nerves. Folate works with Vitamin B12 to help form red blood cells and is needed in the production of DNA which controls tissue growth and cell function. Pantothenic acid is needed for metabolism of food and production of hormones and cholesterol. Riboflavin is B2 and helps the production of red blood cells. Thiamine B1 helps the body change carbohydrates into energy. Choline helps in normal functioning of the brain and nervous system. Carnitine helps the body to change fatty acids into energy. A good multivitamin should help to maintain healthy levels inside the body. Children, men, women, pregnant women and seniors are all required to have different levels to maintain optimum health. You can consult with a nutritionist to ensure that you are eating all the required vitamins in your daily diet or you need to supplement for the lack of. Vitamins help all your body systems perform at their best.

Walk

Walking is one of the main goals of locomotion. Walking is slower than running and jogging. Regular brisk exercise of any kind can improve confidence, stamina, energy, weight control and life expectancy and reduces stress. It benefits the mind by improving memory skills, learning abilities and concentration. Walking has many benefits. It can increase cardiovascular and pulmonary fitness, reduce risk of heart issues, improve management of conditions one is dealing with, strengthen bones and improve balance. Walking is free to do and easy to fit into your daily routine. Walking can help you burn calories. It depends on your waking speed, distance covered, and terrain. Walking daily can improve your immune function and mood, increase your energy and strengthen your mobility. Walking at an average pace will extend your life. Research suggests that walking will improve creative thinking. As you increase your oxygen levels and clear your head it will help you think of new ideas. To ensure your safe walking buy sturdy shoes with good heel and arch support. Or seek orthopedics. Wear loose comfortable clothing, stay hydrated and try new trails to stimulate enjoyment. You can choose your pace. You can try to find a walking partner. Dogs are usually the best animals to get owners to stay in shape.

Yoga

Yoga is a group of physical mental and spiritual practices or disciplines which originated in ancient India. It's more than physical exercise; it has meditative and spiritual disciplines. There are postures connected to flowing sequences accompanied by breathing exercises. There are various types of yoga. Vinyasa is an athletic style of ahstanga, power and prana. Hatha yoga is very physically based. Iyengar is focused on alignment with detailed precise movements. Kundalini is spiritually and physically energetic. Ashtanga is the eight limb path with flowing breath movements. Bikram has a sequence of set poses in a sauna like room. Yin has many seated postures that are held for longer periods of time. Restorative yoga focuses on relaxation. Prenatal is for the moms to be. Anusaea focuses on mind body heart connections and alignments. Jivamukti emphasizes connection to Earth as a living being. Yoga improves strength, balance and flexibility. Yoga can relieve stress and pain from the back and joints. It can improve heart health. Yoga relaxes you and helps you sleep better. It provides you with a brighter mood and more positive energy. It's a great way to connect with a supportive health conscious community. Yoga can improve your quality of life in so many ways. Being able to breathe easy, move gentle and flow into postures feels good and will keep you healthy.

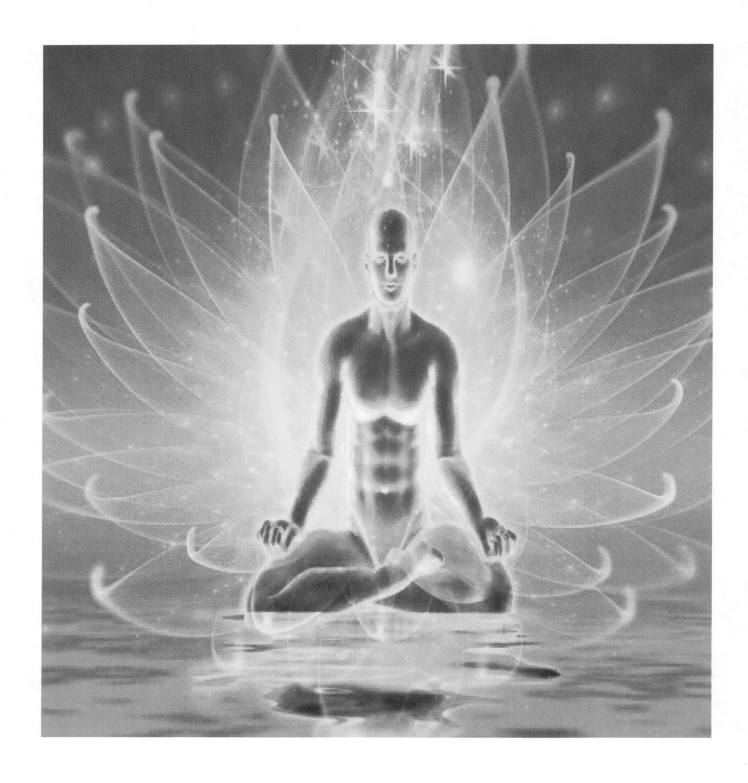

Godly Virtues Oracle
Character Traits with an Action Plan

By Diana Hutchings

Virtue is moral excellence. A virtue is a morally good quality. It is a behavior that illustrates high moral standards. Aristotle says in the Nicomachean Ethics: "at the right times, about the right things towards the right people, for the right end and in the right way, is the intermediate and best condition and this is proper to virtue." The term virtue itself is derived from the Latin "virtus" which means "manliness" or "honor" or worthiness of respect. The Bible mentions virtues such as the "fruit of the Spirit is love, joy, peace, patience, kindness, goodness, faith, gentleness and self control. Against such things there is no law." Galatians 5:22-23 In Buddhism, there are four divine virtuous states. They are metta or a loving kindness towards all, karuna or in English meaning compassion, mudita or altruistic joy in the accomplishments of a person and upkesha or equanimity. Living a moral ethical and virtuous life can be considered as living a dharmic life. As Guru Nanak says in the Sikh's Adi Granth, "truth is the highest virtue, but higher still is truthful living." This 76 card Godly Virtues oracle will lead you to a path of perfection. As you gather and practice the virtues, you will transform your life for the better. In addition, to adding moral value to your life, others will benefit from your righteous choices and behaviors.

1. Acceptance	27. Enthusiasm	53. Modesty
2. Accountability	28. Excellence	54. Optimism
3. Appreciation	29. Fairness	55. Orderliness
4. Assertiveness	30. Faith	56. Patience
5. Beauty	31. Fidelity	57. Peacefulness
6. Certitude	32. Flexibility	58. Perseverance
7. Charity	33. Forbearance	59. Purity
8. Cheerfulness	34. Forgiveness	60. Reliability
9. Cleanliness	35. Fortitude	61. Respect
10. Commitment	36. Friendliness	62. Responsibility
11. Compassion	37. Generosity	63. Reverence
12. Confidence	38. Gentleness	64. Self-Discipline
13. Consideration	39. Grace	65. Serenity
14. Contentment	40. Gratitude	66. Simplicity
15. Cooperation	41. Helpfulness	67. Sincerity
16. Courage	42. Honesty	68. Steadfastness
17. Courtesy	43. Honor	69. Strength
18. Creativity	44. Hope	70. Tact
19. Decisiveness	45. Humility	71. Thoughtfulness
20. Determination	46. Initiative	72. Tolerance
21. Devotion	47. Joyfulness	73. Trust
22. Dignity	48. Justice	74. Truthfulness
23. Diligence	49. Kindness	75. Understanding
24. Discernment	50. Love	76. Wisdom
25. Empathy	51. Mindfulness	

26. Endurance	52. Moderation	

Acceptance

In human psychology is a person's asset to the reality of a situation, recognizing a process or condition without attempting to change it or protest it. For example, someone gives a gift. Acceptance is a positive welcome of belonging, favor and endorsement. One can like someone and accept them due to their approval of that person. This definition overlaps toleration. Acceptance means allowing. Allowing unwanted private experiences thoughts, feelings and urges to come and go without struggling with them. Acceptance is treating whatever happens as overall the best outcome. The term Kabbalah literally means acceptance.

"Acceptance doesn't mean resignation it means understanding that something is what it is and that there's got to be a way through it." Michael J. Fox

Please God help me accept that everything is going to be alright. Amen

What do you need to accept right now?

Hang in there. Things will improve. Go with the flow instead of fighting against the current. Have positive thoughts. Relax.

Accountability

Accountability is this governance in answerability, blameworthiness, liability and the expectation of account giving. In leadership roles, accountability is the acknowledged and assumption of responsibility for actions, products, decisions and policies including the administration, governance and implementation within the scope of the role or employment position. It encompasses the obligation to report, explain and be answerable for resulting consequences. One is being called to account for ones actions. Accountability stems from Latin accomplare "to account" prefixed computare "to calculate."

"Accountability is a statement of personal promise both to yourself and to the people around you to deliver specific defined results" Brian Dive

Dear God help us be accountable in all our actions, decisions, behaviors and results. Amen

Do you have any obligations at the moment?

Be decisive. Work to take ownership. Be consistent. Your results and project completion are your responsibility. Make a chore/to do chart with timelines and rewards for finishing successfully.

Appreciation

Appreciation is a fair, valuation or estimate of merit, worth, weight, recognition of excellent. Its recognition and enjoyment of the good qualities of someone or something. It provides a feeling of gratitude or expression of admiration, approval or gratitude. For example, small token of my appreciation. Appreciation in the value of something is on increase in its value over a period of time.

"By appreciation we make excellence in others our own property." Voltaire

Dear God, give us the gift of appreciation. Let us always be thankful for who and what we have. Amen.

What are 5 things you appreciate?

Take 5 minutes write all the things you are grateful for. Start a daily gratitude journal write three things in the morning and 3 things at the end of the day you appreciate. Pay attention to what others offer, a smile, a service, a product, or a conversation. Treat others with as much appreciation as you can. Host an appreciation party.

Assertiveness

Assertiveness is the quality of being self-assured and confident without being aggressive. It's a communication skill that can be taught. A method of critical thinking where an individual speaks up in defense of their views. Assertive people support creative thinking and effective communication. Training increased awareness, passive vs aggressive, verbal vs nonverbal. It involves respect of boundaries.

"One of the ways you build self-esteem is by being self-assertive when it is not easy to do so." Nathaniel Branden

Dear God, provide us with assertiveness that is honorable and consistent. Amen

In what ways do you show assertiveness?

Work on communication skills verbally, nonverbally and body language. Take a self-assertive class or course, speak boldly and with intellect. Turn on bright lights for alertness.

Beauty

Beauty is the ascription of a property or characteristic to an animal, idea, object, person or place that provides a perceptual experience of pleasure or satisfaction. Ideal beauty is an entity which is admired or possesses features attribute as beauty. To view an entity as balanced, in harmony with nature leads to feels of attraction and emotional wellbeing. Beauty is in the eye of the beholder. Ancient Greek beauty 'kalos' equals good or fine quality. Aristotle said, "Virtue aims at the beautiful" Beauty is not just skin deep.

"Everything has beauty, but not everyone sees it." Confucius

Dear God, help me realize the beauty that's within and around me. Amen

How do you feel beautiful?

Take a spa day. Do something to reward yourself. Dress up, and look your best. See the beauty in everything. For attractive lips speak kind words. Seek out the good and beauty in others. Go to a fashion show. Surround yourself in pink light. Paint something beautiful. Buy something that makes you feel attractive.

Certitude

Certitude is absolute, certainty something that someone firmly believes is true. It's a state of being certain or confident. People who are very religious express certitude about their faith. Certainty is an epistemic (theory of knowledge) properties of beliefs are related to knowledge. Descartes said I think I exist.

"Certitude is not the test of certainty" Oliver Holmes

Dear God, Instill in us certitude for what is right and proper. Amen

What are you certain about?

Be sure. Take Time to express your opinion and state of mind. See a herbologist. Get a cupping treatment. Watch a choir or symphony. Be conscious of your posture.

Charity

Charity is the practice of being benevolent giving and sharing. Charity the virtue is the religious concept of unlimited love and kindness. Charitable organizations are nonprofit and their primary objectives are philanthropy and social wellbeing. An act of feeling kindness or goodwill or a voluntary gift of money or time to those in need. For example giving $10 to the local food bank.

"Give that which is within as charity then all things are clean for you." Luke 11:41

Dear God, let us practice charity and love always. Amen.

In what ways do you show charity?

God grant us the gift of faith, hope and charity. Amen

Devote some time volunteering. Give money to a charitable organization. Fundraise for a cause of your choice. Run or walk for the cure.

Cheerfulness

Cheerfulness is a person or thing that brings joy, humor or good spirits. It is full of cheer, optimistic, bright, and attractive. Promotes a feeling of pleasant cheer.

Proverbs 15:13 "A joyful heart makes a cheerful face."

Dear God, put things, places and people in our lives that bring us high levels of cheer. Amen

Thessalonians 5:16 "Be cheerful no matter what, pray all the time."

What brings you the most joy?

When do you feel the most cheerful?

Find your passion. Look on the bright side. Be optimistic. Meditate. Smile at everyone. Find ways to cheer others on. Make some lemonade. Try a buffest or go on a restaurant outing. Watch cheerleading for inspiration.

Cleanliness

Cleanliness is a state of being clean and free from filth. It is achieved through cleaning. Cleanliness is next to godliness. Cleanliness related to hygiene and disease prevention. Hinduism extols external cleanliness or internal cleanliness or purity. This is cultivated by Vedic students.

Allah loves those who keep themselves pure and clean. Reduces disease, increases the life span, and it feels good to be clean.

"Cleanliness is next to godliness." John Wesley

Dear God, keep us and our lives clean and tidy. Amen.

Do you keep your home, work, and vehicle tidy? Do you have a cleaning schedule?

Bath or shower once or twice a day. Declutter. Organize spaces that need cleaning. Clean off countertops. Buy organizers. Keep a cleaning schedule. Use organic cleaning solutions. Hire a maid for a couple hours. Create an art zentangle using any medium you choose.

Commitment

Commitment is a promise or agreement to do something. It is an official dedication to a long term course of action, engagement or involvement. It is a pledge or obligation. It's the state of being emotionally or intellectually devoted as to a belief, a course of action or another person.

"The quality of a person's life is in direct proportion to their commitment to excellence regardless of their chosen field of endeavor." Vince Lombardi

Dear God, help us follow through with all our commitments. Amen

What are you committed to? Are there expectations with these commitments? If so, what are they?

Set goals. Set routines. Stay inspired. Be loyal. Join a club, be a member or a class with certain commitments to attend. Listen to the mantra Om Shanti.

Compassion

Compassion motivates people to go out of their way to help the physical, mental or emotional parts of another and themselves. It involves feeling as another capacity for better person centered acts. Qualities of compassion are patience, wisdom, kindness, perseverance, warmth and resolve. It's a variation of love.

"Compassion is a necessity not a luxury." Dalai Lama

"I will have compassion on whom I will have compassion." Exodus 33:19

"The Lord is gracious and righteous our God is full of compassion." Psalm 116:5

Dear God, be compassionate towards us as we are to the world. Amen

When do you experience being compassionate and to whom are you the most compassionate?

Purchase a world vision child or sponsor a child from the Compassionate Society. Affirm I am loving, loveable and compassionate. Practice the Ho'oponopono meditation. Do a heart chakra meditation by listening to 528 Hz or get a reiki treatment. Surround yourself with the colors green and pink. Find the fragrance of a lotus. Purchase, wear or carry a green gemstone.

Confidence

Confidence is a feeling or consciousness of one's powers or of reliance on one's circumstances. It is a faith or belief that one will act in a right proper or effective way. It's the quality or state of being certain of your abilities or having trust in people, plans or the future.

"It is confidence in our bodies, minds and spirits that allows us to keep looking for new adventures." Oprah Winfrey

"With realization of one's own potential and self confidence in one's ability one can build a better world." Dalai Lama

Dear God, let us radiate confidence always. Amen

What areas do you exude the most confidence?

Trust yourself. Create the kind of self you will be proud of. Wear yellow or light a yellow candle. Find the fragrance Lemongrass and immerse yourself in it (in a mister, essential oil, incense) Do a guided meditation for confidence with self-affirmations.

Consideration

Consideration is careful thought, typically over a period of time. A factor or a motive taken into account in deciding or judging something. Its thoughtfulness and sensitivity towards others.

"The only true source of politeness is consideration." William Simms

Dear God, grant us consideration when dealing with others. Amen

Who do you find the most considerate in your life? How can you tell they care?

Write a gratitude list of the magical people in your life and why you are grateful for them. Buy a gift for someone. Write a thank you card/notes. Consider other's views and opinions more and seek out their perspective. Join a healing group circle. To some energy exercises like qi gong, tai chi or breath work.

Contentment

Contentment is an emotional state of satisfaction as a mental state of being at ease in one's situation, body, mind and soul. Siddhartha said, "Health is the most precious gain and contentment the greatest wealth." Maslow mentioned the more needs achieved the more easily contented.

"Keep your lives free from the love of money and be content with what you have." Hebrews 13:5

"Health is the greatest possession. Contentment is the greatest treasure. Confidence is the greatest friend. No being is the greatest joy." Lao Tzu

Dear God, provide contentment to us and our loved ones. Amen

Are you content with your life?

Read the book called The Power of Now. Write an appreciation list of all the things you are grateful for. Buy an essential oil mister or humidifier. Try a eucalyptus steam. Smile. Do Breath work and take a few deep breaths. Be happy with what you have and appreciate it.

Cooperation

Cooperation is the actions of someone who is being helpful by doing what is wanted or asked for. Called common effort. Cooperation is the act of working together with someone or doing what they ask of you. Groups of organisms, acting or working together for common, mutual or some underlying benefit. Animal and plant species cooperate both with other members of their own species and members of other species. Language allows for cooperation. There is no I in team.

"Teamwork coming together is a beginning keeping together is progress working together is success." Henry Ford

Dear God, help us be cooperative in all our undertakings. Amen

What examples do you have of cooperation? Are you a team player or do you prefer to do things independently or both?

Respect each other, communication, spend time team building. Create traditions together. Comprise and take turns deciding. Display pictures and capture moments of working together. Have a party and invite others. Do a bake exchange.

Courage

Courage is called bravery and valour. It's the willingness to confront the agony, pain and intimidation. Fortitude is related to courage and portrays aspects of perseverance and patience. Virtue may be defined as a habit of mind (animi) in harmony with reason and the order of natures. It has four parts: wisdom, justice, courage and temperance.

"What would life be if we had no courage to attempt anything?" Vincent Van Gogh

"Be strong and of good courage do not fear nor be afraid of them, for the Lord, your God. He is the One who goes with you." Deuteronomy 31:6

Dear God, help us to face life with courage and bravery. Amen

When do you need the most courage?

Be fearless. Enlarge your comfort zone and make a learning zone. Wear the gemstone carnelian. Build your confidence through self-affirmations. Embrace bravery and do it. Wear the color orange to adapt. Go swim in a pool, hot springs, lake, ocean. Go for a vacation to the ocean.

Courtesy

Courtesy is gentle politeness, courtly manners. In middle ages in Europe the behavior expected of the nobility was compiled in courtesy books. The books covered basic etiquette and decorum but also provided models of sophisticated conversation and intellectual skill. A

polite speech or action especially one required by convention. A polite remark or respectful act.

"Politeness costs nothing and gains everything." Lady Montague

Dear God, teach us how to be more courteous. Amen

Do you appreciate those who give you courtesy and respect?

Look up the best etiquette skills. Say please and thank you as often as possible. Offer a tip of gratuity. Wear silver on a ring, necklace, and bracelet. Smudge with sage or Palo Santo. Go get a manicure or sports pedicure.

Creativity

Creativity is a phenomenon whereby something new is somehow valuable and is formed. Creations may be intangible such as an idea, and scientific theory or musical composition or a joke or a physical object such as an invention, a printed literary work or a painting. Latin creare means "to create, make." Creativity is an innovation.

"Creativity is intelligence having fun." Alberta Einstein

Dear God enable us to express ourselves in more creative ways. Amen

How do you express your creativity?

Make a to do list. Create a music playlist. Draw, color or paint something. Dance to a song. Join an art class or try a new hobby. Play the game called Cranium. Wear bright colors. See a naturopath. Shake and wiggle your whole body for 2 minutes.

Decisiveness

Decisiveness is the state of quality of being decisive. It's having the power or quality of deciding a question or controversy final conclusive. Marked by promptness and decision. One can make decisions, quickly and confidently. The processes to observe, orient, decide and act without regret.

"The way to develop decisiveness is to start right where you are with the very next question you face." Napoleon Hill

Dear God bless us with the ability to make good decisions in a timely manner. Amen

What big decisions are you facing or have you made in the past?

Have patience. Raise your energetic vibration and level of confidence. Research options and seek wise counsel when making big decisions. Take gingko biloba. Attend a sound bath mediation session.

Determination

Determination is positive emotional feeling that involves preserving towards a goal. It occurs prior to goal attainment and serves to motivate behavior. Self-determination theory is a theory of motivation and dedication towards or ambition. Social environments effect intrinsic and extrinsic motivation.

"To all the positions, I just bring the determination to win." LeBron James

Dear God, provide motivation, self-discipline and determination. Amen

Why do you stay motivated and determined? What rewards do you seek?

Listen to Pump Up the Jam. Exercise at a moderate to high intensity. Set goals often. Work for a prize or reward. Have a steam room or sauna. Buy an amethyst or quartz cluster. Believe, achieve and receive.

Devotion

Devotion is the act of devoting. It's a religious piety. It provides feelings of strong affection and dedication. Devoveo is Latin and means, "vow, devote." Daily devotion is a publication in a spiritual reading that happens each calendar day. You may use songs, hymns, prayers or a religious ritual. For example reading the Lord's Prayer.

"To succeed in your mission, you must have single minded devotion to your goal." Abdul

Kalam

Dear God, aid us to be completely devoted to you and faithful to all our commitments. Amen.

What are you devoted to?

Join or attend a church or faith based organization. Create a sacred altar. Pray daily. Start a journal. Try Laughter yoga. Sing your favorite song.

Dignity

Dignity is the right of a person to be valued and respected for their own sake and to be treated ethically. Describes the personal conduct behaving with dignity. Dignitas in Latin means worthiness. Dignity pertains to the worth of human beings. Receiving proper degree of respect.

"All human beings are born free and equal in dignity and rights." United Nations Universal Declaration of Human Rights

"Dignity is the reward of obeying your heart." Wes Fesler

Dear God, Jesus and the Holy Spirit assist us to give and receive the highest levels of dignity and respect. Amen

What brings you dignity?

Pull your shoulders back and down, raise your chin and breath. Sing R-E-S-P-E-C-T. Read your Charter of rights. Everyone is worthy of dignity so foster this principle. Paint a rock to give to someone.

Diligence

Diligence is one of the seven heavenly virtues. Diligent behavior is indicative of a worth ethic. It's a belief that work is good in itself. Its carefulness and persistent effort or work. Diligence in students is correlated to academic performance. Other factors which encourage diligence in students include motivation, discipline, concentration, responsibility and devotedness. Due diligence is the necessary amount of diligence required in a professional activity to avoid negligence.

"Strive on with diligence." Last words of Buddha

"Diligence is the mother of good luck." Benjamin Franklin

Where do you need to be the most diligent?

God, give us strong work ethics and due diligence to do good. Amen.

Treat others as you want to be treated. Know your responsibilities and do them. Write a personal, moral or ethical code you follow and share this with others. Wake up early pray, exercise and set daily goals. Be a good planner and open your calendar on your smartphone to schedule tasks. Take a multivitamin.

Discernment

Discernment is the ability to obtain sharp perceptions of to judge well. In the case of judgment discernment can be psychological moral or aesthetic in nature considered to possess wisdom and be good judgment. In Christianity, its describes as the process of determining God's desire in a situation or for one's life or identifying the true nature of a thing or person. Required tasks while taking time in making the decision using both heart and head, assessing important values. True discernment comes from God.

"Discernment in the Lord guides me in my way of governing." Pope Francis

Do you have discernment? And when do you use it?

God please provide us with the ability to discern and make good decisions. Amen

Share your insight and perspectives often. Listen to others. Create a comic strip. Buy a dubble bubble and have a bubble blowing contest. Wear white of purity and innocence. Take an emotional intelligence test.

Empathy

Empathy is the capacity to understand or feel what another person is experiencing. The capacity to place oneself in others position. Different types of empathy include cognitive (thinking), emotional (emotion), and somatic (feelings). Greek empatheia means "physical affection or passion." It is the ability to feel and share another person's emotional compassion and sympathy associated with empathy.

"So maybe part of our formal education should be training in empathy. Imagine how different the world would be if in fact that were reading, writing, arithmetic, empathy." Neil Degrasse Tyson

When have you felt empathy for another? Give an example of when you used empathy.

God provide us with empathy to understand what it's like to be another person's shoes. Amen

Be honest with your feelings and emotions. Look up an emotion wheel and the coordinated color. Take a color personality test. Cultivate your sense of curiosity with others by asking questions. Practice a loving kindness meditation. Affirm I am compassionate, loving and loveable. Actively listen without judgment. Use LEAPS (listen, empathy, ask questions, paraphrase, summarize) Offer help and assistance, Visualize connecting with a coloring changing LED light.

Endurance

Endurance is the ability of an organism to exert itself and remain active for as long period of time as well as its ability to resist, withstand and recover from and have immunity to fatigue. Used in aerobic and anaerobic exercise. Endurance is a term interchangeably used with stamina. It's the ability to keep going through a tough situation.

"Endurance is patience concentrated." Thomas Carlyle

"To endure what is unendurable is true endurance." Proverbs

When were a few times you showed endurance?

God we pray for endurance, stamina and perseverance. Amen.

Be consistent. Increase your aerobic cardio exercises. Follow a personal training plan and increase speed and intensity. Eat a well-balanced diet. Try a session of breath work from a practitioner. Research Ayurveda and take a body test to find out what body type and diet you need. Participate in a physical challenge like walking for the cure; join a sports team or club. Drink 2 Liters of water. Try alkaline water.

Enthusiasm

Enthusiasm is intense enjoyment, interest or approval, exhibits intense piety, possessed by God. Socrates taught inspiration of poets is a form of enthusiasm. Syrian sects of the 4th century are known as the Enthusiasts. They believed in perpetual prayer, ascetic practices and contemplation that man could become inspired by the Holy Spirit.

"We have to straighten out our country we have to make our country great and we need energy and enthusiasm." Donald Trump

What is an example of enthusiasm?

God please grant us enthusiasm, charisma and leadership. Amen.

Pray for charisma and enthusiasm. Surround yourself with high vibing optimistic people. Force yourself to think positively. Enjoy every second with good company. Get a reiki treatment. Wear neon colors. Try karaoke. Get an acupressure or shiatsu treatment.

Excellence

Excellence is a talent or quality which is unusually good and so surpasses ordinary standards. Most important way to achieve excellence is thru practice, practice makes perfect. It is the quality of being outstanding or extremely good. It means greatness, the very best. People appreciate excellence.

"We are what we repeatedly do excellence then is not an act but a habit." Aristotle

What areas of your life are in excellence?

God help us do everything with excellence and perfection. Amen

Practice and study for perfection. Take a course from the online website called Center for Excellence. Believe in yourself. Make the effort to do your best all the time. Show up and be present. Visualize gold and silver light. Wear gold on your right hand. Run or jog on the treadmill for 5-20 minutes.

Fairness

Fairness is impartial and just treatment or behavior without favoritism or discrimination. It's the quality of treating people equally or in a way that is right and reasonable. Considering everything and making a fair judgment. It means justice and evenhandedness.

"Fairness is what justice really is." Potter Stewart

Is fairness and equality important to you?

God brings fairness to our lives. Amen

Take turns. Tell the truth. Play by the rules and follow the laws and policies set before you. Don't play favorites. Treat all people the same. Live by the golden rule (treat others as you want to be treated.) Do some art and draw the scales of balance. Give to a police, authoritative organization or courthouse charity. Tell someone of authority you appreciate them.

Faith

Faith is allegiance to duty or a person. Its fidelity to ones promises sincerity of intentions, beliefs and trust in and loyalty to God. The belief in traditional doctrines of religion. Faith is something that is believed especially with a strong conviction.

"Now faith is the assurance of things hoped for, the conviction of things not seen." Hebrews 11:1

"Faith can move mountains." Matthew 17:20

What do you have faith in?

God give us a shield of faith. Amen

Pray daily, Read Throne of Heaven by Diana Hutchings. Read devotional or holy scriptures that appeal to you. Wear faith by buying apparel like a rosary, shirt, bracelet or hat. Get involved with a faith based community. Visualize ultraviolet light surrounding you and your aura. Draw a merkaba which in sacred geometry is the light soul body chariot.

Fidelity

Is the quality or state of being faithful. Faithfulness to a person, cause or belief demonstrated by continuing loyalty and support. Sexual faithfulness to a spouse or partner.

"True happiness is not attained through self-gratification but through fidelity to a worthy purpose." Helen Keller

How do you use the word fidelity?

God help us to have fidelity and create fidelity in all our relationships. Amen

Give your partner space. Build and keep trust. Offer love and support. Communicate with honesty and use the love appreciation language. Read the book The Five Love Languages by Gary Chapman. Keep the spark alive by trying new things. Create a fairytale story. Get a couples portrait or pictures together.

Flexibility

Flexibility is the quality of bending easily without breaking. It's the ability to be easily modified and willingness to change or compromise. Flexibility is defined as the ability to change, to bend or to persuade.

"Stay committed to your decisions but stay flexible in your approach." Tony Robbins.

In what ways are you flexible?

God help us to be flexible in all ways. Amen

Practice daily stretching. Download a stretching or yoga app. Try a warm up and cool down stretches after exercising. Take time to change your approach by taking a break or vacation from your daily routine. Get a massage or sometime of body work session. Try a whole body vibration machine. Take a hot bath with Epsom salts.

Forbearance

Forbearance is the patient self-control, restraint and tolerance. It's the quality of being patient or being able to forgive someone or control yourself in a situation.

"The fruit of the spirit is love, joy, peace, forbearance, kindness, goodness, faithfulness, gentleness and self-control." Galatians 5:22-23

What does it look like for us to forbear?

God provide us with reverence and forbearance. Amen

Practice the Ho'oponopono meditation. Say a person's name you need to forgive and forgive them. Be calm and sensible when dealing with others. Focus on things that make you happy. Write 5 things you are grateful for. Buy a lavender plant or purchase some lavender essential oil. Take a few deep breaths and let it go. Try being a vegan for a day. Get an ion foot detox bath cleanse.

Forgiveness

A conscious deliberate decision to release feelings of resentment or vengeance toward a person or group who has harmed or hurt you. Forgiveness brings the forgiver peace of mind and frees him or her from anger. It's the action or process of forgiving or being forgiven.

"For if you forgive other people when they sin against you, your heavenly father will also forgive you." Luke 17:3

Who do you need to forgive and who do you need to be forgiven by?

God please forgive us and help us to forgive others easily. Amen

Say the Lord's Prayer daily. Practice the Ho'oponopono meditation that says I am sorry. Please forgive me. I love you. Thank you. Confront the truth, apologize and forgive. Confess at holy church or temple. Write a letter to God to discuss forgiveness. Seek holy water or rose water to purify and cleanse. Have a shower and let it go. Buy the gemstone called chrysoprase which is the stone of forgiveness.

Fortitude

Fortitude is the strength of mind that enables a person to encounter difficulty with courage. Its mental and emotional strength or courage over a long period of time. In Latin fortitude means, "strength."

"Fortitude is the marshal of thought, the armor of the will and the fort of reason." Francis Bacon.

When have you practice fortitude?

God help us to have more fortitude, strength and courage. Amen

Be aware of your primal fight or flight response. Earn respect by making responsible choices. Take a Vitamin B full complex. Practice mindfulness. Be aware of your emotions and how to maintain calmness and peace. Reflect on your actions, thoughts and behaviors to better them. Buy the gemstone carnelian which is the stone of courage/fortitude and put it in your pocket.

Friendly

Friendliness is the quality of behaving in a pleasant, kind way towards someone. It's being friends with someone. Offering friendly greetings. The quality of open warmth that makes you feel welcome and at ease. Evident in facial expressions, body language and the way you treat other people.

"To be kind, honest and have positive thoughts, to forgive those who harm us and treat everyone as a friend." Dalai Lama

How would you describe your friend's social circle?

God help us to maintain a friendly reputation. Amen

Take time to get know someone. Nurture and maintain your friendships by calling, texting, emailing and writing letters often. Show kindness to others. Be open and honest. Go out for coffee, lunch and shopping dates. Create traditions with your friends. Wear the color pink which creates sympathy and friendship. Buy a gift for a friend. Try cannabis CBD oil or flower.

Generosity

Generosity is the quality of being kind and generous. The tact of being plentiful or large. Showing generosity is happy to give time, money, food or kindness to people in need. It is the willingness to give or to share an act of unselfish giving.

"Gentleness, self-sacrifice and generosity are the exclusive possession of no race or religion." Mahatma Gandhi

How have you shown generosity?

God give us a generous heart. Amen

Fund a cause of your choice. Spend time with people in need. Give a gift from the heart. Be grateful for who and what you have. Celebrate somebody. Be very kind to strangers. Donate and give to a charity. Volunteer your time. Create a photo collage or scrapbook. Buy flowers for someone.

Gentleness

Quality of being kind, tender or mild mannered. It is softness or action or effect, lightness. Describes the way someone acts when they are soft, calm and sweet to other people. It is also termed meekness.

"Do everything with gentleness, with kindness, with reverence. That is how grace moves." Heather O'Hara

When was a time you showed gentleness?

God allow us give and receive gentleness and kindness always. Amen

Be conscious of your feelings. Allow yourself to care for one another. Be sweet like sugar. Use a calm, kind voice and tone. Respond to others with kindness and love. Connect with the gentleness of the animal deer. Connect to other plants and animals. Go to a zoo or sanctuary for a nature walk. Buy a house or work plant to nurture.

Grace

Grace is simple elegance or refinement of movement and courteous goodwill. Its honor or credit to someone or something by one's presence. It's the unmerited divine assistance given to humans for their regeneration or sanctification. It's a virtue coming from God and is the love of God. It's a quality of moving in a smooth, relaxed and attractive way.

"Grace and peace by yours in abundance through the knowledge of God and of Jesus our Lord." 2 Peter 1:2

How has God's grace impacted your life?

God provide us with your mercy and grace. Amen.

Buy, draw or paint something elegant like swans to display. Join a ballet or ballroom dancing class. Walk with the purpose of a relaxed graceful posture. Pick up your feet, look ahead and take graceful strides. Watch a you tube video about proper etiquette. Wear the color white. Go to a ballet, symphony or dinner theater.

Gratitude

Gratitude is the quality of being thankful, readiness to show appreciation for and to return kindness. It's a feeling or quality of being grateful. Similar to appreciation. Latin word gratus means, "pleasing."

"Go outside and turn your attention to the many miracles around you. This 5 minute a day regimen of appreciation and gratitude will help you to focus your life in awe." Wayne Dyer

When are you the most grateful?

God make sure we show gratitude daily. We thank you for everything and everyone. Amen

Smile often. Say Thanks always. Write a thank you card or note to someone. Read the book The Magic by Rhonda Byrne. Read the book Throne of Heaven by Diana Hutchings. Offer a token of appreciation. Take someone out for a treat. Offer praises and encouragement. Create a vision board of everything you are grateful for.

Helpfulness

Helpfulness is the quality of giving or being ready to give help. It's giving or rendering aid or assistance. It means serving or usefulness.

"Every life is meant to help all lives; each man should live for all men's betterment." Alice Cary

In which ways do you offer help? What ways do you need help?

God let us serve and help others willingly and often. Amen

Ask others how you can help. Schedule mindfulness for 5-10 minutes daily. Think how you can be of service to others. Practice empathy. Use positive language. Train in more industries than just one so you have the know-how to help others. Get some sunshine and go for a walk.

Honesty

Honesty is the quality of being honest. It's a facet of moral character that connotes positive and virtuoso attributes such as integrity, truthfulness, straightforwardness of conduct.

Involves being trustworthy, loyal, fair and sincere. Uprightness and fairness by telling the truth.

"Honesty is the best policy." William Shakespeare

Is honesty important to you?

God help us to be open, honest and tell the truth always. Amen

Be open to giving and receiving feedback. Accept others comments without judgment. Accept the consequences and be honest. Start phrases with honesty or truthfully. Be assertive and tactful. Accept the truth for what it is instead of fighting for what you want it to be. Bath with rose quartz and citrine for 20 minutes. Visualize a white light coming in from the top of your head where your crown chakra is.

Honor

Honor is high respect or great esteem. Its adherence to what is right or to a conventional standard of conduct. To regard or treat someone with respect and admiration. Honor relates to a relationship to reputation and fame. Doing what you believe to be right and confident that you did what's right.

"To the king of ages, immortal, invisible, the only God be honor and glory forever and ever. Amen." 1 Timothy 1:17

"Honor your father and your mother." Deuteronomy 5:16

"Honor everyone." Romans 12:10

What do you want to be honored for?

God may you give us honor, glory and power. Amen

Give compliments. Treat others as you want to be treated. Pray. Give food, gifts and advice freely. Draw yourself as a superhero and name yourself. Write a letter to someone you respect and honor. Wear a majestic purple or royal blue color.

Hope

Hope is a feeling of expectation and desire for a certain thing to happen. It is to cherish a desire with anticipation to look forward to with desire and reasonable confidence. To believe, desire or trust in something or someone. Hope is an optimistic state of mind based on an expectation of positive outcomes.

"And now these three remain: faith, hope and love. But the greatest of these is love." 1 Corinthians 13:13

What do you hope for? What gives you hope?

God please give us hope daily. Amen

Focus on the things and people that empower you and raise your vibration. Create a soul collage with goals in mind. Create outings to look forward to. Make a list of your strengths. Engage in pleasurable activities. Have a daily reflection journal to record thoughts. Give to a children's charity. Connect with angel therapy. Buy an angel oracle deck.

Humility

Humility is a modest or low view of ones' own importance. It's the quality of being humble and not being proud. In Latin humilis means, "low."

"Humility is the solid foundation of all virtues." Confucius

When was a time you were humiliated but learned a lesson from it?

God help us remember that in our humility you make us stronger and better. Amen

Try new things that take practice and devote 10000hrs into it. Ask for help when you need it. Review your actions to avoid pride. Avoid bragging. Be grateful. Admit when you are not the best at something and get advice from veterans or others skilled in that area. Give others credit. Paint your emotions. Get a shaman treatment. Buy a musical instrument and learn how to play or listen to it. Pull your shoulders down and back to remember good posture. Take a few calming breaths. Buy some Vitamin C+D to take daily.

Initiative

Initiative is the ability to assess and initiate things independently. It is the power or opportunity to act or take charge before others do.

"Initiative is doing the right thing without being told." Victor Hugo

When were times you took initiative?

God let me take initiative. Amen

Be proactive and action oriented. Collaborate and discuss with colleagues, partners, family and friends. Get a car mister that diffuses peppermint and lemongrass for clarity and focus. Express your ideas in a written logical organized manner. Avoid standing still and delegate duties when needed. Listen to a song that pumps you up and increases productivity and energy,

Joyfulness

Joyfulness is the quality of being very happy. It is a condition of supreme wellbeing and good spirits.

"If you care joy in your heart, you can heal any moment." Carlos Santana

What brings you joy?

God bring us joy, comfort, peace and love. Amen

Prioritize. Set goals and achieve them. Do random acts of kindness for others and see there joy. Donate or give generously. Plan to go on a mini vacation or schedule a fun event in the future to look forward to with someone. Go for a brisk walk in nature. Eat and smell orange foods. Try a banana peel egg yolk face mask. Buy a citrine, rose quartz or sunstone diffuser bracelet and put the essential oil orange, mandarin or bergamot onto it. Connect with friends and family you haven't talked to in a long time. Smile and laugh.

Justice

Justice is the cause of rightfulness or lawfulness to moral conduct. A just individual is someone at the right place doing their best and following the system of laws set in place by their country and community.

"The moral arc of the universe is long, but it bends toward justice." Martin Luther King Jr.

Do you follow the laws of justice in your community?

God serve justice. Amen

Follow the rules, guidelines and laws outlined in your home, work and community. Draw the libra symbol of scales and make it balanced. Seek out and say Maat (the Egyptian goddess), whom rules order, justice and harmony. Vote for bills, actions and be involved in actions taking place in places that affect your community. Support causes you believe in. Have consequences and external and internal rewards for those whom follow your rules.

Kindness

Kindness is the quality of being friendly, generous and considerate. Treating people with care and respect.

"No act of kindness, no matter how small, is ever wasted." Aesop

What random acts of kindness can you do?

God give us the fruits of kindness, gentleness, meekness, reverence and self-control. Amen

Smile at everyone. Offer affection through hugs, kisses and gentle caresses. Invite someone out to treat them. Provide small gestures and gifts admiring someone you care about. Give many compliments. Wear and surround yourself with pink light. Try red light therapy or add a red light bulb to your house to radiate this warm energy. Try a random acts of kindness bingo with yourself, family, friends or associates. Pay it forward at the drive thru. Buy your favorite flowers and give a few away. Drink pink lemonade.

Love

Love is an intense feeling of deep affection. It is a great interest and pleasure in something or someone. Love is something you enjoy very much.

"Love is patient, love is kind." Corinthians 13:4

Can you describe what love is like and how it feels?

God teach us how to love beyond all measure. Amen

Repeat the affirmation I am loving, loveable and loved. You are loving, loveable and loved. We are loving, loveable and loved. Share your affection, attention, acceptance and appreciation with others. Buy roses and have a rose Epsom salt bath. Hang a bunch of dried roses up by a photo frame of people you love. Try a vision board/ soul collage with the theme of love. Try a few drops of 100% rose hip oil on your face. Read the Five Love Languages by Gary Chapman. Call upon angel Jophiel whom beautifies you with love and rose water. Try rose hip tea. Write on post it notes things you love about yourself or your loved ones and leave them all around. Do a heart chakra meditation. Listen to 528 HZ sound frequency. Buy a heart chakra singing bowl. Research other ways to say I love you.

Mindfulness

Mindfulness is the quality or state of being conscious or aware of something. It is a mental state achieved by focusing one's awareness on the present moment, while calmly acknowledging and accepting one's feelings, thoughts, and bodily sensations.

"Our life is shaped by our mind, for we become what we think." Buddha

Do you practice mindfulness? If so, when?

God provide us with the awareness to be more mindful. Amen

Try meditating for 5-10minutes a day. Join a qi gong class. Connect to nature and sit lay down and or go barefoot. Just breathe and focus on your inhales of love and exhales of peace. Put intentions into everything you do, eating, drinking, dressing, driving and walking. Notice the sights, sounds, smells, textures and tastes. Take a mindfulness course or read a mindfulness book. Do yoga. Try sungazing at sunrise or sunset. Use mudras like prayer position (hands together), heart chakra (thumb and index finger palms up), palms flat up on knees opening to receiving energy or palms flat down on knees for grounding. Use mantras and chant them aloud seven times.

Moderation

Moderation is the avoidance of excess or extremes, especially in one's behavior or political opinions. It's the quality of doing something within reasonable limits.

"Never go to excess but let moderation be your guide." Cicero

Do you consider yourself to be moderate?

God, help us live moderate lives. Amen

Follow specific outlines and guides like physical activity, nutrition, sleep. Try the 888 diet. 8 hours to sleep 8 hours to play 8 hours of work. Notice when you feel like that was too much of something and refrain from doing that for a while. Keep a journal that records you diet, exercise, sleep and schedules daily. Buy Throne of Heaven that has lifestyle planning templates to keep your life in moderation. Focus on quality not quantity. Live simple. Try a liquid fast for a day or three to eliminate any cravings. Do an inventory check with items and prices, which can be good for your insurance to keep up to date. Discard, donate or sell items that have not been used in months or years. Do a liver detox with apple juice.

Modesty

Modesty is the quality or state of being unassuming or moderate in the estimation of one's abilities. It is having the behaviors, manners and or appearance of decency.

"Modesty is the highest elegance." Coco Chanel

What does modesty mean to you?

God keep our modesty and reservation for the right time, place and partner (s). Amen

Put the needs of others before your own. Avoid be too revealing in terms of your physical privates. Be modest in your dressing. Lower your gaze if someone is exposed. Be quiet and humble. Try not to brag. Appreciate and compliment others on their skills and talents. Do random acts of awesomeness even when others are not around. Try a few drops of lavender in the bath or a mister. Drink a calming chamomile tea. Go through your wardrobe and donate all clothing you don't wear or need. Wish for modesty.

Optimism

Optimism is hopefulness and confidence about the future or the successful outcome of something. It's the doctrine that all outcomes are for the best and there are favorable conditions.

"I am and always will be the optimist, the hoper of far flung hopes and the dreamer of improbable dreams." Doctor Who

What ways do you show optimism?

God, fix our mindsets and enable us to be optimistic always. Amen

Wear yellow. Cancel, clear and delete any thoughts that are not positive. Rephrase your speech in positive optimistic language. Shift your focus to see the good. Buy rose or yellow colored lenses in your glasses. Journal about the best thing that happened that day. Grow lemongrass and citronella. Try smudging with sage, Palo Santo or mugwort. Cleanse your space. Play some purifying sound frequencies like 741 Hz, or some gongs and chimes. Avoid complaining and blaming. Focus on solutions and joy.

Orderliness

Orderliness is the quality or state of being orderly. It is having things neat and well arranged.

"Good order is the foundation of all things." Edmund Burke

What things do you keep in order?

God create in us order and harmony. Amen

Create a cleaning schedule. Rearrange a room every weekend to move energy. When you take something put it back in the same place. Label items like jars, pantry, totes, drawers and cabinets. Keep a to do list and check it off for accountability. Look up Feng shui and reorganize your work and home in this design. Request a Feng shui master to visit your home or to arrange your wedding or birth of a child. Get a cleaner or nanny if need be weekly or monthly. Grow a garden in a row and review vegetable and herb compatibility. Keep a daily routine with healthy habits. Maintain stable career, relationship and home lifestyles. Download google calendar to review schedules. Set boundaries and expectations to those sharing the house with you about the kitchen, laundry and other shared spaces.

Patience

Patience is a person's ability to wait something out or endure something without getting riled up. It is the capacity to accept and tolerate.

"Patience is the key to contentment." The prophet Muhammad

Do you consider yourself a patient person?

God keep us patient. Amen

Learn to relax and breathe. Take a vitamin B complex to relieve stress. Try coping strategies like counting, listening to your favorite songs, walk it off, repeat I am affirmations. Pick up hobbies to bide the time and keep you focused on productivity and success. Practice positive self-talk. Do a mindfulness meditation. Pray about everything and ask the divine universe, God, creator to deliver you. Call upon Eth the angel of time to assist you. Visualize yourself completing the task you are being patient about with the desired outcome. Do a merkaba light activation and visualize a big bubble of pink light surrounding you. Connect with lavender, grow or buy lavender. Drink a relaxing chamomile, peppermint or passion flower tea blend. Double check your basic necessities and provide for them. Ask yourself have you eaten, drank anything, dressed warm or cold enough, had enough sleep, is it your time of month? Stay calm and munch or drink a healthy snack like kombucha or macadamia nuts or black licorice.

Peacefulness

Peacefulness is a state of being quiet and calm. Being peaceful means being in a state of tranquility untroubled.

"The day the power of love overrules the love of power the world will now peace." Mahatma Gandhi

What brings you peace?

God let us give and share peace. Amen

Create a Zen garden. Buy a Buddha board and doodle in the sand. Enjoy nature. Play and pet an animal or bird. Listen to your favorite music. Try learning an instrument. Chant OM 108 times. Surround yourself in the blue hue. Paint a wall blue or pink to envelope compassion, calm and peace. Do a pranayama breathing exercise. Find a hiking trail in a forested area and sit by the running creek or river. Listen to alpha waves in binaural beats. Maintain a morning ritual to start your day. Say aloud the metta prayer. "I wish all beings were safe. I wish all beings were happy. I wish all beings were healthy. I wish all beings reach their highest potential. I wish all beings were at peace."

Perseverance

Perseverance is to continue to achieve something with effort and determination despite conditions.

"Success is no accident. It is hard work, perseverance, learning, studying, sacrifice and most of all love of what you are doing or learning to do." Pele

When have you showed perseverance in the past?

God give us the perseverance to complete every task necessary for our highest good. Amen

Set clear goals and benchmarks. Have the on a written or typed list and look at it daily for motivation. Exercise for at least 20 minutes daily. See a life coach for a one on one session. Get some phytogreens and make a smoothie. Print off a smart goals template and set the pace for completion of your goals. Have a coffee/lunch date with a friend to discuss your vision and goals. Try a 3-5km walk for a charity organization.

Purity

Purity is the freedom of being pure. Being clean, clear, unmixed and chaste.

"Purity is the gatekeeper for everything precious and blissful in God's kingdom." Eric Ludy

How can you live a pure life?

God help us to keep our lives and intentions pure. Amen

Say God Bless you in all that you do. Repeat the Hare Krishna mantra. Hare Krishna Hare Krishna Krishna Krishna Hare Hare Hare Rama Hare Rama Rama Rama Hare Hare which means you are eternally forgiven, cleansed, purified and attractive. Keep your sexual relations moral and pure. Where and surround yourself with white. Go to church, a mosque or holy temple to attend and request a blessing from the pastor or leader. They may bless you with holy water. Request forgiveness and say the Lord's Prayer daily. Go get baptized. Do a waterfall visualization cleansing yourself. Get some rose water spritz your auric field. Have a long bath and read positive I am affirmations.

Reliability

Reliability is the quality of being trustworthy or performing consistently well. The degree to which the result of a measurement, calculation or specification can be depended and accurate.

"Your personal brand is a promise to your clients, a promise of quality, consistency, competency and reliability." Jason Hartman

Is reliability important to you?

God instill in a solid, stable and reliable nature. Amen

Do what you say you're going to do. Start and finish your commitments. Be truthful. Stick to your promises or don't promise. Maintain a visual schedule with alarm reminders and to do list with rewards. Be proactive. Always be on time or call. Plan to be at least 15 to 30 minutes early for everything and to stay that long if need be. Repeat this affirmation: I am dependable, punctual, reliable and committed. You are dependable, punctual, reliable and committed. We are dependable, punctual, reliable and committed. Appreciate other people's reliability. Wear yellow to remain sharp, focused and have mental clarity. Try a lemongrass diffuser at home or work.

Respect

Respect is a feeling of deep admiration for someone or something elicited by their abilities, qualities or achievements. It is due regard for the feelings, wishes, rights or traditions of others.

"Treat people the way you wanted to be treated. Talk to people the way you want to be talked to. Respect is earned, not given." Hussein Nishah

How can you show respect to others?

God, ensure that we respect you and others. Amen

Sing R-E-S-P-E-C-T. Follow the golden rule which is treat others as you want to be treated. Respect people, places and property by follow rules, laws and guidelines set out by the government and various organizations. Be polite and kind. Pay attention to speakers and listen empathetically. Walk away when needed. Write an acrostic poem with each letter describing what respect means to you. Like Remember basic kindness, encourage others, Stand firm in your convictions, Play fair and smart. Extend a helping hand. Cause no harm. Think before you speak. Listen to 639 Hz to manifest loving relationships. Speak in an optimistic, love appreciation language.

Responsibility

Responsibility is a state or fact of having a duty to deal with something or of having control over someone the state or fact of being accountable to. The opportunity or ability to act independently and make decisions without authorization. The duty or work for or help someone who is in a position of authority over you.

"The price of greatness is responsibility." Winston Churchill

What type of responsibilities do you have?

God help us to keep our responsibilities. Amen

Write a to do list. Schedule things with a reminder to do them. Avoid procrastination. Take a financial budgeting course. Clean up after yourself and put things away with a place to organize them. Take pens and post it note reminders. Light a green candle. Dab a few drops of peppermint oil into your head and massage it. Listen to classical music.

Reverence

Reverence is the deep respect for someone or something. Its regard or to treat someone with deep respect. Its feelings of awe or an attitude of admiration for someone. Could be a holy figure in religious institutions that shares deep reverence for their religion.

"Gratitude bestows reverence, allowing us to encounter every day epiphanies, those transcendent moments of awe that change forever how we experience life and the world." John Milton

What does reverence mean to you?

God, bless us with the Holy Spirit's fruit of reverence. Amen

Share aha moments with others. Research Zen religion and make a Zen garden. Bow in gratitude to others and say Namaste. Try yoga. Connect with God source. Enter holy grounds: a church, temple or mosque. Appreciate and honor the unity in religion. Tell someone how much you admire and respect them. Display a picture of someone whether family, partner or deity you admire. Wear gold and silver. Listen to hymns and sign a spiritual song like Friend of God.

Self-discipline

Self-disciple is putting off your immediate comfort or wishes in favor of long term success. Key to happy, healthy productive work and personal life is discipline. It's the action or inaction that is regulated to be in accordance or to achieve accord with a particular system of governance. Control gained by enforcing obedience or order training that makes people more able to control themselves.

"Respect your efforts, respect yourself." Self-respect leads to self-discipline. When you have both firmly under your belt that's real power." Clint Eastwood

Would you say you are a self-disciplined person? What do you need more discipline with?

God guide us to live a life of self-discipline and self-control. Amen

Set clear smart goals with an execution plan. Build discipline with focus and effort. Create a new good habit. Try making a routine. Reward yourself. Listen to a self-discipline audio book or meditation. Wear the gemstone tiger's eye to create willpower. Join a martial arts or sports team. Take protein and a greens supplement.

Serenity

Serenity is a state of being clam, peaceful and untroubled. It's the quality or state of being serene and tranquil. The goal of meditation is making the mind still and perfectly calm

"God grant me the serenity to accept the things I cannot change courage to change the things I can and wisdom to know the difference." Serenity Prayer

"Radiate an energy of serenity and peace so that you have an uplifting effect on those you come into contact with." Wayne Dyer

How do you practice serenity?

God, grant us the serenity to accept the things we need to. Amen

Make a gratitude list in the morning and at night. Be careful what you drink. Try Chamomile calming tea. Sleep at least 8 hours. Meditation with sound therapy (gongs, crystal singing bowls, chimes, flute) Draw sacred geometry. Immerse yourself in ultraviolet and blue lights. Create a sacred altar. Paint a rock.

Simplicity

Simplicity is the state or quality of being simple. It's something easy to understand or explain in human lifestyles simplicity denotes freedom. Simplicity implies beauty, purity and clarity.

"I have just 3 three to teach, simplicity, patience and compassion. These three are your greatest treasures." Lao Tzu

What do you need to simplify?

God help me simplify and declutter my life. Amen

Declutter your home, room, vehicle and work space. Buy only what you need. If you haven't used it in a year or two give it away or sell it. Buy an essential oil mister to purify space. Dress with a simple wardrobe. Affirm I live a simple life. Color a mandala. Try a detox, fast or juice fast.

Sincerity

Sincerity is the quality of being free from pretense. It's a mix of seriousness and honesty. If you do things with sincerity people will trust you. It is the quality of being honest, true and real. For example, someone who means everything they promise and say.

"To rule a country of a thousand chariots, there must be reverent attention to business and sincerity economy in expenditure and love for men and the employment of the people at the proper seasons.' Confucius

Who do you find the most sincere?

God assist us to be sincere and genuine with others. Amen

Be genuine. Create five daily positive affirmations to repeat three times. Use sincere body language. Research emotional intelligence. Buy a selenite or Himalayan salt lamp.

Steadfastness

Steadfastness is the quality of being resolutely or dutifully firm and unwavering. It's being firmly fixed in a place unmovable. Implies sureness and continuousness that may be depended on. Firmly loyal or constant.

"Through our trials we are to remain steadfast and know that this light momentary affliction is preparing for us an eternal weight of glory beyond all comparison." Hebrews 3:14

How do you use steadfast in a sentence?

God help us acquire steadfastness. Amen

Pray more and never worry. Create a love music playlist. Try a liquid fast for a day and pray 5 times that day. Be firm in your convictions. Stand by your word like gold. Join tai chi or qi gong.

Strength

Strength is the quality or state of being physically strong. It's the capacity to withstand force or pressure, exertion or endurance. The ability to do things with a lot of physical or mental effort. The state of being bodily or muscular power and vigor.

"Only one who devotes himself to a cause with his whole strength and soul can be a true master. For this reason mastery demands all of a person." Albert Einstein.

What are your strengths?

God, keep us strong, flexible and quick. Amen

Focus on mastering your strengths. Try positive self-talk. Do strength training. Hire a person training for a session or two. Commit to a 21 day fit fix. Take a mental acuity supplement. Wear the color red. Get a chiropractor or osteopath treatment. Take a Vitamin B complex to increase energy, destress and metabolize fats, carbohydrates and proteins.

Tact

Tact is sensitivity in dealing with others. A keen sense of what to do or say in order to maintain good relations with others or avoid offense. IT is skill in dealing with difficult situations. Tact is the ability to tell the truth in a way that considers other people's feelings and reactions. Avoid upsetting people by being careful.

"Tact is the ability to describe others as they see themselves." Abraham Lincoln.

What strategies do you use to be tactful?

God give us tact and diplomacy. Amen

Create a healthy, happy, safe and friendly environment. Choose your words carefully. Watch and learn body language. Give honest feedback. Learn to say no. Read a book about communicating with diplomacy and tact. Listen to binaural beats with headphones. See a hypnotherapist for a session. Dress professionally and with class.

Thoughtfulness

Thoughtfulness is the state of being absorbed in thought. The consideration for the needs of other people. The quality of being kind and thinking about other people's needs. Showing consideration for others.

"I'm all about thoughtful gifts. If you put thought behind it-it could be $5 but if there's thought behind it, I think that's what matters." Brittany Spears

Would you say you're a thinker or a doer or both? What do you think about the most?

God provide us with helpful, positive beneficial thoughts. Amen

Brainstorm and write your thoughts. Send messages to people you think about and ask them how they are doing. Buy a gift for someone that you they will use. Write a sweet little note to someone a leave it for them to find. Every morning pick 3 people you are grateful for. Learn what others love and give it to them. Get a tuning fork treatment.

Tolerance

Tolerance is the ability or willingness to tolerate something in particular the existence of opinions or behavior that does not necessarily agree with. Allowing permitting or acceptance of an action, idea, object or person which dislikes or disagrees. It is the capacity to endure pain or hardship.

"I think tolerance and acceptance and love is something that feeds every community." Lady Gaga

What is an example of tolerance that you experienced?

God, be tolerant with us. Amen

Listen carefully without jumping to conclusions. Try to use Leaps when communicating. (Listen Empathy Ask Questions Paraphrase Summarize) Address conflict with calmness and patience. Get a massage to relax. Listen to celestial music. Drink passionflower tea.

Trust

Trust is the firm belief in the reliability, truth, ability or strength of someone or something. To rely upon or place confidence in someone or something. To trust another's honesty. It is a set of behaviors such as action in ways that depend on another.

"Love all, trust a few, do wrong to none." William Shakespeare

Who do you trust the most?

God teach us how important trust and honesty are. Amen

Stay faithful. Say and do what you said you are going to do. Be reliable. Always be open to telling the truth. Look up the 10 commandments of Christianity and follow them. Honor your pinky promises. Join in an interpersonal group. Create a family crest.

Truthfulness

Truthfulness is the fact of being true and realistic. It is an action as well as in words. It's the quality of being honest.

"Truthfulness is the foundation of all the virtues of mankind." Abdu'l Baha

Are you a truthful person?

God help us be truthful, open and honest all the time. Amen

Research the term Satya. Speak your truth. Read the holy scriptures of Upanishads. Nurture your relationships by setting boundaries that require open, honest communication. Find a white ostrich feather and do a sage smudge. Display the Egyptian goddess Ma'at. Find three white feathers as this indicates truth and divinity. Wear the color white. See a spiritual psychotherapist for a session.

Understanding

Understanding is the ability to understand something comprehension. It's sympathetically aware of other people's feeling tolerant and forgiving. It is a psychological process related to an abstract or physical object such as a person, situation or message whereby one is able to think about it and use concepts to deal adequately. Having mental quality, act or state of a person who understands.

"The noblest pleasure is the joy of understanding." Leonardo Da Vinci

How do you know when someone understands you?

God please provide us with understanding. Amen

Look up active listening techniques. Ask questions to check for understanding and comprehension. Recognize different ways of life. Think before you speak. Say less, listen more. Write reminder messages, emails to confirm details on instructions and plans of action. Use simple language. Rephrase details to confirm you know what to do. See an art therapist.

Wisdom

Wisdom is the quality of having experience, knowledge and good judgment. It's the quality of being wise. The ability to think and act using knowledge, experience, understanding, common sense and insight. It's associated with attributes such as unbiased judgment, compassion, experiential self-knowledge, self-transcendence and non-attachment and virtues such as ethics and benevolence.

"Science is organized knowledge. Wisdom is organized life." Immanuel Kant

Who do you consider to be wise and why?

God, teach us your wisdom and knowledge. Amen

Find your self-interests and master them. Eat for your brain; consume omega oils and protein daily. Ask questions if you want to know. Find mentors, guides and teachers. Read and research topics to gain knowledge. Enroll in professional development courses at least once a year. Check out www.udemy.com for online lifetime warranty courses. Take an IQ test. Pray for wisdom and intelligence. Try a vegetarian diet for a week. Listen to a third eye and crown chakra meditation. Decalcify the pineal gland by avoiding fluoride.

Zeal

Zeal is great energy or enthusiasm in pursuit of a cause or an objective. Fervor for a person, cause or object. Its eager desire or endeavor and intense emotion compelling emotion.

"Zeal will do more than knowledge." William Hazlitt

What is your zeal?

God, give us vitality and zeal. Amen

Raise your energy vibration. Rub your hands really fast together for 60 seconds to create friction heat energy. Get a reiki treatment and hot stone therapy massage. Try Acupuncture. Do chakra guided meditations to activate, cleanse and energize your 7 major chakra energy centers. Wear and eat warm colors like yellow, orange and red. Genuinely cheer people on. Do a daily devotion. Commit to a person or object. Drink hot lemon honey water.

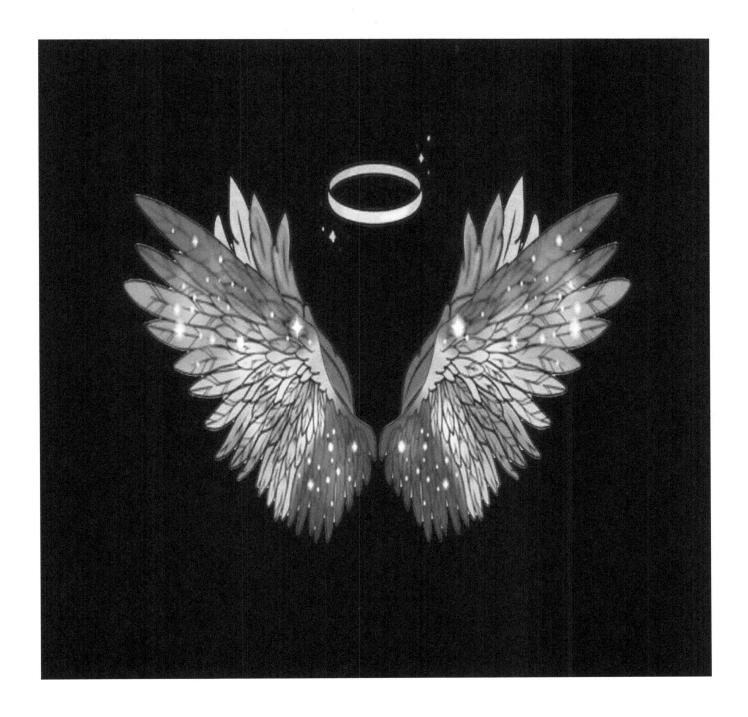

The Book of Angels Oracle

How can I talk to angels? Do you need answers to questions or issues to make life easier? Perhaps you have multiple concerns that you need help with. Whether your concern is getting the answers to your questions or you need direct guidance as to what steps to take. This angel oracle was inspired by Angela McGerr's Book of Angels deck and it will give you positive, uplifting advice and affirmations that will put you on the right path.

Daily pick a number from 1-100 and find your angel alphabetically. You may start at one to get to know your angels or choose where you want to go. Maybe you keep seeing the same numbers pop up. This could be your angel trying to communicate with you. If you are really aware of numbers then look up numerology. You may find your birthday and name have special destiny and life path numbers. This is fun and there are apps you may find for numerology.

Read and invoke the angels three times to request their help. Remember to thank them for their services. They love you and want to guide you. The guidebook will provide you with an extended explanation and format to hear your angel's advice, guidance and support. Once you have mastered all 100 angels, a suggestion is to get a real angel deck by Doreen Virtue. Her oracle cards provide positive assistance, guidance and action. Each message will be perfect for you. You may knock on the deck three times to clear the energy and ask your inner self what is right for you.

Steps in the Guidebook include:

1. Drawing the angel sigil from the back of your card in the sky or on yourself or with a paper and pen (heart, hand, or mind)

   i. Read the angel poem

   ii. Read the number meaning for this angel. Then when you see this number reappearing, it could be a message to you.

   iii. Practice makes perfect. Learn your numbers and your angels. You will notice more synchronicities appear.

   An option for you is to write out all 100 angels and cut them out on equally sized card-stock. Write their name on one side and the number on the other side. Put these written names + numbers into a bag and draw one at a time. Read your message. Enjoy yourself!

1-Achaiel

Is the guardian angel of the secrets of nature

Learn the power and beauty of the fragrance feature

The flower fragrances enhance and delight

Using the beauty of color to heal sight

Nature's symmetry is pleasing to the eye

Shapes, patterns, perfumes, oils recognize and try

Each color carries a different vibration

Harmonizing the chakra system sensation

Gemstone: red beryl

Number Meaning

1-Stay positive and everything you're thinking is manifesting.

2-Adiel

Is the guardian angel of the 14th mansion of the moon

I am the silver light of your intuition trying to attune

The 28 mansions of the moon are the mystical days and phases

I am the guardian of the 3rd moon quarter

Use me to bring something to a conclusion for him or her

I can help you with the loving determination to change

Do meditations to provide guidance on the situation or relationship you want to arrange

Gemstone: garnet

Number Meaning

2-Everything is fine, luck is yours.

3-Adnachiel

Is the guardian angel of November and Sagittarius

I will help bring about new and exciting activities to discuss

Guiding you towards career opportunities and spiritual growth

Giving you energy to set goals to focus on both

Take quiet time to meditate and receive a vision

Move your goals and dreams from concept to reality

Take these steps in a new direction of your destiny

Gemstone: star ruby

Number Meaning

3-The ascended masters are helping you.

4-Ambriel

Is the guardian angel of Gemini and May

I will surround you in powerful silver energy today

Because of your quick brain

Affirm you are healthy and sane

You have sympathetic ears and intuitive skills

Providing knowledge of important wills

Give yourself love and listen to your heart

Say no when you need to depart

Gemstone: jasper

Number Meaning

4- The angels are with you helping you

5-Amnediel

Is the guardian angel of the seventh mansion of the moon

I recharge your dreams and help you attune

Make use of my quarter moon to make something happen

Bringing a project, situation or relationship out in the open

Plan for the matter to come to fruition

Culminating in the full moon your final decision

Gemstone: sunstone

Number Meaning

5-A significant change is occurring

6-Anafiel

Is the guardian angel of the heavenly key

Given the knowledge of truth and keys to be free

The power is within your own heart

Instructing to love is a good start

Pure silver light will show you the way

Your heaven on earth is here to stay

Gemstone: heliotrope

Number Meaning

6-Do not worry about material things. Ask the angels for help.

7-Anahitel

Is the guardian angel of medicinal plants

I lift the seeds of opportunities one supplants

The flowers of fruitfulness gladden the heart with compassionate love

Learn some new era of knowledge inspired by God's dove

The water of life provides a remedy

Heal with plant energy vibrations like chemistry

Gemstone: sardonyx

Number Meaning

7-You are on the right path and divine magic surrounds you. Justice is served.

8-Ananchel

Is the guardian angel of acceptance and grace

All things heal and prayers are answered face to face

It is I who give you the grace to accept what life offers you

Help may be offered to honor something deep and true

Gemstone: topaz

Number Meaning

8-Signifies abundance and prosperity.

9-Aniel

Is the guardian angel of luck and silver rotection

Sending a pure silver energy in high vibration

Wrap yourself in an invisible cloak around you

It's very protective and can help anyone its true

Write my name on paper, on a pendant and place it near your heart

This will guide your dreams and what you do not want will depart

Gemstone: kunzite

Number Meaning

9-Lightworker, take the actions steps to achieve your life purpose.

10-Aradel

Is the guardian angel of beliefs

Shaping your personality and character like chiefs

Making you the person you really are

Invoke me to enfold you in protection from afar

Gemstone: sapphire

Number Meaning

10- Call upon God to perfect you and your life.

11-Aratronel

Is the guardian angel of nature's magic

Mind is the old practical uses and healing benefits antic

Use my natural medicine to heal your life

Sending soothing silver energy to relax and heal your life

Combine old with new remedies

Reveal ancient knowledge of shamanic memories

Gemstone: diamond

Number Meaning

11- Focus on the good within yourself and others.

12-Ariel

Is the guardian angel of earth, Pluto and air

I am the meeting of underworld and over world if you care

You must see with your heart and listen to your soul

Cleansing old patterns of behavior to surge into light is the goal

Use each rainbow color to replenish your energy

Feel the elements of water and fire chemistry

Gemstone: tourmaline

Number Meaning

12-Your positive thoughts influence your positive future.

13-Barakiel 1.

Is the guardian angel of Scorpio and Pisces and February and October

I can help you take calculated chance and risk with people and every adventure

I will provide positive energy and good luck

Power you're thinking pass the buck

You are compassionate and care about many things

Ask your heart to be happy and find its silver wings

Gemstone: rhodochrosite

Number Meaning

13-Female ascended masters are helping you now.

14-Barkiel

Is the guardian angel of February and Pisces

I shield your sensitivity about people and their crises

You are compassionate and care about many things

Ask your heart to be happy and find its silver wings

Gemstone: morganite

Number Meaning

14-Maintain a positive outlook be optimistic and bright.

15- Camael

Is the guardian angel of Tuesday, Mars and 5th heaven

I am divine justice and thank you heaven for 11:11

I guide you to the personal empowerment of light

It takes determinations and stamina to succeed in personal flight

Sending you ruby red rays to boost your root chakra

I am empowered becomes your new mantra

Gemstone: rhodonite

Number Meaning

15- Respect change to manifest the best outcomes.

16-Cambiel

Is the guardian angel of January and Aquarius

Bringing silver water to your heart victorious

Use your gold left brain for decision, logic and action

Apply your silver right brain for a dreamy, less practical sensitive reaction

The moon and water will assist to make decisions with your heart and head

In return you will have increased well being, and a greater balance instead

Gemstone: beryl

Number Meaning

16- Your words are magnetic affirmations so be aware of them.

17-CassieL

Is the guardian angel of Saturday 7th heaven and Saturn

I lead the way to a peace and serenity pattern

I hold the gate of the 7th heaven for those souls who accept opposites

It is a time of optimism, the light is there to look at the positives

Gemstone: bismuth

Number Meaning

17-Keep up the good work you are on the right path.

18-Dabriel

Is the guardian angel of writing

The heavenly scribe records in handwriting

You need to master the art of written communication

To build a clear and honest foundation

Invoke me to give you courage to write your message

Atoning for the past and moving towards a brighter passage

Gemstone: rose quartz

Number Meaning

18-All your material resources will come easily.

19- Diniel

Is the guardian angel of luck and golden protection

Bringing the golden light to help others bring a healing connection

Write my name anywhere, inscribe it on a pendant to bring unconditional love and light transcendent

For protection close your eyes and call my name

Feel the power of your will become your aim

Gemstone: moonstone

Number Meaning

19-Believe in yourself and follow your dreams.

20-Dokiel

Is the guardian angel of work and home balance

Holding the golden scales in a harmonious dance

Use your skills and abilities in the way they were intended

Use your time efficiently to correct the balance its recommended

Take positive action towards a better future

A future harmonious happier and mature

Gemstone: ametrine

Number Meaning

20-Your connection to the creator is strong. Fill your heart and mind with faith.

21-Dumasel

Is the guardian angel of silence

I will give you potential knowledge by keeping noise at a distance

Step back from the noise in a silent meditation

Find your rest and peace for a short time duration

Gemstone: citrine

Number Meaning

21- Your optimism is definitely warranted. The angels are working behind the scenes on your behalf right this very minute. You can help support the angels work by saying positive affirmations and believing that your dream is already manifesting.

22-Ethel

Is the guardian angel of time

Use your powers to guide your memories in prime

I can bend time if the need is great

Like a time traveler through a gate

My love helps you manage your present more effectively

My golden ebb flows to your future for your good collectively

Gemstone: fire opal

Number Meaning

22- The angels can see the positive results of your prayers and they want you to have patience and stay optimistic while the final details are being worked out in heaven.

23-Farlasel

I am the guardian angel of winter

As a time of transition in nature

Cleansing and tidying should be undertaken

Quiet beauty, reflection and peace taken

Gemstone: Mexican opal

Number Meaning

23- You are working closely with one or more ascended masters such as Jesus, Moses, the saints or goddesses. This is a message from your ascended master guided, who can see that the answer to your prayers is within reach.

24-Gabriel

I am the guardian angel of Monday, 1st heaven and the moon

I am the spiritual awakener visiting you in your dreams, helping you attune

My task is to guide you to fulfill your hopes and dreams

Dissolving barriers and expanding your intuitive skills with golden beams

Gemstone: spinel

Number Meaning

24- Additional angels are surrounding your right now helping you stay optimistic no matter what is going on around you. the angels know the magical power of faith.

25-Gazardiel

Is the guardian angel of the rising setting sun

Mine is the golden energy guiding making things fun

Practice the sun salutation

Focus on the power of will and intention

Gemstone: chrysoberyl

Number Meaning

25-As you go through major life changes, expect the best and your optimism will be rewarded.

26-Geliel

Is the guardian angel of the 21st mansion of the moon

I am the fourth and final phase of the journeys moon

This is a time of closure and completion

A project, plan relationship or works complete transition

Gemstone: pyrite

27 Geniel

Is the guardian angel of the 1st mansion of the moon

Make something new happen for your highest good soon

Absorb the silver energy to develop your intuitive powers

Commence a project within a few hours

Gemstone: gold

Number Meaning

27-Congratulations! Your optimism is attracting wonderful situations and relationships.

28-Hadakiel

Is the guardian angel of judgment

Set yourself standards achievable to by adjustment

But judge not and work towards self improvement

Gemstone: chrysoprase

Number Meaning

28-Money comes to you as you keep the faith that you, your loved ones and your beautiful life purpose are all fully supported by heaven.

29-Hagithel

Is the guardian angel of metal

I guide you to creative inspiration and planetary royal

There are seven sacred metals, angels and days of the solar system

They are silver, iron, mercury, tin, copper, lead and gold to name them

Gemstone: jade

Number Meaning

29-Stay positive about your life purpose and put all of your focus on being of service, utilizing your natural talents, passions, and interests. Doors are opening for you. Keep your faith strong.

30-Hahliiel

Is the guardian angel of colors

To enrich and heal your life with colored covers

The creator gave us 12 colors of creation

To empower each energy center station

Red, orange, yellow and green are masculine

Blue, purple, violet, magenta and feminine

Gemstone: quartz

Number Meaning

30-You are fully supported by God and the ascended masters. Step forward confidently in the direction of your dreams.

31-Hamaliel

Is the guardian angel of August and Virgo

To put relaxation, tranquility and harmony in turbo

Both at home and at work I want to enhance your interactive skills

Meeting new people developing character and personality while sharing wills

Gemstone: sulfur

Number Meaning

31-See the perfection within you, other people and your current situations. As you see divine perfection in your mind, it manifests externally in your relationships, career, health and other life areas.

32-Haniel

Is the guardian angel of Venus and third heaven and Friday

My message is of love and light as it heals eternally everyday

My golden love and emerald magenta rays begin the process of healing

If you look in the mirror and practice using your heart by feeling

With all the beauty and love surrender

Brings the power of compassionate love to representer

Gemstone: Vesuvianite

Number Meaning

32- The ascended master Jesus reminds you to apply his affirmation about the power of faith.

33-Hariel

Is the guardian angel of animals tame

Mine is the energy of creatures same

Your love for animals will lead to guidance from them

Ancient souls can be compared to a diamond gem

Your animals will contact the right people and help heal you

To learn a lesson in life and animals are sacred and true

Gemstone: serpentine

Number Meaning

33-You have a strong and clear connection with one or more ascended masters who have answered your call and your prayers. Keep talking to them.

34-Haurvatatel

Is the guardian angel of rivers that flow

Enjoy a long cool drink invigorating your glow

I protect you, go with the flow

Helping direct how to move to win

Be successful smile and grin

Gemstone: amazonite

Number Meaning

34-Your prayers are heard and answered by the angels and ascended masters who are with you now.

35-Hermes Trismegistusel

Is the guardian angel of spiritual alchemy

I am the thrice great master of masters with the master key

We are all part of the universal mind

The world above and below are one kind

The yin and yang element that can be found

Balance is attained safe and sound

Gemstone: malachite

Number Meaning

35- A positive change is coming about for you, with the assistance and protection of the ascended masters.

36-Iadiel

Is the guardian angel for dispelling worry

Insuring all your earthy cares to victory

You are on the right path and track

Avoiding concerns about what you may lack

I bring you silver strength of love and light

Asking you to be patient every night

Gemstone: bloodstone

Number Meaning

36- The ascended masters ask you to keep your thoughts focused on spirit.

37-Icabel

Is the guardian angel of fidelity

Giving unconditional love without judgment so free

I counsel you in loyalty and faithfulness

Showering lovers, friends, and family with forgiveness

I will lift your soul

Sticking to your promise is goal

Gemstone: alexandrite

Number Meaning

37- You are on the right path and the ascended masters are encouraging and helping you along the way.

38-Isdael

Is the guardian angel of food and nourishment

Its subtle energy of nutrition God sent

Urging you to a suitable diet with sufficient exercise

Supporting you in attaining harmony wise

Respect your mind, body, and spirit like a friend

Feel the love of nourishment to defend

Gemstone: dalmation jasper

Number Meaning

38-The ascended masters are helping you with your financial situation.

39 -Isiaiel

Is the guardian angel of the future

Guiding your present building it bright for sure

Put the past behind you

Be open to warm golden rays of love true

Attracting beneficial new people, situations, and opportunities for abundance

Sending positive energy back in time, past and future with reliance

Gemstone: chrysocolla

Number Meaning

39- You are being helped by the ascended masters, who are strongly encouraging you to work on your life purpose right now.

40-Israfel

Is the guardian angel of poetry

Creating living beauty with words so mote it be

Inspired at the soul level to express

Write a book or poem to impress

Gifted with the ability to heal others

Poetry is a gift to all sisters and brothers

Gemstone: diopside

Number Meaning

40- God and the angels are surrounding you with heavenly love and protection.

41- Ithuriel

Is the guardian angel of your true self

It is time to embrace truth and freedom for yourself

The path of your life can be viewed from a crystal mountain

As you ascent you have the ability to feel, love and accept the knowledge fountain

When you reach the golden crown

Look how far you've come around

Gemstone: emerald

Number Meaning

41- The angels as you to keep very positive thoughts as everything you say and think is manifesting into form rapidly.

42- Jofiel

Is the guardian angel of jobs and roles

Take time to understand you lessons and goals

Accept your position and learn from it

Be patient, new opportunities will come in a bit

Gemstone: fucsite

Number Meaning

42- The angels are urging you to keep the faith.

43-Kadmiel

I am the guardian angel of good fortune

Inscribe my assistance on the Nordic rune

I will provide good luck, protection and healing

You will be surrounded by a golden auric feeling

Ask me to assist you in sealing love and light

Inscribe me on a bracelet or paper to give insight

Gemstone: moldavite

Number Meaning

43- Both the angels and the ascended masters such as Jesus, Quan Yin or a saint are helping you right now.

44-Machidiel

I am the guardian angel of Mars and Aries

Guide your decision making and goals please

You will completely understand your hearts desire

Think carefully and clearly on what you admire

I will balance your body, spirit and mind

Building your skills and resources benefiting you'll find

Gemstone: prasiolite

Number Meaning

44-The angels are giving you extra comfort, love, and support right now. Ask them for help with everything and listen to their guidance through your intuition.

45-Manakel

I am the guardian angel of dolphins and whales

The voice of the sea herself swimming ancient trails

Holding ancient knowledge and special power

Tune into my aeons old vibrations on a sound tower

Bringing much healing in a deep spiritual way

Commune with dolphins and whales in play

Number Meaning

45- The angels are helping you through a positive life change.

46-Matriel

I am the guardian angel of rain

Bringing showers on every road and lane

Wash clean your heart and reopen your heart

Be clear on what you want is a good start

Let my silver tears flow into your heart to heal

Receive this precious gift, be cleansed and feel

Gemstone: peridot

Number Meaning

46- The angels are saying to you: keep your thoughts focused upon your spiritual self and your divine source for everything.

47-Metatronel

I am the twin guardian of the tree of life

The pure white dove of peace is like a husband or wife

Silver white rays shine as the radiant light of the crown

Shekinah helps you to secure your foundations in every town

Reconnect with all life through sacred geometry

You will send and receive love and light free

Gemstone: sphene

Number Meaning

47- The angels say that you are on the right path.

48-Melchisadecel

I am the guardian angel of peace and spirituality

Holding the chalice of life and the key to tranquility

Your quest is to find my rainbow palm in center of the labyrinth of peace

Heal mind, body and spirit with rainbow colors please

Explore my spiritual violet ray

In sacred geometry visualize pure white and play

Gemstone: unakite

Number Meaning

48- Your prayers about money have been heard and answered by the angels.

49-Michael

I am the guardian of Wednesday Mercury and the 4th heaven

Traveling to strengthen and protect you on earth in heavens seven

Truth, wisdom, and freedom light your way

Building your confidence with powers of speech and my blue energy ray

Gemstone: zoisite

Number Meaning

49- The angels urge you to get to work on your major goals and life purpose now. Ask them to help you with ideas, courage and motivation.

50-Mumiahel

I am the guardian angel of energy and well being

Golden light sparkles to cleanse, purify and balance your being

Imagine your body as a vessel of pure crystalline light

Overflowing with golden light protecting your aura with strong might

Gemstone: tree agate

Number Meaning

50- God is helping you to change your life in healthful new ways.

51-Muriel

I am the guardian angel of Cancer and June

I will aid you to find empowerment for the future soon

Now is the time to speak up and be honest

Silver energy will boost your confidence and rest

I am the voice of your heart pure and clear

Expressing your thoughts, feelings and decisions dear

Gemstone: blue chalcedony

Number Meaning

51-Keep positive thoughts about the changes you're desiring and experiencing.

52-Mupiel

I am the guardian angel for mending a broken heart

I send a clear green water of life to flow in to soothe and heal

Imagine bright pink lotus of unconditional love help you to deal

Reopen your heart to heal the past for real

Gemstone: azurite

Number Meaning

52-Accept that the changes you're considering or experiencing are for the best.

53-Nadiel

I am the guardian angel of December and Capricorn

I will build your self-esteem with bright rays of golden yellow like corn

My love brings you a real vision

Arriving at a perfectly derived decision

Gemstone: aquamarine

Number Meaning

53- Ask for their help with any aspect of these situations, such as additional ideas, opportunities, courage and so forth.

54-Nathaniel

I am the guardian angel of passion

Like the phoenix reborn on a mission

Emerge triumphant from the ashes of your past

With more vitality, enthusiasm and joy at last

Gemstone: apatite

Number Meaning

54- The angels are guiding and supporting you as you make healthy and necessary changes in your life.

55-Ochel

Is the guardian angel of crystal alchemy

Generating crystal power of light you see

A whole world of knowledge rests in each mineral

Rainbow colors of various vibrations are contained with each crystal

Gemstone: benitoite

Number Meaning

55- This is a period of out with the old in with the new. Welcome these changes as they bring about new blessings.

56-Ofaniel

Is the guardian angel of the wheel of the moon

Providing pure silver light power we can attune

I will help you achieve balance and clarify your purpose

Set an intention and light a white candle to be of service

Gemstone: star sapphire

Number Meaning

56- As you go through changes with your home life, career and relationships stay focused on your growth. Find the blessing within each change you're experiencing.

57-Oriel

Is the guardian angel of destiny

Free choice is your reality

Is the guardian angel of the hearts desires

I bring you love and support to fulfill your dreams and desires

You will meet someone new and be invited to attend

These are synchronicities on your journeys that will mend

Gemstone: iolite

Number Meaning

57- The changes you are experiencing are for the best. Trust these changes to lead you where you want to go.

58-Padiel

Is the guardian angel of good luck and silver protection

I teach you that silver combined with love brings healing and protection

Inscribe my name on a piece of paper or a pendant

This will magnify the energy of peace, love, light, power and wisdom sent

Gemstone: labradorite

Number Meaning

58- Your finances are improving, and there will be a positive change in your financial flow. This could also signal a job promotion or career change, with an increased salary.

59-Pagiel

Is the guardian angel of the heart's desires

I bring you love and support to fulfill your dreams and desires

You will meet someone now and be invited to attend

These are synchronicities on your journeys plan so intend

Gemstone: lapis lazuli

Number Meaning

59- The changes you are going through are bringing you closer to your divine life purpose. You can calm yourself by spending time on activities related to your interests.

60-Parasiel

Is the guardian angel of hidden treasure

I shine the silver light of your true talents in due measure

All knowledge is held within your own heart and soul

Experience this prize that leads to wisdom as a goal

Number Meaning

60- This number is a call for you to balance and always remember that spirit is your source and the force behind everything in your life.

61 - Pedael

Is the guardian angel of deliverance

My role is to help you let go with reliance

On a certain situation, object or person

Ask me to help you release this soul to the light of God's son

Say goodbye and breathe in golden rays

Invoke the power of love into your heart for all your day

Gemstone: kyanite

Number Meaning

61 - Keep your thoughts about your material life such as home, work, body and possessions very positively focused.

62 - Phalegel

Is the guardian angel for managing and refocusing anger

Directing your passionate feelings in positive ways like Jesus in manger

As I send you unconditional love in golden waves

Breathe it in to your heart soothing and calming energy saves

Gemstone: petersite

Number Meaning

62 - Keep believing that the details of your life are working out in miraculous ways.

63 - Phanuel

Is the guardian angel of atonement and forgiveness

Through me seek repentance and selflessness

Invoke me to surround you with golden wings

Ask to be forgiven and forgive amongst helpful things

Gemstone: blue topaz

Number Meaning

63 - Ask for help and then be open to receiving the assistance that they bring to you in the form of ideas, guidance and unexpected gifts.

64 - Phuel

Is the guardian angel of the waters of Earth and Neptune

Waters of earth and the tides of the moon

Mine are the powers that rule the waters and breathe my loving golden energy

My waters soothe and balance bringing peace and tranquility

Submerge yourself in gentle water

Washed clean and pure let yourself be reborn in order

Gemstone: sodalite

Number Meaning

64 - You are fully supported by the angels in every area of your life.

65 - Pitis Sophiael

Is the guardian angel of wisdom and faithful heavenly and earthly mother

I am the celestial star fire that brings new faith like a godmother

I connect you to wisdom and spiritual sustenance

Pure energy will open your meridians you will feel your chakras expanse

Gemstone: turquoise

Number Meaning

65 - Congratulations! This is an excellent time to make changes at home, work, or within relationships. Follow your inner truth.

66 - Rachiel

Is the guardian angel of sexuality

Reciprocated between two persons brings riches and vitality

Infuse passion with true love

Pleasing each other like heaven above

The powerful orgasmic energy released from your head and heart

Assists in healing your loved one through the power of love smart

Gemstone: amethyst

Number Meaning

66 - This is a message for you to spend time in prayer and meditation. Ask for spiritual intervention and open your arms to receive the help that always follows prayers.

67 - Rachmiel

Is the guardian angel of compassion

Help all living creatures giving them attention

Compassions will heal any despair

Reopening your heart to the serenity and hope repair

Sit quietly and breathe in loving golden energy

You will receive comfort as a guarantee

Gemstone: charoite

Number Meaning

67 - Well done! You're on the right path at home and at work.

68 - Radueriel

Is the guardian angel of artistic inspiration

The master of heavenly song, patron of the artist station

Whatever medium you use

Interplay color texture, light and sound in the ideas you introduce

You are an expression of the human spirits power

Allow your soul to flow with intuitive knowledge that does empower

Gemstone: corundum

Number Meaning

68 - Remember that spirit is the source of your income.

69 - Ramiel

Is the guardian angel of clarity

I help you see your true self in true familiarity

My light helps you to clarify purpose, motivation vision

Light my silver light shine through to enlighten every decision

Infinite love with support, and motivate you

Make your goals clear and follow them through

Gemstone: lepidolite

Number Meaning

69 - As you spend time working on activities related to your spiritual passions and interests, every part of your life automatically improves.

70 - Rampel

Is the guardian angel of mountains

My sacred breath directs glaciers, snow and rains

Find peace, tranquility and plenty

My still pools of water provide hope in a time of need

I support you with unconditional love as my peaceful deed

Gemstone: sugilite

Number Meaning

70 - This is a message from god that you're on the right path. Keep up the good work.

71 - Raphael

Is the guardian angel of Sunday the second heaven and the Sun

I bring you a glorious energy and joy that enlightens life with fun

My task is to guide you towards self-healing

You require balance and harmony

I will aid your decisions and feelings to free

Absorb my silver and gold rays

Visualize your chakras color gaze

Gemstone: tanzanite

Number Meaning

71 - You are on track with your manifestations. Stay positive and optimistic and all of your dreams will be right there for you.

72 - Raziel

Is the guardian angel of the celestial secrets

I am the secret wisdom and mysteries of all god angel sets

They contain universal laws and astronomy

Revealing secrets of angel hierarchies sacred geometry

I counsel you to the path of my celestial book

Unlock its wisdom, find the truth and take a look

Gemstone: Botswana agate

Number Meaning

72 - Have faith that you're taking the right steps toward the manifestation of your desires because you are.

73 - Rikbiel

Is the guardian angel of the power of love

I drive the light chariot of the holy spirits dove

Love is faster than the speed of thought and light

Focus on the situation you need the help and gods might

Send golden love through every in and out breath

Feel the pure love of every deep golden breath

Gemstone: fire agate

Number Meaning

73 - The ascended masters are guiding you, and you are listening to them accurately. Stay on your present path as it is illuminate with blessings and gifts.

74 - Rochel

Is the guardian of lost things

Invoke me to retrieve anything on golden wings

If it is possible it will be refound

Whether it's a physical thing, aspect of yourself to be found

Invoke my name three times and ask, will and command with all your heart

Have faith, trust and gradually things will come and start

Gemstone: mahogany obsidian

Number Meaning

74 - The angels surround you and walk beside you every step of the way. You're on the fast track to the manifestation of your dreams, so stick to the ideas and activities you're involved with now.

75 - Ruhiel

Is the guardian angel of the winds

Bringing a new perspective with westerly winds

Invoke my help to improve programming your mind

My east wind invigorates bringing clarity of every kind

South winds will guide you

Blowing the light true

Gemstone: leopard jasper

Number Meaning

75 - The changes you're considering are exactly right for you.

76 - Sachluphel

Is the guardian angel of plants

My light shines a foliage, ferns, and desert slants

My plants protect mother earth in many ways

Assisting you to cultivate plants, and flowers all your days

Gemstone: picture jasper

Number Meaning

76 - You're on the right path, and your material needs are fully supported by your choices and actions.

77 - Sahaqiel

Is the guardian angel of the sky and doves

Our celestial secrets revealed, the spirit is free and loves

Look up see white birds and a cloud of white wings

See three white feathers amongst things

Focus your energy, commit to your guest

Surrender and let spirit radiate love and light best

Gemstone: tigers eye

Number Meaning

77 - Keep up the great work. Everything you're doing right now has the Midas touch.

78 - Sandalphonel

Is the guardian angel of prayer

Gathering your prayers when you think, speak or share

I hear all your words when you hear me

It is for your highest good so mote it be

Listen to my guidance and try to meditate

I will give you signs from nature, books, a song, and dreams great

Gemstone: black diamond

Number Meaning

78 - Your present focus and actions have tapped into the universal financial flow of abundance. Stick with your current plans as they're right on the money.

79 - Savatriel

Is the guardian angel of sunlight

I will illumine your heart and mind to be light

Protecting you with love, picture me above you

Breathe deeply and visualize golden light filling you through

This light will bring divine angelic comfort and healing

Your own will power receives this golden energy feeling

Gemstone: onyx

Number Meaning

79 - You're on the right path for your divine life purpose.

80 - Seraphiel

Is the guardian angel of cosmic spirit quintessence

I am the music of spheres, the light of source from creator's essence

My celestial music empowers your spirit and resonates within your soul

Magnify your diamond energy by sacred breathing

Connecting your heart to sacred geometry

Will bring universal harmony

So mote it be

Gemstone: star diopside

Number Meaning

80 - God is supporting you in all areas, including your financial life. Let go and let god help you.

81 - Shekinahel

Is the guardian angel of the tree of life

I guard the tree as it grows in the earthly kingdom with wildlife

Invoke me to bless your choice of a life partner

And to build a life happy and secure with your co-partner

You deserve love and must affirm positive fulfilling relationships

When love is given to the right partner it heals, strengthens our divine companionship

Gemstone: black opal

Number Meaning

81 - The more you stay positive about money the greater your financial flow will be.

82 - Sofiel

Is the guardian angel of earth's bounty

The richness, beauty and fruitfulness of mother Earths County

Choose food which builds bodily strength and power

Drink water, wash and shower

Breathing properly helps correct energy centers

Respect Mother Nature, go outside and on adventures

Gemstone: black tourmaline

Number Meaning

82 - Keep the optimistic that your financial situation is taken care of.

83 - Spugliguel

Is the guardian angel of spring

Causing the beauty of a new season swing

I bring you the same opportunities to make a fresh start

Nature chooses the strongest seed with heart

Make plans, determine your best options and watch it grow

Sunshine rain help develop your joyful life with the seeds you sow

Gemstone: snowflake obsidian

Number Meaning

83 - The ascended masters have heard and answered your prayers about your financial needs.

84 - Tabrisel

Is the guardian angel of free will

And many are the doors to light still

The creator gave you many choices and doors in all things

Find your golden path of true wholeness with your spiritual wings

Invoke my loving support to help you choose the way of love and light

Receive this dazzling golden love so bright

Gemstone: rainbow obsidian

Number Meaning

84 - The angels are helping you increase your financial flow so that you attain a state of security and abundance.

85 - Tagasel

Is the guardian angel of music

I resonate your soul to the melodies of love like cupid

Let your soul be lifted by vibrations of harmonic sound

Bring melody into your life and healing will be found

Musical notes and cards provide harmony

Let sound and light be your duty

Gemstone: hematite

Number Meaning

85 - Hooray! You're experiencing positive changes in your financial situation.

86 - Thuriel

Is the guardian angels of wild animals and birds

Admiring these wild creatures in migration and herds

They inspire your thoughts and dreams

Achieve ecological balance in lakes, forests and streams

A white dove or three white feathers communicates peace in teams

Gemstone: smoky quartz

Number Meaning

86 - The higher your thoughts, the better the outcome.

87 - Torquaretel

Is the guardian angel of autumn

Look at the beauty of color and farm your lawn

It is your harvest to reap and you are the harvester

Ensure all is well supporting your efforts for winter

Gemstone: cat's eye

Number Meaning

87 - You're on the right track with respect to your career and finances. Flow with the seasons.

88 - Tuael

Is the guardian angel of April and Taurus

As my season awakens new life for us

You give your word and deal in certainties

Learn to say no and balance your responsibilities

Decide where to hold on and when to let go

Create calm and focused flow

Gemstone: tourmalinated quartz

Number Meaning

88 - This is a favorable sign about your finances. Your actions, prayers, visualizations, and manifestations work have resulted in a large inflow of abundance. Open your arms to receive.

89 - Tubiel

Is the guardian angel of tame birds and summer

You may keep them as pets and let them chirp, sing and hummer

Birds can comfort you and lighten your day

Visualize a golden summer while the birds play

Use color to assist

Understand your color meaning list

Gemstone: calcite

Number Meaning

89 - Your divine life purpose is key to opening the door to abundance. Take steps daily beginning now to work in areas elated to your spiritual interests.

90 - Umabiel

Is the guardian angel of astrology

Study the stars and the celestials of cosmology

All knowledge is written in my heavenly bodies and stars

Wisdom and secrets unfolds relating to planets even Mars

Gemstone: danburite

Number Meaning

90 - God is calling upon you to work on your divine life mission now. You are ready! Take action today.

91 - Uriel

Is the guardian angel of fire and alchemy

I can cleanse and purify fire of lightning you see

And offer the power of creativity, innovation and transformation

Replenish with my colors of powerful imagination

My alchemy flames bring the mystical phoenix

Finding glorious new beginnings with a color hue mix

Gemstone: optic calcite

Number Meaning

91- Stay positive and optimistic about your divine life purpose. You and your missions are needed in this world.

92 - Vasariahel

Is the guardian angel of finances

You will have joy and abundance in finances

Take ownership for your money situation

Put your affairs in order to receive a golden transformation

Your financial situation is now resolved

Tackle money issues so golden energy is rekindled

Gemstone: rainbow quartz

Number Meaning

92 - As you keep the faith that everything is unfolding perfectly with your divine life purpose you more clearly see and understand the steps that are best for you to take.

93 - Verchiel

Is the guardian angel of Leo and July

I bring you the confident leadership ability to live by

You can inspire the hearts of others with your power of vision

Spark enthusiasm and passion

Accept and believe your potential

You inspire the group with love for every individual

Gemstone: rainbow aura quartz

Number Meaning

93 - You have listened to the guidance of your guides even unconsciously you are now on the right path for the fruition of your dreams and life purpose.

94 - Yusaminel

Is the guardian angel of fertility

Carry silver seeds of fertility

I have the power of a love and light ability

To aid conception you can invoke me

To illuminate fertility of the mind, body and spirit so mote it be

Speak your truth clearly

This will aid your well being completely

Gemstone: shaman stone

Number Meaning

94 - Your actions are guided and supported by the angels who say that your doing great keep up the good work.

95 - Zadkiel

Is the guardian angel of Thursday, the sixth heaven and Jupiter

Mine is the golden light of wisdom everyone looks for

Abundance of all kinds can flow to you

I guide your prospects for success too

You have a personality people admire

Keep your integrity, compromise and inspire

Gemstone: spodumene

Number Meaning

95 - The changes that you are currently considering are taking you in the right direction for the manifestation of your divine life purpose.

96 - Zephonel

Is the guardian angel of vigilance

My secret armor enfolds love protects with reliance

My eyes of watchfulness see all

Invoke Zephon and call

I urge you to pursue a path of integrity, honesty and respect for others

Treat others as you want to be treated between all sisters and brothers

Gemstone: goshenite

Number Meaning

96 - With respect to your divine life purpose put all of your focus onto the spiritual aspects such as helping others, asking for heaven to support you and coming from a place of love.

97 - Zeruchel

Is the guardian angel of strength

You are stronger than a thousand eagles at wing length

You have the power to pull yourself free

Reflect calm in your heart so let it be

I aid you with mental and emotional courage

Gemstone: quartz

Number Meaning

97 - Keep trusting and following your intuition its accurate.

98 - Zikiel

Is the guardian angel of comets and meteors

I will give you brilliant inspiration through seers

Galactic wisdom is held in the crystal moldavite tektite

So hold this magical crystal with the intent of love and light

Gemstone: clear diamond

Number Meaning

98 - The more that you focus, the more that the gateways of opportunities open up for you.

99 - Zuphlasel

Is the guardian angel of trees

Slender, tall, mighty all are trees

My trees stabilize earth and produce oxygen

Beneath the ancient oak is wisdom

Enjoy all four seasons

Fir roots, clean air and sunshine are good reasons

Be calm, walk in the woodlands

You'll feel healing energy in your hands

Gemstone: howlite

Number Meaning

99 - The spirit world has an urgent message for you. Ask them to show you signs, symbols and messages.

100-Zuriel

Is the guardian angel of Libra and September

Mine is the pure golden energy of the scales sober

I will help balance and guide your decisions

Relationships will work and home are happy visions

Gemstone: pearl

Number Meaning

100 - This is a strong message from God to help your loved ones and check in on them.

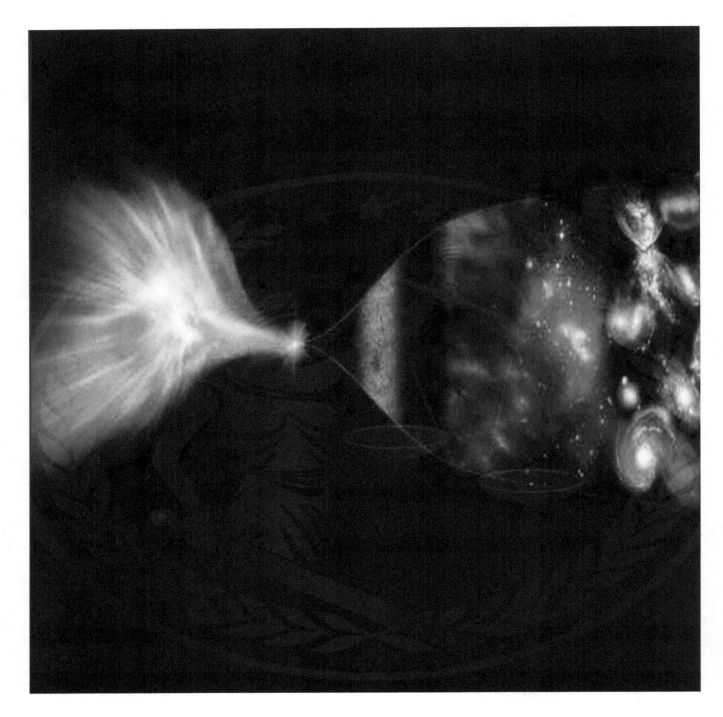

UNIVERSAL AUTHORITY

Sacred Awakenings Oracle

What is spirituality? It involves finding the meaning and purpose of life. Having a spiritual experience is sacred, transcendent and connects one to self, others, nature and source. Spirituality can be referred to as a religious process that involves practices, rites and rituals to achieve the highest sacred dimension. Some people refer to themselves as being spiritual and not religious. Whether spiritual or religious, this oracle defines spiritual practices that lead to the journey of moksha, liberation and freedom. This Sacred Awakening deck will bring you awareness of self, discovery of higher truths and awaken your higher consciousness. These practices are intended as a way of knowledge and devotion that assist you in perfecting your higher self. The more work you do on this spiritual path the more enlightened you will be. You will have a better understanding of your purpose. You will explore your life meaning. In this 62 card Sacred Awakening oracle you will discover your path to enlightenment; which can be translated into connecting to God and becoming more aware.

Golden Enlightenment

Enlightenment is the full comprehension of a situation

Moksha is a concept for all human creation

To be awake is to have spiritual insight

Golden energetic liquid light

Feeling vibrations of nirvana and bliss

Cuddling with our lover giving a soul kiss

Pure true knowledge is attained

Our righteous souls are entertained

Higher love and higher spiritual states

Twin flames, companions and soul mates

All these things are interconnected

Because golden enlightenment can be perfected

My intention is this oracle will awaken and enlighten you more; which will guide you to live better lives and reach higher dimensions.

1. Altars and Shrines	22. Chant	43. Music
2. Ancestors	23. Confess	44. Nature
3. Animals	24. Community	45. Names of God
4. Art	25. Dance	46. Offerings
5. Awareness	26. Divination	47. Oracles
6. Adab	27. Dream	48. Prayer
7. Akido	28. Drum	49. Symbols
8. Amulets	29. Fast	50. Rituals
9. Angels	30. Food	51. Sacraments
10. Aromatherapy	31. Garden	52. Sacred texts
11. Astrology	32. Journal	53. Self-care
12. Bathing	33. Hymns	54. Solitude and silence
13. Bible study	34. Intentions	55. Tantra
14. Bodywork	35. Labyrinth	56. Tea ceremony
15. Bowing	36. Laughter	57. Travel
16. Brush meditation	37. Mandalas	58. Vows
17. Breathwork	38. Mantras	59. Walking
18. Candle	39. Meditation	60. Worship
19. Caregiving	40. Mentor	61. Yoga
20. Celebration	41. Mindfulness	62. Writing
21. Chakra	42. Mudras	

Altars and Shrines

Altars and shrines are external representations of interior mysteries. Shrines and altars are a way of showing what's happening in our hearts and spirits. Creating them gives us opportunities to remember, reflect, honor and heal. A personal shrine can be established in a private place to reflect, meditate, and engage in a ritual and honor. Shrines can be portable, can help to maintain a needed connection with your loved one. You can use anything for your basic memorial like personal objects (pictures, photos, jewelry, books, natural objects, flowers, rocks, shells, candles, chimes, spiritual religious objects).

What would your ideal altar shrine be like?

Create an altar. Pick a deity, angel or ancestor that you associate with and display an image of him or her. Gather some sacred items you want to charge on you altar. Burn incense to communicate with your deity, angel or ancestor.

Ancestors

An ancestor also known as a forefather, fore elder or a forebear is a parent or the parent of an antecedent (grandparent, great grandparent, great grandparent and so on). An ancestor is any person from whom one is descended. They share a genetic relationship. Some cultures confer reverence to ancestors both living and dead. Some people seek providence from their deceased ancestors honor, love, respect are given in ancestor worship.

Who and what do you know about your ancestors?

Get your family history through genealogy records and or ancestry.com. Research your family tree to discover origin and importance. Create a family crest. Pray to your ancestors.

Animals

It is essential to be a good animal communicator. Journeys are guided by animals, birds and other creatures. Learning to listen to animals opens realms of magic. It's the foundation of spiritual practice that can change our perception. Animals vary in their spiritual awareness, understanding, experience and evolution as do humans. Animals vary in understanding of past lives, soul purpose and tasks for this lifetime. Animal's spiritual awareness will match with their owners. They can be great master teacher s for humans. Animals evolve and grow and need to be understood.

Do you have any spirit animals?

Do an animal oracle reading. Go to a zoo and or pet shop to connect with the animals. Adopt a pet and learn its language. Take an animal therapy course.

Art

The delights of creative expression including paint, markers, collage, poetry, movement, words and sound. Introduce art making in context of prayer. As it says in the Lord's Prayer, our father who art in Heaven. Cultivating the arts as a spiritual practice is a way of freeing our imagination and developing valuable skills for vital living in the world. By making the arts a spiritual practice we discipline ourselves to make time for our relationship with God through the conscious act of creating. Art can be playful and encourage wonder and joy.

What do you like about art?

Set a timer for 20 minutes weekly/daily and create art. Go visit an art gallery. Take an art class. Put on some music and start painting, doodling and drawing.

Awareness

Purpose of spiritual practice is expressed in 3 streams of awareness. One purpose is to reach full awareness of who and what your truly are. Two is to reach full awareness of what God or truth or source is. Three is to reach full awareness of the relationship between the previous two to see what is real. Attentive observation and mindful meditation help in transcending and witnessing consciousness.

Do you consider yourself as being aware and why?

Each day pick a new meditation to bring your awareness to. Be conscious of your breath and bring aware to your body. Do a full body scan. Bring attention to your senses.

Prayer

Prayer is a simple way of keeping attention focused on God's presence. Our thoughts and intentions are in openness with God. Prayer helps us empty inner chatter to create a space for being with God. Set a regular time and place for your centering prayer. Prayer communications our love to God in a faithful relationship. It is powerful, efficient and worthwhile.

Do you know any prayers off by heart?

Start with the Lord's prayer reciting it daily. Pick a topic and pray aloud. Create a prayer journal and write all your wishes and requests.

Adab

Adab is the context of behavior refers to prescribed Islamic etiquette, refinement, good manners, moral decorum, decency and humanness. To exhibit Adab would be to show proper discrimination of correct order, behaviors and taste. It's an ethical code involving every aspect of life. Covering acts like entering and exiting a washroom, posture when sitting, cleansing oneself, saying Bismillah before eating and drinking. Using right hand for drinking and eating.

Do you have your own ethical code?

Create a moral code. Repeat daily rituals. Try by putting your right shoe on first all the time. Wash your hands before you eat.

Aikido

Aikido is spiritual practice because the technical application of Aikido is nested within a universal humanistic philosophy. Practicing Aikido activates growth and development. The soul's journey from ego manifestation to divine spirit is the very process of Aikido itself. Way of unifying with life energy to defend oneself. Ai means joining, unifying combing. Ki means spirit energy mood morale. Do means way or path.

Have you tried any martial arts before?

Draw Aikido in calligraphy. Watch and attend an aikido class. Join an aikido club. Do an Aikido energy meditation.

Amulets

Known as a good luck charm is an object believed to have protection upon its possessor. Anything can function as an amulet items commonly used include gems, statues, coins, drawings, plant pots and written words. Amulets drive their extraordinary properties and powers from magic or luck from folk religion or paganism whereas amulets or sacred objects of formalized mainstream religion. Amulets can include hamsas, calligraphy, bells, tablets or holy books.

What amulets do you have?

Go to a metaphysical store and purchase an amulet. Wear an amulet on your wrist or neck always. Create an amulet out of clay. Display amulets in your car, home and work.

Angels

Angels are supernatural beings in various religions and mythologies. In Abrahamic religions often they are depicted as benevolent celestial intermediares between God or heaven and humanity. Other roles include protectors and guides for humans and servants of God. Some angels have specific names such as Gabriel or Michael or titles such as Seraph or archangel. Angels in the art world include birdlike wings and halos, divine light. Angelus in Latin means messenger.

Which angel do you associate with?

Purchase an angel oracle from the bookstore or online. Ask the angels to help you and give them permission. Before going to bed ask the angels to visit you and offer guidance and deliverance. Carry a pocket angel and or angel visor for the vehicle. Take an angel course to learn how to communicate with them.

Aromatherapy

Aromatherapy is a holistic treatment that uses natural plant extracts to promote health and well-being, sometimes called essential art therapy. Medically used to improve the health of the body, mind and spirit. It enhances physical and emotional health. Thought to be art and science. It's been around for thousands of years in resins, balms, oils. Aromatherapy works through the sense of smell and skin absorption using in products like diffusers, spritzers, inhalers, bathing salts, oils/creams/lotions, facial steamers, clay masks and hot/cold compresses.

Explore, what are your favorite essential oil smells?

Buy a mister with lavender. Try some arnica drops in your shampoo. Try rose water as a facial toner. Buy some peppermint oil to smell, put on your temples, wrists and top of your head. Try making your own volatile oil. Get an aromatherapy treatment or raindrop therapy.

Astrology

Astrology is a pseudoscience that claims to divine information about human affairs and terrestrial events by studying the movements and relative positions of celestial objects. It has roots in calendrical systems used to predict seasonal shifts and to interpret celestial cycles as signs of divine communication. Used to predict significant events can explain personality and relationship patterns and consisting of horoscopes. Astrologia in Latin means star divination. There are zodiacs in Chinese and Western culture, along with Vedic astrology.

What is your astrological zodiac?

Download an app to find your astrology. Find your galactic birth chart online. See a psychic to offer information about your astrology. Read your daily horoscope. Look into other astrology systems like Vedic, Mayan, Chinese Natal, relationship and western.

Bathing

Bathing is the washing of the body with a liquid usually water. It may be practiced for personal hygiene religious ritual or therapeutic purposes. Water can be warm to cool in a bath rub, shower, river, lake, waterhole, pool or ice. Rituals religious baths are referred to as immersion or baptism. Treatments include hydrotherapy. You can combine herbs, salts, and oils, stones in a bath as a spiritual practice to rejuvenate body, mind and soul and removed obstacle.

Are you a water person?

Soak in the tub with a ¼ cup of Epsom salts. Cold plunge in the lake. Enjoy a hot tub. Soak your feet with Himalayan salts. Go to a float house. Buy some roses to soak in a 20 minute bath with a candle and meditation music.

Bible Study

Bible study is when we study and apply scripture we find ourselves in accord with God. The mission of bible study is to produce passionate commitment to God his word and fellowship and church temple or mosque. It magnifies God and matures his people as they cultivate a deeper relationship with Him. Valuing dependence on God, compassion for people, excellence, integrity and humility.

Can you think of anytime where the bible was referenced?

Get a bible and read the good news. Pick a holy scriptures to study like Adi Granth, Four Teachings of Buddha, The Qur'an, The Kabbalah, The Holy Bible, The Vedas, The Sutras or any you are drawn to. Read the instructions given and put them into practice. Use a paper and pen or pencil to study verses of interest and skepticism.

Body Working

Body work is the metal outer shell of a body vehicle. Therapies and techniques in complementary medicine that involve touching and manipulating the body. Body is a part of a larger holistic umbrella that encompasses massage therapy much as does other forms of herbal and even energy therapy. From Reiki to cupping, acupuncture, Thai massage, shiatsu and even mediation and yoga. Thera are benefits to getting your body worked on like increased circulation, resets digest activation which speeds up body's healing process and overall general health and happiness.

What types of body work have you tried?

Book a massage once a month, try reflexology, get a Thai massage, see an osteopath, look into health benefits for dentist, acupuncture, chiropractor to explore for the year, do a partners massage and therapeutic touches, give yourself a foot rub and try stretching or yoga.

Bowing

People bow their heads in prayer or kneel as a sign of submission before Go. Bowing is linked to adoration and reverence for God. Bow has a particular moving in each tradition. Bowing is meant to call us to greater awareness of our thoughts, motions and intentions. It is physical prayer can be your private informative practice or can be used in sync with others in community worship. One teaches said when you hit the floor in the morning do 3 bows. Before anything bow. Zen style is formal and repeated bows.

When would be appropriate to bow?

Take a trip to Japan. Go out to a traditional monastery to attend a meditation, visit the Mecca or a Muslim mosque, attend a Catholic mass, try a Muslim sutra, bow and say the Lord's Prayer.

Brush mediation

The mindful use of brushes into paper as a method of depending the spiritual journey has been employed throughout the centuries and by numerous traditions. In the Japanese tradition this technique is reformed to as Shodo or the way of the brush, a mindful method that brings great peace, balance, and harmony into our lives via patient brush strokes.

Has there been a time you have used a brush? If yes, what did you brush?

Take Japanese language course. Use a brush and create something. Research Japanese Reiki. Get some red paint and brush Cho Ku Rei healing symbol 10 times. Look at Shodo art and videos.

Breathwork

Breathwork refers to any type of breathing exercises or techniques. People often perform them to improve mental, physical and spiritual well-being. During breathwork you intentionally change your breathing pattern. Many people find breathwork promotes deep relaxation or leaves them feeling energized. It aids positive self-development, boosts immunity, develops life skills, self-awareness, enriches creativity, increases joy and happiness, and improves relationships'. Types of breathwork includes shamanic, transformational, clarity, rebirthing,

When are conscious of your breath?

Take 5 deep breaths. Consult a breathwork practitioner. Register for a breathwork session. Research Wim Hof breathing. Research breathing techniques. Consciously breathe while you eat. Take a 5 minute break from work and focus on breathing. Inhale for a count of 5 and exhale for a count of 5. Do this 5 second breathing for a minute which is 6 breaths.

Candle

Candles are traditional element of several rituals. They can be lit near statues, shrines as a mark of respect. The lit candle flame represents the light of the teachings and is symbolic of the state of enlightenment. Candles add an element of ceremony and create an atmosphere of reverence. One candle can illumine empower enlightened wisdom, symbolizing inner light.

Are there special occasions you light candles?

Light a candle and set an intention for your day then blow it out. Buy gold and silver candles to bring in wisdom and riches. Go to a candle making workshop. Buy a rainbow selection of candles to enjoy. Gift a candle to a loved one. Candle gaze and look for the flickers, bright and dimness. Have a candlelit dinner. Go to church during Christmas for a candle lighting ceremony.

Caregiving

Caregiving is a discipline a paramita that packs surprise for caregivers. Caregivers should extend generosity to themselves in self-care. Caregiving is a bringing of care and compassion to a person in need. Taking care of someone can be volunteer or paid work. It can include family, friends, neighbors, the elderly and other people's children.

Who have you been a caregiver for?

Offer to babysit someone's children. Go volunteer with a senior's complex. See about helping the handicapped. Offer support and caregiving services to your family.

Celebrations

Celebration brings joy to others and enhances our worship. Celebration connects us with friends and family when we share together in jubilations. With joyful spirit of festivity people become excited and life giving.

When were a few celebrations that you remember?

Celebrate a birthday, anniversary, special holiday, wedding, birth or any other day you like. Plan and host a party. Get tickets for a celebration outing. Go to a dinner theatre. Plan a celebration for your birthday or a loved ones birthday. Go to more parties.

Chakras

In the science of chakra the yogi focuses on the aura which permeates his physical body. This aura creates the spinning vortexes of energy oath the specific places of the endocrine glands. These vortexes of energy look like spinning wheels chakra. The body has seven major chakras that account for our overall health mental emotional and physical. Chakras reflect the levels of consciousness, colors and lessons of life, body, mind, senses and identity. They are root, sacral, solar plexus, heart, throat, third eye and crown chakras.

What do you know about chakras?

Get a reiki treatment. Research chakras. Wear one chakra color everyday for seven days. Try a chakra meditation, Book a chakra balancing treatment. Get your level one Reiki. Draw and color the chakras. Print off a chakra chart to bring into your awareness.

Chanting

Chanting is a century old practice that connects us to ourselves our teachers our community and our universe. It is a mantra a sound and a symbol deeply rooted in Hinduisms yoga traditions. The vibrations we feel when we chant Aum have rich spiritual and creative benefits that clear our mind and bring happiness and contentment to our soul. When we chant Aum our voices become one and reconnects your body, hear and place in this world.

Do you know any chants?

Chant om for 3 minutes straight. Research common chants. Try an chanting meditation. Pick a one word intention and chant it. Try chanting the Hawaiian phrase hu sitting, standing and laying. Go to a chanting circle or temple.

Confession

Confession is a spiritual practice that can happen along, between you and God or a community with other followers. When confession happens privately we are coming before God and owning up to what's inside us and accepting the forgiveness we have in Christ. When confession happens, it allows us to release by God's grace and have the opportunity to repent.

Can you think of a few things you would like to confess?

Go to a Catholic church and confess. Confess to a loved one something you need to tell. Write a letter to God and confess then burn the paper. Make a list of things you would like to confess.

Community

Community is churches temples mosques a place of gathering. Participation in community is not about membership. It's about discipleship and participation as a form of spiritual practice. True community is marked by quality of collaboration and flourishing. Energy levels rise and people enjoy being together. It is thru community that we hear God speaking to us.

How are you involved with your community?

Look up meet ups in your community. Attend an event that your community is hosting. Go to a church, mosque or temple for a service. Volunteer for a good cause. Become a member of an organization your passionate about. Participate in a poll and vote. Donate to a community organization.

Dancing

Sacred dance as a daily or regular practice provides a holistic workout of body, mind and spirit. Dance is the oldest form of prayer or direct connection to the divine. It's designed for religious or spiritual purposes in a space or environment connecting you rhythmical to the divine source. Dance is the ultimate surrender. It can by mystical, rhythmic or folk.

When have you danced in the past?

Join an ecstatic dance group. Go out to the bar and dance. Put on your favorite song and dance. Pick a song to create your own dance. Find a friend and create a short fun dance. Take a dance class. Find a partner and learn to ballroom, salsa or tango. Go to a music festival and dance all weekend to different genres.

Divination

Divination in Latin divinare "to foresee, to foretell, to predict, to prophecy." Or to be inspired by a God to gain insight into a question or situation by way of an occult ritual. Diviners ascertain their interpretations of how a querent should proceed by reading signs, events or omens or through alleged contact with a supernatural agency. Oracles were the conduits for the God's on earth; their prophecies were understood to be the will of the God's.

What divination tools do you know of?

Get an oracle reading. Try dice divination. Grab some rocks and great a Nordic rune set. Buy an oracle card deck and practice asking questions. Try a tea leaf reading. Research divination tools. Go see a psychic.

Dreaming

A dream is a succession of images, ideas, emotions and sensations that usually occur involuntarily in the mind during certain stages of sleep. Dream interpretations I the attempt at drawing meaning from dreams and searching for an underlying message. Scientific study of dreams is called oneirology. Dreams mainly occur in the rapid eye movement (REM) stage of sleep when brain activity is high and resembles that of being awake.

Are there any dreams you can recall?

Buy a dreamcatcher to hang over your head while you sleep. Call on your spiritual guides to provide you with guidance as to a certain issue before bed. Create a dream journal. Do a dream interpretation of various objects that you can remember from your dreams. See a shaman to assist. Read the book Dreamhealer by Adam. Play theta lucid dreaming sound therapy on low volume while you sleep.

Drumming

Drums have been used in every culture for many purposes form religious rituals, and other ceremonies to sporting events and as a way to communicate or signal. Shamans used drumming as a means of reading an altered or trance like state so that they can connect the spiritual dimension. Drums can make you smarter by accessing your entire brain. Research shows that physical transmission of rhythmic energy to the brain actually synchronizes the left and right hemispheres. The sound generates new neuronal connections.

Have you connected to drums before?

Attend a drumming class. Go to a pow wow. Take a drum making workshop. Play Native drumming music while going about your day. Attend a shaman meditation circle. Go to a music store and play the drums.

Fasting

People fast collectively at certain times in order to pay homage to God or to be granted some grace. Today that spirit maintained in practices such as Catholic Lent or Muslim Ramadan. Fasting is an act of voluntary austerity and increase concentration. Greater self-controls is experienced and this increases confidence and self-esteem. The regular practice of fasting prolongs life expectance, increases cognitive abilities and reduces heart risks.

What kind of fasts have you done?

Try liquid fasting. Try water fasting for a day. Try juice fasting. Try intermediate fasting. Look up different faiths and join in on their way of fasting and praying. Do a 72 hour fast like the master cleanse.

Food

Clean food leads to a clean body. Simple wholesome food helps the body to function. The ritual of shopping or growing foot, the ceremony of preparation, the act of feeding oneself and others is an active mediation. Show your good love, gratitude and beauty. Try to eat meals with fewer chemicals and the least harm on living creatures. Take only what you need. Reduce waste. Choose foods with the least plastic and packaging. Arrange food by textures, shapes and colors.

What are your favorite foods?

Look up your local food guide for age and gender. Try eating a whole food based diet for a diet. Eat a raw food diet for a day. Try veganism or vegetarianism. Avoid white flour and sugar for a day. Make a rainbow with your food. Create skewers with your favorite things. Create a charcuterie board.

Gardening

Gardening connects us to life's natural rhythms, each season in the world. Everyday go out and thank the ground. Gardening enhances our relations top the earth. Through cultivating we glean patience, appreciation, anticipation, interdependence and acceptance of the cycles of life, death and rebirth. The tasks of weeding, seeding, watering and other tasks of cherishing and nurturing the miracles of life is sacred.

Where have you connected to gardens?

Go to your local botanical garden. Grow your own garden. Try indoor gardening. Visit a greenhouse. Take a gardening class. Read a gardening compatability book. Buy fresh from your local farmer's market.

Journaling

Journaling can enhance your well-being on every level. When it comes to self-growth and spiritual maturation journaling is in the top five. Your intentions and attitudes matter. Journaling is the practice of writing down your thoughts and feelings for the purpose of self-analysis, self-discovery and self-reflection. It's about exploring ones thoughts, feelings, impulses, memories, goals and hidden desires. Explore who you are, what you think and how you feel. Journaling can strengthen your immune system, enhance and promote mental well-being and emotional recovery.

When do you journal?

Create a daily gratitude journal. Make a reflection of your daily work or at the end of your day. Journal your eating, sleep and exercise. Have a journal for your brain dump about all your ideas and brilliant thoughts. Try bullet journaling for productivity.

Hymns/Psalms

Let the word of Christ dwell in you richly in all wisdom, teachings admonishing one another in psalms, hymns and spiritual songs singing with grace in your hearts to the Lord. (Colossians 3:16) Spiritual because it's inspired by the Holy Spirit. Scripture psalms may be sung, used at church and in worship.

Have you heard of any hymns and psalms?

Go to a see a church choir. Attend a sermon. Get a bible and read a few psalms. Join a choir to sing hymns. Play the music sheet from the hymnal.

Intentions

An intention is a guiding principle for how you want to be, live and show up in the world. Ask yourself what matters most. An intention is an aim, a purpose or attitude you'd be proud to commit to. Setting an intention is a way to bring your heart and mind into alignment. You can set them before meditation, yoga or even your day. As Wayne Dyer said our intention creates our reality. Keep your intentions positive, simple and clear.

What kind of intentions do you have?

Create an intention daily. Be mindful and use the power of intention throughout your day as to what you want the result. Set intentions every new moon. Read Power of Intention by Wayne Dyer.

Labyrinth

Labyrinth walking is an ancient practice used by many different faiths for spiritual centering, contemplation and prayer. It is not a maze; it has only one path to enter and back out making it a unicursal cone. The labyrinth symbolizes a journey to a predetermined destination or the journey through life from birth to spiritual awakening. It is used as an act of repentance. Walk slowly, calm and clear your mind and repeat your prayer or chant.

Have you ever done a labyrinth?

Walk a labyrinth. Get a picture of a labyrinth and follow the path in and out with your finger. Say everything you want to release and let go while walking into a labyrinth then say everything you want to manifest on the way out, Go to a labyrinth retreat. Draw a labyrinth maze. Play pac man.

Laughter

Laughing is very important and sacred. Laughter is good for us physically, emotionally and spiritually. It helps us release our tight grasp on how to see things. The practice of laughter helps reawaken us to the wonder and delight of seeing things in new ways. As we learn to laugh we begin to appreciate the deep diversity of the sacred. Laughter is medicine, activating the immune system. Incorporate humor watch comedies and read jokes.

What makes you laugh?

Watch a funny movie. Try laughter yoga. Go see a comedy show. Play with children. Go out with some friends and have a good time. Read a joke book. Listen to the comedy channel. Hang out with the funniest people you know.

Mandalas

Mandala is the Sanskrit word for sacred circle. Has been used by many different faith traditions. Mandala means to have possession of one's essence. Its sacred circle with center, a universal image that has been a source of experience of oneness and wisdom. It uses symbolic forms to draw out truth from the unconscious. These symbols help connect our inner life to our outer life. A mandala maybe drawn, painted, sculpted and ever danced.

Where have you seen a mandala?

Draw a mandala. Paint a mandala. Get a mandala coloring book. Buy apparel with a mandala on it. Check out mandala art online. Watch a you tube video on Tibetan mandalas.

Mantras

A mantra is a syllable, word or phrase that is repeated during meditation. Mantras can be spoken, chanted whispered or repeated in the mind. Mantra recitation is used to focus the mind, heart and connect with divine both within and without. Mantra serves to evoke positive qualities and confidence rather than external duty. A favorite Christian mantra is the ancient Aramaic prayer maranaka come lord. Om shanti is another peace mantra.

Which mantras do you know?

Chant Om 108 times. Get a mala bead necklace and chant om mani padme om. Create your own mantra daily. Get a mantra journal and learn a new mantra to chant weekly. Write your mantra in the language its in. Go to a chanting temple or circle.

Meditation

Meditation is the mindful practice of connection to something that is great and deeper than the individual self. There are many meditation techniques that increase spiritual awareness. Practicing meditation to achieve superpowers such as telepathy, the ability to heal oneself and others, knowledge of past lives, visions of the future, levitation and so on. Helps you turn inwards to your spirituality for answers. Metta is a lovingkindness meditation.

What types of meditations have you tried?

Try sitting and laying down in silent breath meditation. Send lovingkindness to yourself and others for 3 minutes. Do a walking meditation and try body awareness. Listen to a guided meditation. Lay down for a chakra meditation and visualize the colors of your chakras.

Mentoring

Spiritual mentors are people who are invested in our spiritual health, personal growth and in us reaching our fullest potential. They may help us learn new skills or knowledge, provide guidance and wisdom for decision making or hold us accountable in the ways we engage with ourselves and the world around us. They should be warm, loving, authentic, encouraging and approachable. They should be accessible and willing to provide mentorship.

When have you been mentored in the past?

Find someone to mentor and coach you. Find a peer that you look up to and spend some quality time with them. Search social media for a spiritual mentor in your field of expertise to follow. Hire a personal growth life coach. Join a group focused on achieving their highest potential.

Mindfulness

Mindfulness was introduced into medicine in the 1970's. Seven core attitudes drawn from Buddhist teachings: non judging, patience, a beginner's mind, trust, non-striving, acceptance and letting go. Mindfulness is compassionate and intentional awareness of the present moment; sometimes called mindful breathing. It involves paying attention to thoughts, physical sensations and the environment without judgment and complete acceptance of reality in the here and now.

What does mindfulness mean to you?

Try mindful breathing for five minutes. Be mindful and thankful for what you eat and drink in a day. Put intentions into why you do what you do throughout the day. Try to be your own narrative and describe your moment with all your senses. Take a mindfulness course.

Mudras

Yogis refer to hand signs as mudras. In the stages of yoga, these symbolic body postures appear in many forms (not just the hands and their mastery is essential to becoming a yogi and reaching enlightenment. They are used to achieve higher states of consciousness. The Sanskrit mudra definition translates to gesture or seal. They are used to create an energetic seal of energy existing between two or more points in the body. Mudras are found in Asian martial arts. Hand mudras manipulate the flow of prana by connecting different meridians with different elements.

Which hand mudras do you know?

Research mudras and practice them. Read a mudra book. Learn the chakra mudras. Start a mudra session by washing your hands and rubbing them together 10 times then hold your hands on your navel chakra. Try om chanting then your thumb and index finger together.

Music

Music is the sound of spirit. Beautiful music can inspire, calm and uplift us, as it connects us to our innermost nature of our being. Music bridges material and spiritual realms. Music directly vibrates cellular receptors. Our ear hearing frequency is 20-2000Hz. Everything vibrates matter, sound, light and energy. Singing, playing and composing music as an expression of the divine. It's a means to moksha (liberation). Music is the root of all power and motions there is music and rhythm the play of patterned frequencies.

What are your favorite types of music?

Look up the solfeggio frequencies and listen to them. Learn how to read notes. Find an instrument to play. Listen to 3 different music genres. Create a music playlist. Sing your favorite song. Go to karaoke. Get tickets to a concert. Attend a music festival.

Nature

Nature reminds us of our connection with spirit with the earth and with everything. In indigenous cultures the Earth is seen as our sacred birthplace, our holy temple our sacred ground. The earth has a living soul, the Amina Mundi. The earth herself is a vivacious entity, breathing her great seasonal breaths in and out with vibrating energy.

What do you love about nature?

Go on a nature walk. Plan a camping trip. Visit a nature attraction like waterfalls, a bridge, healing pools or mountain peaks. Go on trail hikes once a week. Enjoy a picnic near a natural body of water. Go to the ocean or the mountains for a retreat.

Names of God

There are various names of God which enumerate the various qualities of a supreme being. One God is a monotheistic view. Exchange or names is sacred. Same say El Yahweh Om Krishna. The Kabbalist states there are 72 names of the lord. The nature of a holy name can be described as either personal or attributive; El comes from a root word meaning might, strength, power. YHWH is the proper name of God in Judaism. Jesus Iesus Yeshua Shongdi King above is used to refer to the Christian God in Chinese union.

Do you know any of the names of God?

Research the names of God. Make a list of God's names. Call upon God and all His almighty names aloud. Meditate on God's names and pronounce them properly. Display the name of God in your home, office and vehicle space. Call on God and make a request. Listen to a breath prayer praising all of God's divine names. Open and close each day by thanking God.

Offerings

In traditional culture like Thailand believers will put offerings of food or gifts out as a means of thanks or respect. Spiritual offerings capture the practice of hope and faith. Each offering is an indication of financial status. Offerings can be placed on a street corner, a place of worship and occasionally in an area where a loved one has died.

What type of offerings have you made or heard of?

Research Buddha's shrine offerings. Make an offering of flowers, incense, lamps, perfume or food to a Buddhist temple. Make an offering at a place of worship. Plan a trip to Thailand to explore their temples and understanding their offerings. Try a cleansing smoke offering called a sang puja. Pick a deity and offer something to the altar to them.

Oracles

An oracle is a person or agency considered to provide wise and insightful counsel or prophetic predictions or precognition of the future, inspired by the God's. It's a form of divination. Latin vern orare means to speak and refers to a priest or priestess uttering the prediction. They are portals in which the Gods speak directly to the people. Most important Greek oracle of Dione and Zeus at Dodena in Epirus. Dione or dios meaning godly literally means heavenly.

What do you know about oracles?

Get an oracle reading. Buy oracle cards to use for guidance and divine intervention. Call upon your spirit guides to present you a dream oracle while you sleep. Research the oracles of God. Read the oracle of Delphi. Watch the movie Immortals 2011. Use oracle cards when you need assistance or higher help.

Prayer

Prayer is an invocation or act that seeks to activate a rapport with an object of worship through deliberate communication. Prayer can have the purpose of thanksgiving or praise. It can be part of a set liturgy or ritual, take the form of a hum, incantation, or formal creedal statement.

What have you prayed about?

Pray about what you want. Learn the Metta Prayer off by heart. Create a prayer journal. Read the Najavo prayer aloud. Go to church to pray and confess. Find a loved one and do a collective prayer. Join a prayer group. Set a fixed time daily to incorporate prayer. Research and practice a centering prayer.

Symbols

Symbols are a significant part in yoga, reiki and our life's journey. Symbols help direct access to forces, elevations, higher states of consciousness while developing positive qualities and insight on one's path. Aum is the most common sacred symbol for the yogis. We use symbols to represent feelings, beliefs, relationships, events we want to remember. Sacred symbols represent spiritual lineages, unspoken communication with mystical significance.

What symbols come to mind right now and what do they mean to you?

Look up spiritual symbols and draw one. Draw an Egyptian Ankh cross and inside it draw what you want to manifest. Display a Hamsa in your home. Read a book on sacred symbols. Do a sacred imagery and visualization meditation and envision what symbol(s) come. Draw the midas star symbol of abudance in green and red. Draw some symbols with a calligraphy pen and try a different language like light language, Japanese, Atlantean or Nordic.

Rituals

A ritual is a ceremony in which actions are preferred in a specific order to achieve a goal. Ritual is both a ceremony and daily practice. It's done with intention and awareness. When you transform your day into a series of rituals it brings you closer to spirit. Spiritual rituals strengthen and support your soul and they clear and open your mind to receive higher guidance. Rituals are a space in which shamans cure disease. They bring greater mental clarity, physical awareness and emotional stability. You can create a ritual for cleaning, writing, eating, bathing and so on. Use right intention, right effort and right concentration.

What kind of daily rituals do you do?

Create and maintain a morning and or evening ritual. Find a new or full moon ritual to complete during that time. Take 5 deep breaths upon waking up and shake your body daily. Find a traditional ceremony to attend. Try rituals for waking, eating, drinking, skin care, exercising, sleeping and meditating.

Sacraments

Sacraments are a means in which god uses to show his grace and help us achieve salvation. The word sacrament means a sign of the sacred. Three sacraments of initiation are baptism, confirmation and Eucharist. Each is meant to strengthen your faith. There are two sacraments for healing; they are penance and anointing the sick. Also through marriage and holy order, couples and the clergy promise to serve and build up the church community.

Which sacraments have you tried?

Get baptized and display your baptism certificate. Gather around with loved ones for a meal and bless it with the blood and bread of Christ. Be confirmed into your church to delve deeper in a relationship with God. Buy some anointing oil to anoint yourself. Request the blessings of God in matrimony.

Sacred texts and Scriptures

A scripture is a subset of religious texts considered to be authoritative, sacred and special to the religious community. Sacred texts serve a ceremonial and liturgical role, particularly in relation to sacred time, the liturgical year, the divine efficacy and holy service. Some religious texts are categorized as canonical which connotes a sense of measure, standard, norm rule. The oldest known text is the K'esh temple Hymn of ancient Sumer. The Rig Veda of Hinduism. The Holy Bible for Christians. The Holy Quran for Muslims. The Buddhist Teachings for Buddhists and the Kaballah for Jews.

Which sacred scriptures are you drawn to?

Pick a sacred text to study from front to back. Focus only on the good news of the messages. Memorize and write one verse weekly to self-interpret. Try bibliomancy by asking a question to God then knock on the text and open up to a passage to read. Listen to a sermon from a world reknown pastor, monk or high priest. Join a bible study group. Look up sacred texts on google.

Self-Care

Self-Care is taking proper care of ourselves; make deliberate effort to prioritize our well-being. Spiritual self-care is comprised of actions we take to deepen our connection with our higher self. It leads to great inner peace and helps us align with our core values. Some strategies include" meditation, gratitude, spend time in nature, attend a religious service, treat yourself, cleanse your space, practice forgiveness, unplug from technology.

What is your self-care routine?

Get a health tracker app. Exercise daily. Drink 2 liters of water. Take a self-care trip and retreat. Eat a wholesome meal. Try a skin care routine. Get into meditation daily. Practice gratitude. Go for a walk. Create a self-care checklist.

Sexuality

Sex is the most common way people connect to their spiritual selves. We long for experiences that are uplifting, pleasurable, and expansive and that brings life force. This helps not only the physical level but the mental/ energetic, spiritual bodies in order to have optimal recovery and health. Erotic spirituality refers to body based sensual and sexual practices that function to support spiritual evolution. In practice tantra is about enlightenment. We arouse sexual energy when we engage in deeply meditative sexual practices.

What are your thoughts on sexuality?

Join a masculine or feminine circle. Research where your g spot is. Go to a passion store and pick a sex toy to use. Get yourself off and visualize one goal as already achieved when coming. Affirm that your sexuality is healthy and pleasuring. Choose partners that meet your expectations and don't settle for anything less. Find articles on how to keep the passion alive.

Solitude/Silence

Solitude and silence are two of the main disciplines. Solitude and silence make space for God to do deep work inside us. Get alone with God to be quiet in a quiet place for hours or days. Do nothing. Don't try to make anything happen. You stop entertaining and pleasing others.

Refrain from speaking and move away from the voices of others, turn off technology and be still. Know God.

Do you get opportunities for solitude?

Take 10 minutes daily to be in silent solitude. Try a Vipasanna meditation at home or in a retreat. Find a quiet area to draw your attention inward. Find a mirror to observe the good qualities you see in yourself. Sit down breath and focus on calm and tranquilitiy.

Tantra

Tantrics realize that sex awakens a powerful source of energy which is used for personal and spiritual growth. Sex can be a dance between Shiva and Shakti a soul merging experience. Tantra in Sanskrit literally means, loam, warp, and weave. Atma trantra means doctrine or theory of Atman (soul, self). Sexuality has been a part of tantric practices; sexual fluids have been viewed as power substances. Shiva is manifest as the great linga, Shakti essential form is the goal. Rituals are the main focus of Tantras. There are initiations, mantras, visualizations, mandalas involved.

What do you know about tantra?

Research tantra. Prepare a space for tantra with the perfect temperature, light candles and incense, cleanse your body and play romantic music. Learn the yab yum position and gaze into your lovers eyes. Foreplay with your partner and take turns massaging each others arms, legs, neck and other parts. Try synchronized breathing. Put your hand on your lovers heart before you get sexual. Try controlling your orgasm three times before full explosion. Try the kama sutra tantra sex positons.

Tea Ceremony

Begin the tea ceremony by setting an intention that acknowledges your cup of tea. Consider brewing your tea and bring your attention to the present. Only the awareness of the present, can your hands feel the warmth of the tea. Savor the aroma, taste the delicacy, feel the energy. Dedicate the mug of tea to the present, to awaken all beings, to peace on Earth. Move the mug in all four cardinal directions. All this opening with you. Call on Archangel Metatron for tea.

Have you experienced a tea ceremony?

Buy a beautiful tea cup set. Watch a Japanese tea ceremony on you tube. Visit Japan and attend a tea ceremony. Look up tea ceremony etiquette. Enjoy your favorite tea after blessing it. Find local tea ceremonies to attend in your community. Incorporate a wedding tea ceremony.

Travel

Travel embarks on a sacred journey of a lifetime. Journeys provide unique opportunities for self-discovery and forging relationships in a magical world. We facilitate learnings of ancient traditions and cultures. Egypt, Peru, India, Italy have many ceremonial sites. Sometimes a long road trip or a secluded retreat away from home unlocks a new spiritual quest. Reaching a destination has an ability to change people and their level of joy. It broadens our experiences perspectives and value on community.

Where have you traveled?

Research the wonders of the world and heritage sites. Make a day trip to a new place to visit an attraction. Travel to an enlightened destination. Watch a video on the most spiritual places on earth. Plan a vacation in a year or two to visit a ceremonial site. Go on a spiritual retreat that includes rituals, ceremonies, and other holistic treatments. Travel by a different mode of transportation like plane, jet, helicopter, boat, cruise ship, bike, trike, quad, snowmobile, etc...

Vows

A vow is a promise or oath. Marriage vows are binding promises each partner in a couple make during a wedding ceremony. Within the world of monks and nuns a vow is sometimes a transaction between a person and a deity where the former promises to render some service or gift or devotees something valuable to the deity's use. The deity being both the witness and recipient of the promise. They are conserved acts of sacred character. Bodhisattva's vows taken by Mahayana Buddhists liberate sentient beings. You can also renew vows.

What type of vows have you made?

Make a pinky promise with someone. Vow to God that you will love him. Vow to your partner something you promise to do forever. Research traditional vows. Create honest marriage vows. Renew your marriage vows.

Walking

Walking is a spiritual practice that holds many dividends like uplifting of the soul, connection with the natural world, problem solving, self-esteem, health and healing and heightened attention. Movement encourages dialogue, leads to richer conversations. Prayers and mantra practice while walking, pilgrimage to sacred sites, walking the labyrinths. Other routines include walking the dog, taking a breath, walking around the block. Muslims have five pillars and one pillar is to go to Mecca and walk back and forth seven times.

Where do you like to walk?

Go on a nature trek. Walk for a cure. Try a walking meditation. Create a daily walking schedule. Get a partner to go for walks with. Do a walking/hiking camping trip up a mountain. Do the pilgrimage in Mecca. Go to a mall and walk the mall. Find a track and do a bunch of laps. Get your favorite music on and walk down the most popular streets in your community while window shopping.

Worship

In worship we remember who God is a who we are in God. Worship embraces the mystery and focuses on God's Majesty. The word worship originated from an old English word wothscope meaning worthiness and conveys the desire of an individual to give worth to God. Christian worship involves praising God in music and speech, readings from scripture, prayers and holy ceremonies. Go to a church and hear the choir sing worship songs.

Who do you worship?

Attend a choir that worships and praises God. Personal worship through daily devotionals. Listen to worship songs. Go to a place of worship like a temple, mosque or church. Find yearly sacred seasons for times and places of worship and follow this fellowship.

Yoga

Yoga is a group of physical, mental and spiritual practices or disciplines which originated in India. The word yoga in Sanskrit means to attach, join, harness, yoke. The ultimate goal of yoga is Moksha (liberation). The goal of practicing is to achieve a state of Samadhi (pure awareness). There are various types classical, Buddhist, Jain, and Vedanta, tantric, hatha, kundalini and more. Many people practice yoga as a means to a toned body, developing strength and stamina, this practice is designed to bring the individual into harmony and at one with all that is. Practicing Yoga has many benefits like give you a sense of peace and energy meanwhile removing blocks.

What kind of yoga have you tried?

Go to a yoga class in person. Look up Yoga with Adriene on you tube. Become a yoga teacher. Take a yoga teaching class. Try yin yoga. Incorporate yoga into your daily routine. Do 3 sun saluations. Try a 30 day yoga challenge. Research types of yoga and try one you haven't tried.

Writing

Through writing you reformulate important life lessons. A written expression exploring many avenues and interests. Writing is a form of illumination, therapy, art and meditation. When journaling or writing it engages our whole being and moves our feelings. Words are a powerful way to express ideas.

What do you usually write about?

Create a reflection journal. Maintain a daily gratitude journal where you write three things you are grateful for daily. Look up self-reflective life coaching questions and answer one daily. Do a brain dump and write down all your ideas. Join a writing class. Try bullet journal for scheduling. Get a white bulletin board to use for your visual schedule and to do list.

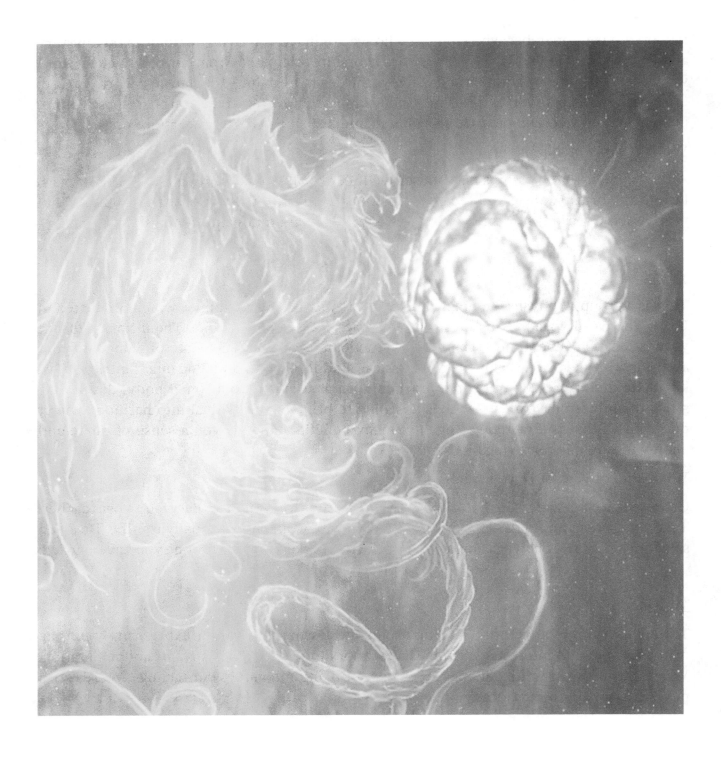

Monthly Recording Sheet

Date:	
Vitamins and Supplements:	
Resting Heart Rate:	
Blood Pressure:	
Body Mass Index:	
Waist Measurement:	
Upcoming Goals/Achievements Made	

Notes:_____
_____

Weekly Food Diary

Date:_____

Day	S	M	T	W	T	F	S
Breakfast:							
Lunch:							
Dinner:							
Snacks:							
Drinks:							
Calorie intake:							

Notes(bowel,bladder,appetite,cycles):_____
_____

Monthly Exercise Recording Sheet

Date:	
Activities+Duration:	Time+Day
	am pm Sunday
	am pm Monday
	am pm Tuesday
	am pm Wednesday
	am pm Thursday
	am pm Friday
	am pm Saturday

Notes(mood,energy):_____

_____

My Goals (look at this daily)

Goal(s):_____

_____

(**S**pecific, **M**easureable, **A**uthentic, **R**ealistic, **T**imely)

It is important I will achieve this goal because:

_____

_____

Steps I need to take to achieve my goal.

_____

_____

The skills, knowledge and resources I need to be successful are:

_____

When will this goal be achieved and how will I know I am successful?

_____

_____

A quote that inspires me and helps me stay motivated:

_____

Any questions or concerns or anything else you want to add:

_____

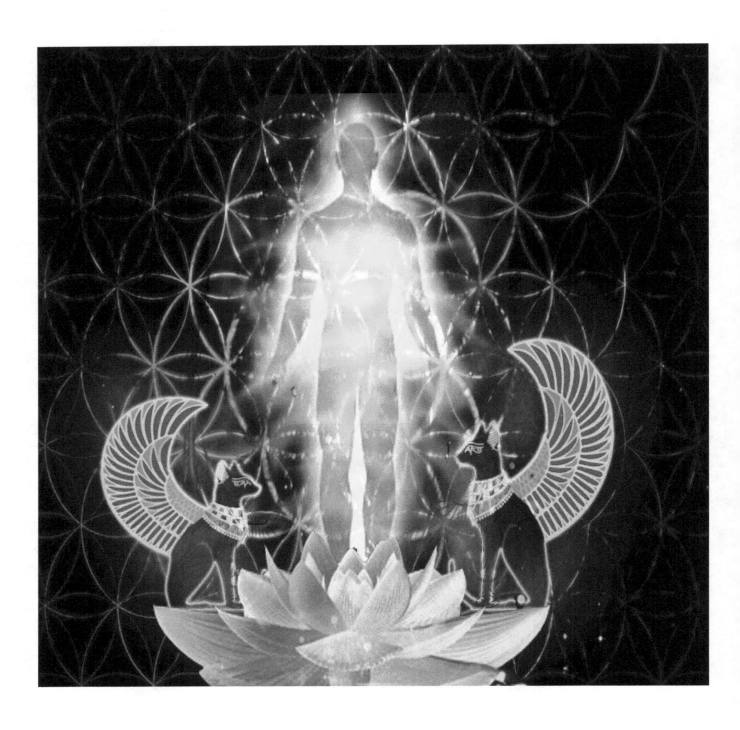

Ascension to Heaven

by Diana Hutchings

I'm climbing. Below me are hills, valleys, aqua blue ponds. I see cotton candy clouds and a rainbow. It's a double rainbow so bright and big. There is a sweet smell of jasmine rose flowers. Above me I hear celestial music. It appears as though there are three realms lower, middle and upper worlds. A golden eagle flies overhear. I ask him who are you? I am Aetos Dios a creation of the 7 D Gaia. You can call me EA. Shaman drumming starts to beat quietly and EA drops a feather from his wings span. I said what's that for? EA explained this is a sign of guidance, respect, truth and freedom. Pick it up the creator has answered your prayers. Creator Spirit is guiding you on this shamanic journey. Thank you for this gift. I am honored and humble. Aetos Dios soared higher and higher up the side of the mountain out of sight. Realizing I needed a staff for this steep climb. I uttered the Egyptian one word spell Haqat and a mighty oak staff appeared on the trail in front of me. There was a perfect hand grip close to the animal head that looked similar to a dolphin and lizard. It was a long straight staff with a shape shifting top. It appeared as though a fairy map was inscribed along the staff. A huge gardner snake came out of the rosehip bush and wrapped itself around from the bottom to the top. The staff's name is Asclepius; named after the Greek Alkepius. God of truth, medicine and prophecy. The snake transformed into pure iron on the mighty oak staff. Surprised we continued on, climbing higher on the rugged dirt foot trail. Time seemed to disappear. A huge royal hawk swooped in and landed on the rod. Hawks are symbols of the great mother Amentil and are great messengers. The Hawk dropped a wrapped up scroll on the trail. The biodiversity and blessings of the hawk, eagle and snake were signs of the second dimension. The scroll was titled Daphne the Map Ascension to Heaven. There was a legend, a star with dotted lines that said please follow to reach the Celestial Kingdom. WOW! Is this actually happening? The adventure keeps getting better. Noticing all the sweet smells of pine, spruce and evergreen on the forest trail. The music gets louder with every magic footstep. Water was flowing in the distance. The sun rays were getting brighter. I am thinking I must be close to the top. One foot after the other. In nearsight I could see the waterfall with a big pool of clean, clear water above these dazzling pyrite snow white quartz rocks. A big wolf slinks in. The wolf stood on the biggest rock that appeared to have the symbol of peace on it. Like in the Jungle Book all the animals and creatures of the land must follow the code of the Peace Rock. The code states that everyone who comes to the pools of water to drink are free and safe without worry of any attack from others. Hakuna Matata. This massive wolf star gazed into my eyes with lime amber eyes. I asked who are you? What do you want? Where am I? The shewolf said I am Lupa. I am here to take you to the next dimension of ascension. You must shower in the pool of Bethesda to prepare you for the journey ahead. This golden healing shower will cleanse, purify and level you up. Then you can meet your messianic guides. You must walk thru the waterfall to find the rainbow bridge. I walked thru the waterfall, my clothes turned bright white. I felt so pure and holy. The sky became a night horizon. The milkway was visible and spiraling with this bright north star. While Lupa lead me across the Rainbow Bifrost to Asgard. Lupa explained the collection of stars is Odin's horse which is called the Little Dipper. With each magic footstep I took towards Asgard a cosmic force was pulling me forward and upward. It had a floating levitating effect. Suddenly my clairsentience (clear feeling), clairaudience (clear hearing), clairgustance (clear tasting), clairalience (clear smelling), clairvoyance (clear seeing) and intuition were amplified. I could feel, hear, taste, smell, see and know with accuracy and strength. I can see the lower and middle worlds from the other side of the Bifrost and knew I we were in the troposphere. The bright light of the stars lit up the sky. Above us were huge pearly white clouds and sun beam like paradigms. I could hear an angel choir playing celestial music. Looking up to see Zadkiel, Haniel, Cassiel, Camael, Raphael, Gabriel and Michael. They were a radiant rainbow hue and playing many golden and silver instruments. There was a piano, trumpet, trombone, clarinet, drums, harp and a guitar. Beethoven is the composer for Heaven. A burst of Jasmine, Rose and Frankincense filled the air. Lupa ran over to the throne. Odin was sitting on the throne with EA overheard. Odin was clothed in a blue cloak with gold trim and a gold headdress. Odin raised his deep loud voice to say, Welcome to Asgard. Glad you made it to the upper world. You shall pass through the gate. I thanked and bowed before him. I happily skipped through the golden gate to be amazed. The vision before me was of a golden temple with pearls and sparkling crystals decorated everywhere around giant pillars and a golden ladder. Hearing laughter in the courtyard. Paramahansa, Yogananda, Guru Nanak, Saint Germain, Hari Krishna, Kuan Yin, Saint Peter, Ahura Mazda, White Tara, Mohammad, Goddess Athena and St. John the Baptist all dressed in luminiou white clothes. They were all doing the sun saluataions of yoga. All their faces were golden, radiant and happy. The courtyard was full of gemstones. The walls were made of Jasper. The floor was pure orange reddish carnelian. There were emerald tables. In addition to the sunflowers and a golden tea set on the emerald table with two lotus meditation cushions. The golden Buddha appears as though he teleported. I smile and bow in reverence while saying aloud Namo Amitabhaya Buddhaya. This means Hail Buddha of Infinite Light. We both bow and he motions me to sit. We both sit facing each other cross-legged on those beautiful lotus cushions. His eyes were like solar sun beams of gold, amber and hazel. He has the most beautiful rainbow above his head. It looked like a giant rainbow orb merkaba chariot. Noticing as out vibration grew higher and higher during our majestic interaction. My physical, emotional, mental and spiritual body was in union with these divine, heavenly frequencies. Our collective consciousness was in tune with each other. I could read the Buddha's mind as he prepared to serve tea. His hands were over his heart as he motioned silently to pick up the tea. Bowing to his grace, I grabbed the golden goblet and peered inside to see the solution. Smelling this musky wood fragrance I took a big gulp of the golden tea. It tasted just like enlightenment should. So pure, fresh, clean and powerful. Every sip was smoother and easier to drink. The tea was finished. The yoga crew gathered around us in a horseshoe style stance singing Hallelulaja. Instantly universal love appreciation vibrations filled the atmosphere; it was all about joy, empowerment, knowledge, beauty, love and gratitude. Each ascended master greeted me politely with various bows, handshakes, hugs and eye gazes. Some stated they were so glad I made it. Pure gold and silver light filled me. The last was Eros. It was Cupid the God of love. Eros had the biggest smile with his pearly white teeth and his bow and arrow. He pointed up to the golden ladder. I could see the numbers 1-30 on the ladder stairs. Each ancient step was identified with a virtue. Virtues included: sincerity, contentment, kindness, justice, patience, faith, truth, victory, wisdom, royalty, lightness, beauty, serenity, mercy, purity, love, power, self-awareness, vitality. By the eighteenth step I could tell we reached the stratosphere. The celestial kingdom below shimmered of pearly golden glows. Every step was surged with more power, confidence and cosmic force. The virtues continued divinity, security, blessings, spirituality, peace, glory, righteousness, freedom, intelligence, self-realization and step thirty was enlightenment. Holy! When I got to the top there were three flags symbolizing the Egyptian nefertum of the union of gods and goddesses on a silver platform. A pure white throne laced with gold and silver trim was embedded on the platform. A beautiful triple velvet layered gold crown rested on the throne with a ring of keys. These were the keys of Heaven. There was a silver and a gold key crossed over a brass one. On a holster buckled into the side of the seat was a giant chakra scepter with a shiny type kaleidoscope looking orb. The orb shimmered a rainbow prism. I grasped the scepter and beautiful, neon sacred geometric shapes appeared all over. The sun rose above my head with a golden liquid light ball. Great Spirit announced with a loud mysterious voice. This is your prize. You have done good Sun. We give you a new spiritual name Muad Dib. Which means the right hand of God.

Congratulations

You officially completed the Book of Life. Happy for you! By going through the pages, you hopefully had insight into your higher self and how to communicate better with source, Holy Spirit, God, universe. You are rewarded.

You are rewarded for doing the inner and outer work needed to align with your mind, body and soul. Nourish yourself and always connect, breathe, discover, create and explore.

I would love a testimonial about your experience, epiphanies, stories about how this book affected you.

Congratulations on saying yes to ascension. You have earned the golden light ascension codes and will receive this divine download these gifts for you. Sign and date your certificate and magic cheque. To receive more light codes, receive a personalized and customized oracle reading, healing session, life coaching package or masterclass, SUBSCRIBE CONFIRM and book at www.throneofheaven.com for more goodies. Stay blessed and connected. God Bless!. Namaste. Peace and love from my heart to yours. We bow to the divinity, beauty, wisdom, truth and love in you that's also in me. We pray you reach your highest potential.

Would love to hear how your experience is going. Feel free to contact us. Stay Tuned for the Book of Truth, Book of Love, Book of Secrets they will be coming out soon.

Thank you all for your time, consideration and effort into connecting with God, higher self, and the creator within. We bless you with love and light, truth and beauty, grace and gratitude, health and wellness, strength and vitality, abundance and prosperity, patience and kindness, joy and forgiveness. God bless you. Believe in Heaven on Earth!

Magic Cheque

THE BANK OF UNIVERSE	Date	D D M M Y Y
FEEL GOOD REMITTANCE ADVICE		

PAY _____ OR BEARER

DOLLARS _____ $ _____

_____

MEMO _____ NON-NEGOTIABLE: THE POWER OF BELIEF

DRAWN ON THE UNIVERSAL ACCOUNT:
UNLIMITED ABUNDANCE

The Universe

CHECK NUMBER ⦂‖ 000 333 444 111111 ‖⦂

SIGNATURE

by Special Delivery

Mastermind Abundance Plan

1. Write a list of everything you want with brands and prices.

2. Total the amount of items

3. Write a cheque to yourself for the total amount.

4. Sign and Date it

5. Carry this in your wallet and purse.

6. Look at it monthly

What do you want?	What specific brand type?	How much is it?	Total

BOOK OF LIFE

ASCENSION COMPLETION CERTIFICATE

GOLDEN LIGHT ASCENSION
CODES PRESENTED TO:

_____

DATE:_____

Book of Life and Secret Oracles
365 Day Devotional Self-Mastery Guide to Ascension
Guided by Diana Hutchings
SUBSCRIBE @ www.throneofheaven.com

In this book you will discover, create, explore and perfect your life. Invest in yourself, do the work, follow the blueprint and practice daily.

You will access akashic fields of knowledge. There are ascension guides for mastering the universal laws, acquiring godly virtues, communicating with the holy angels, attuning to abundance and healing codes. In addition, to provide spiritual awakening practices that will help. Daily devoting half an hour a day will transform your life. Experiment with the spiritual practices and expand your awareness. Have fun doing the activities! Find faith, peace, love and security. Align with your goals, desires, dreams, visions and aspirations.

BONUS: PAIR WITH LIVE COACHING to keep your whole year accountable. Includes: oracle card set, healing sessions, numerology, and soul tribe private group invite and more! Book of Truth coming soon.

INVEST IN YOURSELF!

GOD BLESS!

CPSIA information can be obtained
at www.ICGtesting.com
Printed in the USA
BVHW011452230822
645255BV00006B/54

9 781958 554869